Osteopathy and the Treatment of Horses

Osteopathy and the Treatment of Horses

Anthony Pusey

Julia Brooks

Annabel Jenks

WILEY-BLACKWELL

A John Wiley & Sons, Ltd., Publication

This edition first published 2010
© 2010 Anthony Pusey, Julia Brooks and Annabel Jenks

Blackwell Publishing was acquired by John Wiley & Sons in February 2007. Blackwell's publishing programme
has been merged with Wiley's global Scientific, Technical, and Medical business to form Wiley-Blackwell.

Registered office
John Wiley & Sons Ltd, The Atrium, Southern Gate, Chichester, West Sussex, PO19 8SQ, United Kingdom

Editorial offices
9600 Garsington Road, Oxford, OX4 2DQ, United Kingdom
2121 State Avenue, Ames, Iowa 50014-8300, USA

For details of our global editorial offices, for customer services and for information about how to apply for
permission to reuse the copyright material in this book please see our website at
www.wiley.com/wiley-blackwell.

Library of Congress Cataloging-in-Publication Data

Pusey, Anthony, 1951–2007.
Osteopathy and the treatment of horses/Anthony Pusey, Julia Brooks, Annabel Jenks.
p. ; cm.
Includes bibliographical references and index.
ISBN 978-1-4051-6952-3 (pbk. : alk. paper)   1. Horses–Diseases–Treatment.   2. Horses–Wounds and
injuries–Treatment.   3. Osteopathic medicine.   I. Brooks, Julia, 1960-   II. Jenks, Annabel.   III. Title.
[DNLM: 1. Horse Diseases–therapy.   2. Manipulation, Osteopathic–veterinary.   3. Massage–veterinary.
4. Musculoskeletal Diseases–veterinary.   5. Osteopathic Medicine–methods. SF 951 P987o 2010]
SF951.P97 2010
616.1′0895533–dc22

2009048324

A catalogue record for this book is available from the British Library.

Set in 10/12.5 pt Sabon by Aptara® Inc., New Delhi, India

Printed and bound by CPI Group (UK) Ltd, Croydon, CR0 4YY

C9781405169523_220224

Contents

Foreword

Having inherited the 'horse addiction' gene, I've always consumed horse books with alacrity. In the early days it was Black Beauty, moving on to the Pony Club Manual of Horsemanship, and eventually to the classical veterinary texts. University era textbooks still inhabit my bookshelves but over the years they've been joined by new books describing the latest technologies and techniques. *Osteopathy and the Treatment of Horses* will certainly find a place among my favourites.

The contents of my bookshelves are a testament to how much the world has changed within this one lifetime – a time of incredible scientific and technological advancements that have affected all aspects of our lives and our horses' lives. Horses are no longer utilitarian servants; they enrich the lives of their owners and trainers as valued companions and highly trained athletes. Breeders responded to the demand for high quality equine athletes, different breeds became highly specialized for specific sports and, consequently, competition performances improved dramatically. At the same time, equine sports medicine developed as a specialty area that caters to the special needs and problems of athletic horses. Veterinary practices acquired sophisticated diagnostic equipment and practitioners learned to use new therapeutic techniques including the application of complementary and alternative treatments. Many techniques that are now applied routinely in animals were learned from colleagues trained in the human medical specialties and it became obvious that collaboration between veterinary surgeons and human health care professionals could yield great benefits.

Having experienced the benefits of osteopathy at first hand, it was easy to appreciate the potential value of osteopathic treatments in horses. In fact, I've been eagerly awaiting the publication of *Osteopathy and the Treatment of Horses* for several years and am pleased to see that the final product exceeds even the highest expectations of a comprehensive text on equine osteopathy. The contents represent the collective knowledge and experience of three highly trained osteopaths, all of whom have a special interest in horses, and a renowned veterinary specialist in equine orthopedic surgery. The reader is taken on a journey that encompasses a historical background of osteopathy, a tour of the basic sciences of equine anatomy and physiology, some helpful advice for setting up an animal-oriented osteopathic practice and regulations governing diagnosis and treatment of animals. The later chapters describe the essence of osteopathy with detailed descriptions and copious illustrations of the osteopathic evaluation and therapeutic techniques.

We learn in these pages that Andrew Taylor Still is known as the father of osteopathy – surely the title of father of animal osteopathy belongs to the first author of this book. I regret that I never met Anthony Pusey. I certainly knew of his reputation and had hoped that one day our paths would cross, but it was not to be. It is a great shame that Anthony could not have seen this book in print but it is gratifying to know that his substantial contribution to animal osteopathy has been recognized in the publication of *Osteopathy and the Treatment of Horses*.

Hilary M. Clayton, BVMS, PhD, DACVSMR, MRCVS
Mary Anne McPhail Dressage Chair in Equine
Sports Medicine

Preface

It is many centuries since Hippocrates advocated the use of physical treatment and over 100 years since Dr Still formalised a system of manual medicine known as osteopathy. Since then, osteopathy has developed into a wide-ranging discipline touching the lives of many, from childhood to old age, through sports and in the workplace. The treatment of animals is a natural extension to this field. In essence, it is hoped that this book will highlight the role of osteopathy in the care of animals, and stimulate interest and discussion both between disciplines and within the profession.

Despite having a dedicated and enthusiastic following, very little has been written on osteopathy for animals. This book is the distillation of the experience of a number of practitioners over an extended period. It covers aspects of the history, theory, ethics, diagnosis and treatment of horses under conditions ranging from work in the field to the clinic-based environment.

It seeks to stimulate those already working in the field to analyse the way they practise and to contribute to the body of knowledge. Equally, it aims to provide a framework for practitioners just dipping a tentative toe into the waters of animal osteopathy. In addition, for allied professions such as veterinary surgeons, physiotherapists, chiropractors, saddlers, farriers and equine dentists, to name but a few, it is an opportunity to look at osteopathy with a view to working with osteopaths to provide the best treatment for the horses in their care.

Dedication

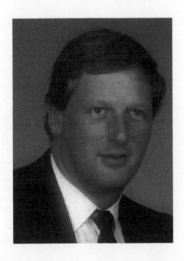

Anthony Pusey was an osteopath of international renown who was instrumental in linking the many different strands of academia, medicine and veterinary science with his great passion, osteopathy.

He was born on 22nd January 1951 and entered the British School of Osteopathy in London in 1969. After qualification with the Clinical Prize, he maintained his links with the school through undergraduate teaching. He infected generations of students with his enthusiasm for his subject, through lectures and demonstrations. His commitment to education was to continue throughout his career and his crowning achievement in this area was the development of a Master of Science degree for osteopaths in the application of osteopathy in the treatment animals.

In the 1970s he moved his practice from Harley Street to Haywards Heath in Sussex, where he was able to develop his osteopathic skill in treating families. This family connection was further extended when he was asked by a patient to

look at his large German Shepherd Dog. He combined forces with the veterinary surgeon to treat the dog. They went on to set up an osteopathic clinic for small animals, presenting the results of this collaboration to the British Small Animal Veterinary Association's congress in 1986.

Whilst developing his human practice, one of the largest in Britain, his work with small animals inevitably led to larger species ranging from prize pigs to racing camels. This interest focused on horses in the 1980s when he met Dr Chris Colles, a vet with a research background at the Animal Health Trust, who was by then a partner in a large equine veterinary referral centre. Chris had noted that a proportion of cases referred to the hospital, with complaints such as stiffness and poor performance, had no demonstrable disease despite extensive tests. This exactly mirrored the cases Anthony was seeing in the human practice. The two of them decided to work together to investigate this phenomenon at Avonvale Veterinary Centre. This clinic had patients from the top echelons of the horse world including Olympic competitors from a number of different nations.

Dr Colles was interested in using infra-red thermography as an objective tool to identify problems and evaluate the effect of treatment. Anthony realised the value of researching the effect of treatment on animals in countering the placebo argument that had been levelled at human osteopathy. This resulted in a number of papers presented to international audiences.

In 1998 a lecture at the Army Remount Centre at Melton Mowbray led to an invitation to treat the horses of the Household Cavalry at Knightsbridge Barracks. Anthony loved working with these magnificent horses, and enjoyed the hospitality of the officer's mess. It also led him into contact with the Crown Equerry, and his clinics came to include the horses at Buckingham Palace Mews and Windsor Castle. He often continued 'case conferences' over dinner at the Cavalry and Guards Club, which he considered affectionately as his London home. In 1999 he became a liveryman in the Worshipful Company of Farriers and a freeman of the City of London.

His infectious enthusiasm and his ability to listen and respect the ideas of the key players in many different walks of life meant that he was able quietly and inexorably to advance his ideas on the role of osteopathy in the medical and veterinary fields.

He died on 30th March 2007 of adenocarcinoma of the oesophagus. His memorial service was held in the Guards Chapel.

Adapted from obituaries in
The Daily Telegraph 6th April 2007

Acknowledgements

This book is the distillation of years of osteopathic treatment applied to animals. None of this would have been possible without the significant input from the many veterinary surgeons, both at home and abroad, who were open to the idea of a different approach to musculoskeletal problems. These include Graham De Baedemaecker with whom the initial foray into working with dogs was made, and Dr Chris Colles whose knowledge, insight and enthusiasm for the subject have resulted in the continued evolution of osteopathic treatment in horses.

Alongside the vets, the efficiency and professionalism of the staff at Avonvale Veterinary Group and in particular Trish Thornton have eased the strain of busy clinics.

Working as part of a co-ordinated team brings innumerable benefits. Multidisciplinary clinics with professionals such as physiotherapist Amanda Sutton and vet acupuncturist Sue Devereaux as well as the many farriers, saddlers and equine dentists encountered along the way have led to the exploration of new ideas together in a clinical setting.

The variety and colour of the osteopathic experience have been greatly enhanced by working with the officers, men and horses of the Household Cavalry and the Royal Mews, especially Major Jo Holmes and Colonel Mark Morrison.

The input of fellow osteopaths such as Tony Nevin, Dr Tony Wahba, Steven Choy, Hilary Hubbers, Chris Fielding and Jonathan Cohen has proved invaluable. Unstinting support from nearer home in discussing the content and endlessly proofreading chapters was provided by Dr Bernard Brooks, Georgina Brooks, James Brooks, Rupert Pusey, Antonia Pusey and Commodore Richard Bridges. My thanks also go to the staff at Awbrook Lodge, particularly Brenda Keerie, Gillian Oldfield, Jill Guard, Susan Elliot, Betty Dann, Janet Saunders and Phil Ashman.

Annabel would also like to acknowledge and thank the following people for their assistance in the making of this book: osteopaths Sarah Howells DO, David Powers DO, Tony Nevin DO and Alison Tyler DO; international dressage rider and trainer Jill Day; Jessica and Stuart Jeffrey for their IT expertise; her sister Caroline for proofreading; her partner Tom Craig and the staff at the stables for all their patience and support; her horse Merlin who modelled for the photographs; and all the patients, horses, vets, riders and owners over the years who have helped her develop her osteopathic skills.

Finally, thanks go to the staff of Wiley-Blackwell and especially Katy Loftus for great patience and encouragement in bringing this book to its conclusion.

About the Authors

Anthony Pusey, an osteopath of international renown, has been instrumental in establishing the role of osteopathy in the treatment of animals. Qualifying from the British School of Osteopathy in London in 1971, he developed a large human osteopathic practice whilst also forging links with veterinary practices where he treated horses from the top echelons of the horse world, including Olympic competitors of many different nations. He also treated the horses of the Household Cavalry, The Royal Mews and Windsor Castle. He lectured nationally and internationally, as well as developing a Master of Science degree in the application of osteopathy in the treatment of animals. This book is a distillation of over 35 years of his work in this field.

Julia Brooks MSc DO qualified from the British School of Osteopathy in 1983 before joining Anthony Pusey in a practice that encompassed both human and animal osteopathy. She has lectured nationally and internationally at postgraduate level and has presented research papers on this subject as well as contributing to a number of veterinary and osteopathic textbooks. She has been involved in Masters programmes and postgraduate diplomas in both the development stages and as an external examiner for the University of Wales.

Annabel Jenks DO ND is an osteopath with over 25 years' experience. She has a private practice in Essex, UK, treating a full spectrum of patients both human and equine, from Pony Club to Olympian. She graduated in 1984 from The British College of Osteopathic Medicine in London, where she has been a governor since 1997. She is a faculty member on the Masters Degree in Animal Osteopathy at the University of Wales. She has previously ridden in all disciplines but now concentrates on dressage, training and competing with her own horses from novice through to advanced level.

With contribution of Chapter 15 from **Christopher Colles** BVetMed, PhD, Hon FWCF, MRCVS, RCVS specialist in equine surgery (orthopaedics). Dr Colles qualified from the Royal Veterinary College, London in 1971. After spending 4 years in general practice, he joined the Animal Health Trust, Equine Clinical Unit (formerly the Equine Research Station) in 1975. He carried out research into orthopaedic conditions of the horse, and was awarded his PhD in 1982. In 1988, when head of the equine clinical department, he returned to equine practice since when he has been carrying out referral work at the Avonvale Veterinary Practice, a specialist equine practice in the Midlands. He was recognised by the Royal College of Veterinary Surgeons as a specialist equine surgeon (orthopaedics) in 1996, and was awarded an honorary fellowship of the Worshipful Company of Farriers in recognition of his research and teaching in farriery in 2000. Dr Colles has published widely in the scientific veterinary literature, and lectured on equine orthopaedic topics world wide. He is co-author of seven veterinary textbooks.

Disclaimer

The information in this book is distributed on an 'as is' basis, without warranty. While every precaution has been taken in the preparation of this book, neither the authors nor the publisher shall have any liability to any person or entity with respect to any liability, loss or damage caused or alleged to be caused directly or indirectly by the information contained in this book.

Introducing Osteopathy for Horses

Anthony Pusey and Julia Brooks

On a blustery Friday evening in the depths of a particularly long winter, I had just finished an afternoon's list of patients when the telephone rang. I lifted the receiver.

'It's Jack', said someone urgently. 'He's lying on the kitchen floor, howling with pain. Can you come out to him?'

I recognised the voice of a patient whose family I had seen intermittently over years and, following the directions given, I arrived at the threshold of a terraced cottage. There was indeed an awful racket coming from inside and my concern for poor Jack deepened. As I was ushered hastily into the kitchen, I was confronted with a very large, shaggy German Shepherd dog obviously in considerable pain!

In response to my questioning gaze, Jack's owner looked apologetic and confessed that he had not been entirely frank on the telephone as he doubted that, if he had, I would have consented to the visit. He added in flattering tones that as I had treated the rest of the family *so* successfully, he was sure that I would be able to help his dog.

It transpired that Jack had suffered recurrent bouts of back pain over a number of years, which had reached a crisis point that afternoon after he had leapt down from the back of the car. The pattern of presentation was one that I recognised from human practice.

I called for help. By chance, the family vet was also a patient of mine and, after talking about Jack's problem in particular and musculoskeletal problems in general, he readily admitted that all he would offer in such cases was symptomatic relief in the form of painkillers and anti-inflammatory drugs. We decided on a combined approach to Jack's treatment. In the following years there were many other animals that benefited from our shared experience on a kitchen floor all those years ago.

After Jack, my experience of using osteopathy with animals broadened, to include a variety of species including a prize-winning pig and a film-star camel.

The animal work has brought innumerable benefits to my human practice. It has sharpened my observational skills of the body both at rest and in motion. It has taught me to rely on the findings of my fingers. It has refined my diagnostic reasoning. I have benefited from contact with other professions whose skills and ideas provide an added dimension to my work as an osteopath. It has also brought the friendship of other osteopaths working in the field, whose dedication and enthusiasm have been palpable.

For many osteopaths, much of their animal work involves horses, apparently heedless of the warning issued by a well known farrier that horses are 'dangerous at both ends and uncomfortable in the middle'. We decided to write this book to introduce the subject and encourage contributions from current practitioners and future generations as knowledge and expertise in this field develop.

It is therefore the intention to provide a theoretical and practical framework for students and practitioners with an interest in the osteopathic treatment of the horse. It will also be helpful to allied professions such as veterinary surgeons, other musculoskeletal specialists, farriers, equine dentists and saddlers to introduce some of the concepts underlying osteopathic treatment and enable them to identify the cases where osteopathy may benefit animals in their care.

A history of the development of animal treatment has been included, as well as the legal and ethical aspects to be considered when working in this field. Anatomical, biomechanical and neurophysiological principles on which osteopathic treatment of horses is based have been discussed and a diagnostic and therapeutic approach has been proposed.

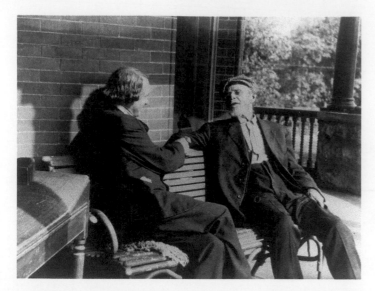

Figure 1.1 Andrew Taylor Still (1828–1917), father of osteopathy (right) with author Mark Twain.

This approach is by no means prescriptive. Each practitioner will develop their own diagnostic routines and therapeutic techniques, according to training, experience and preference. In this diverse and challenging field there is a place for everyone.

HISTORY OF OSTEOPATHY

To begin at the beginning is to take a leap back into antiquity. Over 2500 years ago, Hippocrates advised that 'a physician must be experienced in many things, but assuredly in rubbing'. Over the centuries that followed, many forms of physical treatment have been shown to be beneficial.

Osteopathy as a medical philosophy was developed in the 1880s by Andrew Taylor Still, a doctor from the American mid-west (Figure 1.1). Dr Still became disillusioned with the medicine practised at that time, which included bleeding, purgatives and other equally unpleasant forms of treatment. Instead, his anatomical studies led him to envisage a system of medicine that placed chief emphasis on the structural integrity of the body as being vital to the well being of the organism. In other words, if the structure is fine, then the body can function normally. Over the years, a number of definitions of varying length and complexity have been proposed for osteopathy, but Dr Still's original concept has largely been preserved.

LEGISLATION

If human medicine was basic in the time of Dr Still, then the care of animals was also less than satisfactory. In early years the treatment of horses was the responsibility of far-

riers, regulated in England by the Worshipful Company of Farriers established in 1674. However, they competed with cow-leeches and horse doctors in applying uncomfortable and invasive treatments such as oiling, firing and rowelling, and prescribing toxic substances, of which antimony and sulphur were particularly popular. In 1844, the Royal Charter for the Royal College of Veterinary Surgeons advocated that horses should be treated by veterinary surgeons. Over the following decades, farriers reverted to specialising in the craft of shoeing horses, and those trained at the new veterinary colleges undertook the treatment of animals.

In the 20th century, all professions moved towards the regulation of training and practice. For osteopaths in America this meant merging with the medical profession in the 1960s. In England, osteopaths preserved their identity as an independent profession, and the Osteopaths Act of 1993 restricted the title of osteopath to those who had fulfilled the necessary training required by the General Osteopathic Council.

Similarly, the Veterinary Surgeons Act of 1966 made it illegal for anyone other than a veterinary surgeon to treat an animal. An exception to this was physical therapists. This category included physiotherapists, chiropractors and osteopaths, who could treat an animal under the direction of a vet. This recognised the contribution of physical treatments made by these disciplines. It also provided protection for animals in terms of early diagnosis of pathological processes and preventing inappropriate treatment.

HISTORY OF OSTEOPATHIC TREATMENT OF ANIMALS

Recognition of osteopathy as a healing system spread and it soon became clear that a treatment apparently so successful in humans could be applied with equal success to the treatment of animals.

Many of those regarded as forerunners in the field were osteopaths practising in the first half of the 20th century. The stories of the way they started will reflect a common experience in the generations that followed. Some began after a request from a patient to look at a family pet; others began in response to the suffering of their own animals. Colin Dove, a former principal at the British School of Osteopathy, remembers applying his cranial expertise to treat a colleague's dog that was crippled after an afternoon cavorting with his children! Osteopaths in rural areas were approached by farmers concerned about their various animals. Practitioners such as Greg Currie in Epsom were inevitably drawn into the racing world.

For some these will have been one-off or infrequent experiences, but for others it was a launching pad into an exciting, challenging and rewarding field. One of the pioneers

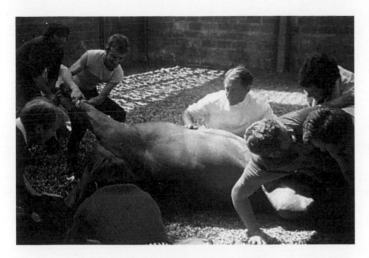

Figure 1.2 Arthur Smith (centre): a pioneer in the osteopathic treatment of horses under general anaesthetic.

in the field, working alongside vets, was Arthur Smith (Figure 1.2). Arthur qualified in 1951 from the British School of Osteopathy and set up practice in Leicestershire. One of his patients was a vet who, having felt the benefit of osteopathic treatment for himself, asked whether the principles could be applied to horses. Initially reluctantly, he took time out to study horse anatomy at a local museum and decided that it might be possible. After successes with the first few cases, veterinary surgeons referred hundreds of horses to him over subsequent years. In his retirement he described vividly techniques that involved a general anaesthetic and six strong men!

Society of Osteopaths in Animal Practice (SOAP)

In the early 1980s, in response to increasing interest from the general public and the profession itself, Mr Barry Darewski, the registrar of the regulating body, the General Council

and Register of Osteopaths (GCRO), asked for a list to be compiled of osteopaths with a special interest in treating animals. This list formed the core members of the special interest group, Osteopaths in Animal Practice (OAPs) which was to become SOAP (Society of Osteopaths in Animal Practice) in 2004.

This group and the osteopathic schools have assisted in sharing knowledge in this field through postgraduate education. Interdisciplinary communication with vets, physiotherapists, chiropractors, farriers, dentists and saddlers has flourished in this environment. Institutions such as zoos, the army and the police have also come to appreciate the contribution osteopathy can make to animals in their care. More recently, the advantages of research in this area have become evident in demonstrating the effectiveness of osteopathy in subjects not susceptible to placebo.

With the growth and development of this field, osteopathy has been shown to make a valuable contribution as part of a multidisciplinary team devoted to the care of animals. It is also an exciting and rewarding part of the rich tapestry that is osteopathy.

BIBLIOGRAPHY

Hunter P (2001) Researching the past: archival sources for the history of veterinary medicine. In: Rossdale PD, Green G (eds) *Guardians of the Horse II*. Romney Publications, Newmarket, pp. 34–39.

Osteopaths Act 1993. HMSO, London.

Prince LB (1980) *The Farrier and His Craft*. JA Allen, London.

Still AT (1902) *The Philosophy and Mechanical Principles of Osteopathy*. Hudson-Kimberly, Kansas City.

Veterinary Surgeons Act 1966. HMSO, London.

Horse Anatomy for Osteopaths

Julia Brooks and Anthony Pusey

The anatomy of the horse is a huge subject. It is certainly not possible to squeeze it into a few pages, which is why this chapter will concentrate on some of those aspects that may be useful in osteopathic practice. For the rest, it is a case of studying some excellent but weighty anatomical tome, of which there are many. Another useful way of extending anatomical knowledge is to beg a body part from a knacker's yard and dismember it with the aid of a dissection guide. Care should be taken with storage, however. A colleague who was to have provided a horse's head for a study group had it dragged from his garage and away over the fields by a gourmet fox. Fortunately, he was able to provide 'an old one' from his deep freeze!

This text will concentrate on the basic structure, the surface anatomy and the regional anatomy insofar as these have clinical and osteopathic relevance.

OVERVIEW

If some of the anatomical volumes seem a little daunting, there should not be cause for complete despair. Those who still remember human anatomy will appreciate the remarkable similarity in the basic structure between the species (Figure 2.1). The differences are mainly those of scale, proportion and orientation. Also, horses do not have clavicles and have fewer fingers and toes.

The main structural difference is in the legs. It is as though someone has grabbed hold of the third metacarpal and third metatarsal where they join the carpal and tarsal bones respectively, and pulled them out, so elongating them and losing most of the fingers in the process. This means that the carpal bones, instead of being situated towards the end of the limbs as in the human, actually end up towards the middle of the limb. Many of the bone and joint names will sound familiar (Figure 2.2). However, one trickier vagary of nomenclature is that vets refer to the carpal joints in the middle of the forelimb as the knee, which is actually the wrist in human terms. The human idea of the knee, complete with patella, is actually found tucked up at the upper end of the hindlimb and is called the stifle. 'A knee in the groin stifles all comment' may help as an *aide-mémoire*!

Ossification rates of bones are also different. Growth continues up to 4 years and some adjacent ossification centres do not unite until 30 years old, if at all. This should be borne in mind when looking at X-rays to avoid the classic mistake of thinking that an epiphyseal plate or suture is a fracture line.

Muscles that will be recognisable from human studies may be better developed in the horse and have a different orientation to reflect its function as a grazing quadruped. Anatomists have managed to make things slightly more awkward by naming a few things differently, and a number of these names have been changed over time. Some of the muscles are called by alternative names, but as the terminology generally describes the origin and the insertion this should not prove to be too much of a problem.

Body orientation is also different in quadrupeds. The horse stands with around 60% of its body weight through the front limbs, with recent texts indicating a centre of mass at the level of the 13th rib along a line extending between the points of the shoulder and buttock. This explains the observation that, while resting one or other of the hind limbs may be normal, not weight-bearing through a forelimb is usually an indication that there is something wrong.

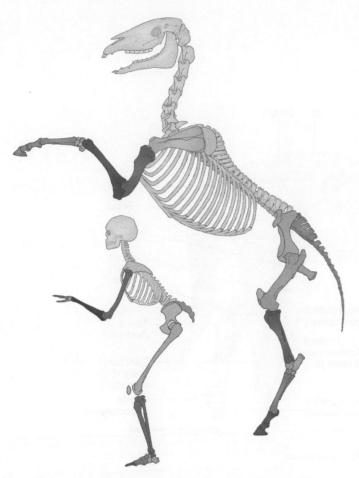

Figure 2.1 Horse and human skeleton: similarities are remarkable and differences are largely of scale, proportion and orientation.

ANATOMICAL DESCRIPTORS

With all four limbs in contact with the ground, some of the anatomical positional terms will be different and so a quick review of descriptive terms may be helpful (Figure 2.3). Planes that face towards the ground, such as the abdominal surface, are described as ventral while those directed skywards are dorsal. Anything facing forwards is referred to as cranial, and backwards as caudal. This also applies to the legs until, below the carpals and tarsals, the forward-facing part of the limb is the dorsal surface and the backward-directed parts become palmar and plantar surfaces respectively. At the head, structures towards the nose are considered to be rostral.

Proximal parts of the limb are located towards the trunk, while distal parts are found at the end of the limb. Other terminology to be aware of includes medial (directed towards the median plane) and lateral (towards the outside of the body).

Descriptions often refer to anatomical planes. The median plane describes a slice taken through the midline of the body from poll to tail, dividing the body equally into left and right halves. Sagittal planes are those running parallel to the median line. The dorsal or frontal plane divides the body into dorsal and ventral portions. Transverse planes are slices at right angles to the median plane of the body or to the long axis of a limb.

When it comes to describing planes of movement, flexion is where opposing surfaces approximate and extension is where surfaces separate. Sidebending, familiar in human terminology, is referred to as lateral flexion.

The following text outlines the regional anatomy of the head, neck, back and limbs with reference to surface features and structural components and touching on areas susceptible to dysfunction and pathology.

THE HEAD

Overview

The head is a large, elongated structure. It provides a considerable surface area for muscle attachments and to accommodate teeth so that horses can do efficiently what horses like doing best: eating. The head is also heavy, which means that, by moving up, down and side to side, it can be used very effectively as a kind of weighted bob to change the horse's centre of gravity and induce momentum during movement (Figure 2.4).

Surface Anatomy

Observable and palpable features include the poll (nuchal crest) from which runs the external or parietal crest. Laterally, the facial crest gives an attachment for the powerful masseter muscle, and the infraorbital foramen conveys a branch of the maxillary nerve to the upper lip. Medially, the nasal peak lies between the nasoincisive notches. On the mandible, rostral and medial to its angle, is a vascular impression that carries the facial artery, vein and parotid duct and is a site often used for taking a pulse. Further along, the mental foramen carries branches of the alveolar nerve to the lower lip.

Anatomical Components

The skull can be divided into two regions by a transverse line through the orbits: the cranium and the face.

The Cranium

The cranium, forming only a small part of the skull, contains a brain of about 600 g, which compares unfavourably with the 1300 g human organ. It lies in the area between the poll (nuchal crest) and the temporal fossa and consists of the same elements that are found in the human skull: occiput, frontal, sphenoid, ethmoid, temporal and parietal bones, in addition to an interparietal bone that is separate only in horses and cats (Figure 2.5).

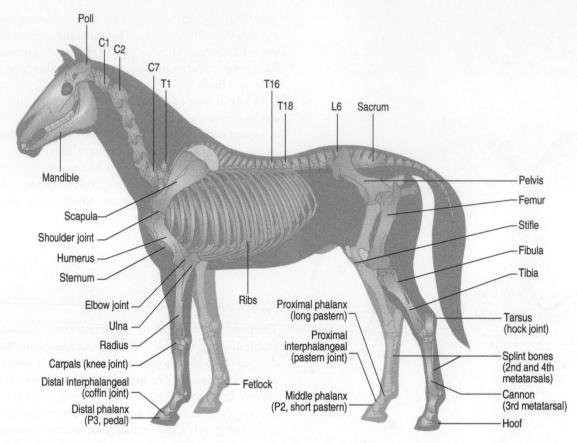

Figure 2.2 Joints and bones: many of the structures are familiar to human anatomists.

As with human skulls, the union between the bones depends on whether ossification occurs in membrane or cartilage. The membranous bones of the vault are joined by sutures which are generally closed by the age of 7 years. The main cartilaginous unions ossify at 4 years between the body of the sphenoid and the basiocciput and 3 years between the pre-sphenoid body with its orbital wings and post-sphenoid body with its temporal wings and pterygoid processes.

An interesting departure from this pattern of progressive ossification is the occipito-mastoid sutures which do not fuse until the horse is in its twenties. From the osteopathic viewpoint, this may be an area where dysfunction can be identified and this is often corroborated by infrared imaging where the site appears as a 'hot spot' (see Chapter 3).

The occiput, at the back of the skull, is the strongest and thickest of the bones. It is topped with the ridge of the nuchal crest which has a central bony eminence, corresponding to the external occipital protuberance in man, to which the nuchal ligament is attached. This crest or poll is the highest part of the head and is often hit if the horse rears and falls backwards. The occiput is not, however, as frequently fractured as the smaller bones of the cranial base.

The caudal part of the occiput bears the occipital condyles which lie either side of the foramen magnum and articulate with the first cervical vertebra. These are very susceptible to compression injuries as a result of falling, which will affect the flexion/extension range of movement of the head on the neck.

Cranially, the brain is protected by the frontal bone with its sizeable sinus. It is this sinus, lying between the temporal fossae, which allows a direct approach to the brain when humane destruction is necessary. The frontal bone also forms the supraorbital ridge, which, together with the zygomatic process of the frontal bone and the zygoma itself, form part of the orbit.

The ear

Rising above the nuchal crest but attached around the external auditory meatus of the temporal bone are a series of cartilages which form the ear. Unlike the human ear, it is freely mobile in order to turn towards the source of sound. This requires an extensive network of voluntary muscles. Lying on the temporalis muscle and in front of the auricular cartilage, which forms the visible outline of the ear, is a small, quadrilateral plate termed the scutiform cartilage.

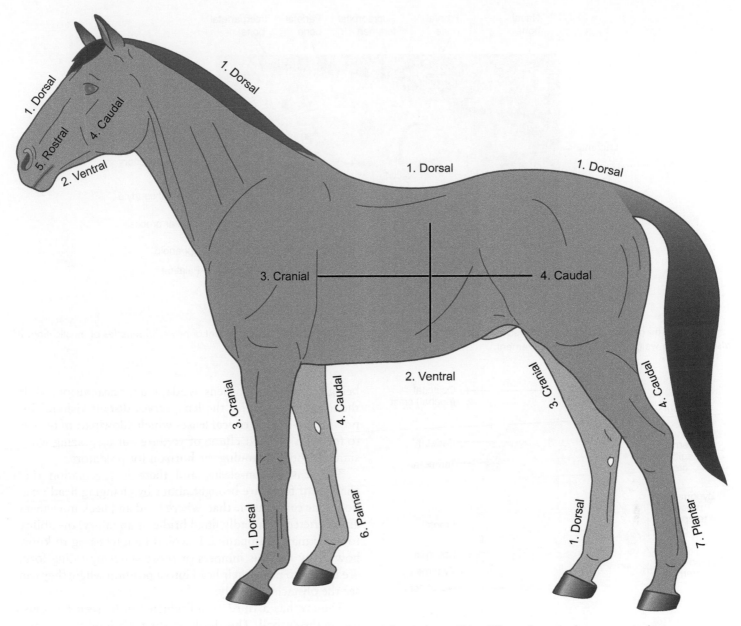

Figure 2.3 Anatomical descriptors: with all four feet on the ground, some descriptions will be different from the human equivalent.

This can be regarded as a kind of sesamoid bone acting as an insertion for muscles such as the interscutularis, scutuloauricularis, frontoscutularis and cervicoscutularis which, as the names suggest, run in many different directions.

In osteopathic terms, this complex arrangement allows the ears to be used in fascial and functional techniques to give a handle on the temporal bone and access to the tissues of the cranium and suboccipital region.

The eye

This is a good point at which to look at the structure of the eye. The orbit is placed laterally on the head so that, although this gives a good range of all-round vision (215°),

the amount of binocular vision to the front is limited. This problem is compounded by the obstructing presence of a substantial nose. Furthermore, the ciliary muscle which, in the human, contracts to make the lens rounder in order to see close to (accommodation), is relatively weak in the horse. This combination means that a horse cannot see directly in front for a distance of about 110 cm, which is a good reason for always approaching a horse from the side.

In addition the eye does not have a regular shape. Rather than the round eyeball of the human subject, a horse's eye is slightly flattened cranio-caudally. This flattening is not even consistent from above to below. The upper part of the retina,

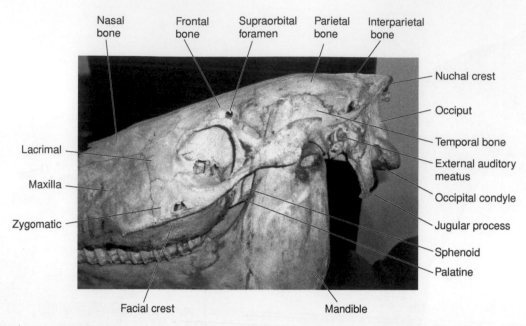

Nasal bone — Frontal bone — Supraorbital foramen — Parietal bone — Interparietal bone

Nuchal crest

Occiput

Temporal bone

External auditory meatus

Occipital condyle

Jugular process

Sphenoid

Palatine

Lacrimal

Maxilla

Zygomatic

Facial crest — Mandible

Figure 2.4 The head: this large, elongated structure provides a large area for teeth and the attachment of powerful muscles of mastication. It also acts as a weighted bob during movement.

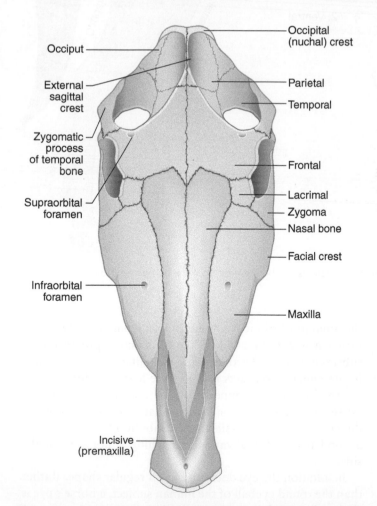

Occiput

External sagittal crest

Zygomatic process of temporal bone

Supraorbital foramen

Infraorbital foramen

Incisive (premaxilla)

Occipital (nuchal) crest

Parietal

Temporal

Frontal

Lacrimal

Zygoma

Nasal bone

Facial crest

Maxilla

Figure 2.5 Cranium: components resemble those of the human skull with a number of additions.

being furthest from the lens, is adapted for near vision, while the lower part, nearer the lens, serves distant vision. This provides in-built varifocal lenses which allow part of the eye to focus on the next clump of verdure during grazing while simultaneously scanning the horizon for predators.

The lens is non-elastic and there is speculation that changes of focus are brought about by changing head position. One can imagine that, where head and neck movement are restricted by a badly fitted bridle or an injury, the ability to focus may be impaired. It would be interesting to know how many nervous jumpers or those suddenly losing form are unable to bring their head into a position where they can see the obstacle properly.

The eye has a third eyelid which can be seen by pressing on the eyeball. This displaces the fat behind the eye and pushes the lid across. The muscle spasticity of the extraocular muscles in tetanus produces the same effect and is in fact a diagnostic sign of the disease.

Above and behind each orbit is a hollow area that houses the coronoid process of the mandible. As the jaw closes, the coronoid forces the fat up from the orbit into the fossa which causes a bulging in this space, an effect readily seen when the horse is feeding.

Running rostrally from the orbit, the zygoma continues as the distinctive zygomatic ridge, referred to as the facial crest, which provides an insertion for the masseter muscle.

The Face

The face is made up of the maxilla, premaxilla, nasal, lacrimal and zygomatic (malar) bones, turbinates, vomer, mandible and hyoid. It is dominated by the elongated oral and nasal cavities and a number of sinuses. The sinuses have a functional role to lighten the large skull area adapted for mastication. They also have a clinical significance in that they can become infected. With unresolving discharge, the frontal, superior and inferior maxillary sinuses can be drained by drilling a small hole (trephining). The sphenoidal part of the sphenopalatine sinus is difficult to access and may be a site of continuing infection.

Osteopathically, some of the cranial techniques can influence the sinuses, an effect which is observable post-treatment when the horse, particularly when sedated, will drop its head low and discharge copious amounts of mucus from the nasal passages.

Laterally, the maxilla bears the infraorbital foramen containing a branch of the maxillary division of the trigeminal nerve to the upper lip, which can be compromised by an over-tight noseband.

Oral cavities

The teeth divide the mouth into the outer vestibule, bounded by the cheek and lips, and the central oral cavity. The main support for the vestibule is the buccinator muscle, which holds the cheek close to the teeth, pressing food through into the oral space. This arrangement is disrupted in facial paralysis when food collects laterally, pouching the cheeks.

The lips are mobile and sensitive musculomembranous folds surrounding the orifice of the mouth. The concentration of sensory nerves in this area is utilised when using a twitch as a means of restraint. A twitch, usually a loop of rope, is placed around the horse's upper lip and then twisted to tighten. A horse will usually go into a trance-like state, dropping the head and closing the eyes, presumably as centrally acting endorphins are released.

Rostrally and centrally, the frenula labii (superioris and inferioris) are made up of two small mucous membranes running from the lip to the gum. The frenulum is sometimes used in osteopathic treatment to achieve general relaxation, presumably using similar endorphin-mediated pathways as those involved when using a twitch.

Tongue

The central oral cavity is filled with the tongue running in the floor of the mouth from the root at the hyoid and pharynx to the free spatula-shaped apex (Figure 2.7).

The tongue is supported in a sling formed by the mylohyoideus muscle running between the horizontal parts of the jaw. The extrinsic tongue muscles, the hyoglossus, the laterally placed styloglossus and the fan-shaped genioglossus, blend with the horizontal, vertical and transverse fibres of the intrinsic muscles to form a highly mobile structure. Under general anaesthetic, the tongue can be used as a tool to relax the intermandibular structures around the hyoid.

Nasal cavities

Horses are obligate nasal breathers. The air is warmed and hydrated as it passes through the large spaces of the nasal cavities. The cavities are roofed by the two triangular-shaped nasal bones, whose bases unite at the frontal and lacrimal bones and then run down to form a sharp apex (nasal peak) with a notch on either side (the nasoincisive notch).

Osteopathic direct inhibition techniques may be used either side of this peak, and appear to reduce tone in the facial musculature and that of the upper cervical spine.

The cavity is divided into two halves by the nasal septum. Projecting into the hindmost part are the ethmoids which have a role in the sense of smell. Rostrally are the turbinates (conchae) whose large, vascular surface warms and moisturises the inhaled air.

Hard and soft palates

The nasal cavities are separated from the oral cavities by the palate (Figure 2.6). The hard palate is made up of the premaxilla, or incisive bone, containing the upper incisors, and the maxilla which accommodates the cheek teeth (molars). This is continuous behind with the large musculomembranous soft palate which extends backwards to contact the epiglottis, so closing off the oral cavity during breathing.

A frequently mentioned condition is dorsal displacement of the soft palate (DDSP). This occurs typically in 2-year-old thoroughbreds during fast work, where the soft palate is displaced above the epiglottis and into the nasopharynx causing turbulence of airflow and giving rise to a characteristic gurgling or choking sound. This anatomical rearrangement resolves on swallowing, when the larynx, poking upwards

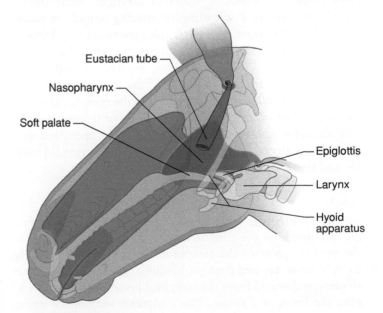

Figure 2.6 The face: nasal and oral cavities form a significant part of this region.

through the soft palate into the nasopharynx, is drawn down and forwards. This movement allows the epiglottis and soft palate to re-establish their normal relationship.

Guttural pouches

Other anatomical features in this region are the guttural pouches, which are large air-filled invaginations in the eustachian tube connecting the nasopharynx and the middle ear cavity. These may become infected.

Intermandibular space

Between the mandibles lies the intermandibular space. This is an interesting area for both veterinary surgeons and osteopaths. Clinically, by palpating the medial edge of the mandible about 7 cm from the angle of the jaw, the facial artery may be used to measure the pulse, which should be about 35 beats per minute at rest.

In the centre of the space lie the elongated mandibular lymph glands. These become swollen in upper respiratory tract infections and are often the site of abscesses in strangles, a highly infectious respiratory disease caused by *Streptococcus equi*.

Larynx

Centrally, at the back of the intermandibular space and protecting the lower respiratory passages from food and liquids, sits the larynx, which is suspended from the cranial base by the hyoid. The epiglottic, thyroid, cricoid and paired arytenoid cartilages are the five articulated components of the larynx which join the nasopharynx with the trachea. A condition which may be apparent by 6 years old or older horses over 16 hands is recurrent laryngeal neuropathy, which presents as a whistling or roaring sound on inspiration. Usually affecting the left side, the vocal fold lying in the opening of the larynx, the glottis, becomes flaccid and obstructs airflow. Two operations, sometimes undertaken together, are performed to tighten these folds and open the glottis. The Hobday operation involves the removal of either the left or both the ventricles either side of the vocal cord. The abductor muscle prosthesis or 'tie-back' operation uses a band of material to replace the wasted cricoarytenoid muscle and tie the left side of the larynx open.

Hyoid

The hyoid provides a framework for the larynx and an origin for much of the tongue musculature. It is attached to the petrous parts of the temporal bones by approximately 2 cm of bone, termed the stylohyoids or great cornua. These structures descend from the temporal bones on both sides to take the form of a swing. The transverse seat of the swing is represented by the basihyoid from which the lingual process projects rostrally, penetrating deep into the muscles of

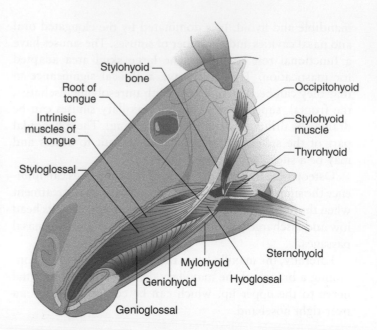

Figure 2.7 Hyoid: the hyoid provides a framework for the larynx and an origin for much of the tongue musculature.

the tongue. Directed back from the basihyoid, the paired thyrohyoid bones attach to the thyroid cartilage.

From the hyoid, muscles radiate in many directions. They project rostrally, attaching to the mandible (mylohyoideus, geniohyoideus) or as part of the tongue (styloglossus, hyoglossus) (Figure 2.7). They attach to the sternum (sternohyoideus), the scapula (omohyoideus) and even the occiput (occipitohyoideus).

It is these multiple relationships that make the region important when assessing the neck function and the patency of the airway within the intermandibular space. An effective functional osteopathic procedure performed under general anaesthetic uses the tongue to assess and resolve abnormal muscular and fascial tone in the supra- and infrahyoid region (Chapter 13).

The Mandible

The mandible is a large structure which houses the lower arcade of teeth, provides a large surface area for the attachment of the muscles of mastication and articulates with the skull at the temporomandibular joint. This area is clinically important for a number of reasons, which will be mentioned below.

Running from the angles of the jaw, the left and right sides of the mandible are fused rostrally at between 1 and 6 months to form the body which bears the lower arcade of teeth. The mandibular ramus extends up from the angle to end caudally in the condyloid process lying in the mandibular fossa of the temporal bone and cranially in the coronoid process lying in the temporal fossa.

Temporomandibular joint

The mandible, slung below the skull, articulates with the temporal bone at the temporomandibular joint. The articulation is formed by the incongruous articular surfaces of these two components. On the temporal surface, the long axis of the glenoid cavity is directed laterally and somewhat forwards. It is continued in the postglenoid process behind and the temporal condyle in front. This receives the transversely elongated condyle of the mandible.

An articular disc lies between these surfaces, attached to the circumference of the joint capsule. It divides the joint into a lower compartment and a more roomy upper compartment. This gives congruency and facilitates more complex joint movements. External and posterior ligaments reinforce the joint.

The chief movement is around a transverse axis through both joints to give a hinge-like action for opening and closing the mouth. As the mouth is opened, the condyle moves forwards in the glenoid cavity, carrying the disc with it. On closing the mouth, the disc returns to rest under the glenoid cavity. Protrusion and retraction of the lower jaw, such as occurs when dropping and lifting the head, involves the forwards and backwards glide of the disc. The lateral movements, employed in eating, take place about a vertical axis through the condyles, while the disc glides forwards on one side and backwards on the other. This grinding movement is associated with rotation at the atlanto-axial joint.

Not only is the temporomandibular region related to the neck functionally, but there is also a neurological link. The joint is innervated by the spinal trigeminal nerve, whose nucleus stretches from the brain stem down as far as the first cervical segment. Here, the nerve nuclei intermingle with those fibres supplying the upper neck, and changes in signals from one structure will often affect the function of the other.

The state of the muscles operating over the articulation often give a clue as to the symmetry and effectiveness of joint function. The main muscles are the masseter, running from the facial crest to the mandible, and the temporalis, originating in the temporal fossa and inserting on the coronoid process of the mandible. Both muscles act with the medial pterygoid to close the mouth. Other less bulky muscles, the digastric and lateral pterygoid, open the jaw. Where the temporomandibular region is compromised by injury or dental problems, the temporalis and masseter muscles often look and feel flattened and fibrotic.

Dentition

This is a subject in its own right. The state of the dentition is important not only for the condition of the horse through nutrition, but also for ensuring optimum function of the temporomandibular joint, the structures of the intermandibular space and the upper cervical spine.

The table of the teeth is worn down by abrasion at a rate of about 3 mm per year. This is replaced as the alveolar cavity, where the root lies, gradually fills with bone and slowly pushes the tooth out beyond the gum line to compensate for attrition at the masticatory surfaces. The erosion exposes different elements of the tooth structure over the years, which gives a way of ageing a horse on the basis of the cross-sectional appearance of the teeth (Table 2.1).

The lower arcade of three pairs of incisors is used to age a horse (Figure 2.8). Owners are sometimes a little vague about dates of birth and it may be helpful to distinguish a 5- from a 15-year-old for prognostic purposes.

Ageing is a somewhat inexact art, particularly after the age of 6 years. Points to look for are the presence of deciduous or permanent teeth, whether they are fully erupted, if they are in wear, if they have cups and the shape of the teeth. The principal landmarks are the age at which the permanent teeth replace the deciduous teeth ($2^1/_2$ years) and the age at which they start to grind on the surface of the teeth above (in wear).

By 4–5 years, the full complement of permanent teeth on each side is comprised of three incisors, one canine in the male which may be absent or rudimentary in the female, three premolars and three molars. Between the incisors and premolars is the interdental space or diastema where there are no teeth and where the bit of the bridle sits.

In these spaces, there may be supernumerary first premolars called wolf teeth, appearing in the upper jaw between 6 and 18 months of age. They may not erupt through and can be felt as bumps under the gum. These can cause bitting difficulties and behavioural problems when ridden. Removal is a common operation under standing sedation.

As the tooth is pushed down from the root and wears at the crown, different features of its cross section will be exposed, depending on the years of wear. One useful feature is the presence of a fold in the enamel to form an infundibulum or cup on the surface of the tooth. This becomes filled with rotting foodstuff and appears as a black slit in the middle of the tooth surface, which disappears around 8 years old.

On the upper arcade, Galvayne's groove can be seen appearing in the upper corner incisors at around 10 years old and will extend halfway down the tooth by 15 years of age.

Whereas the incisors are used for cutting verdure, the cheek teeth or molars provide a broad surface for grinding. Important in this process is the type of feed given. Feeding on the ground is preferable as the mandible comes forward into protraction as the head drops and occlusion between upper and lower surfaces is better.

As the lower jaw is narrower than the upper jaw, the teeth do not exactly cover each other and so the wear on

Table 2.1 Ageing a horse using the lower incisors

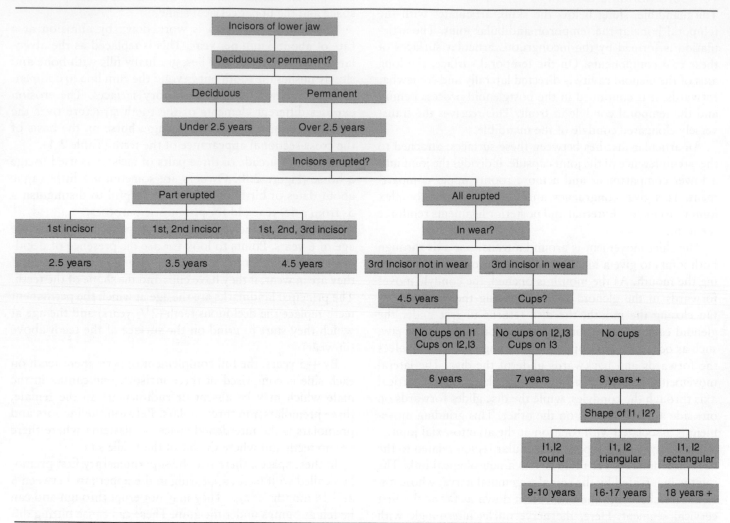

the upper and lower arcades of cheek teeth is not even. This is less of a problem if the horse is at grass as there is less lateral movement. However, if uneven wear results in the development of sharp edges, the upper teeth may irritate the labial (near the lips) surface, and the lower teeth may irritate the tongue. Not surprisingly, the horse may change in temperament, alter feeding habit and be very uncomfortable with a bit in its mouth. Referral to a qualified equine dentist is helpful in these cases.

THE VERTEBRAL COLUMN

The regions of the spine are named in the same way as for humans but there are some variations in the number of vertebrae making up each section. The cervical spine is composed of seven vertebrae; the thoracic spine has 18; the lumbar has six (except breeds such as Arabs, which have five vertebrae); the sacrum is formed from five fused vertebrae;

and, at the tail, there are approximately 18 coccygeal vertebrae. The outline of the horse is rather misleading when it comes to locating vertebral position for palpatory examination. Those practitioners used to the accessible human spinal structure conveniently close to the surface of the back will need to appreciate the bulk of some of the ligaments and muscle groups and the size of some of the spinous processes and will have to shift their sights ventrally in the horse (Figure 2.2).

The Neck

Overview

The neck controls the position and movement of the head and provides important information concerning balance. It is the initiator of that sinusoidal movement of the back which produces smooth forward propulsion. From an injury point of view, when a horse falls at speed it will fall on the head and neck: 500 kg at 30 miles an hour falling on to a mobile structure will undoubtedly have some undesirable

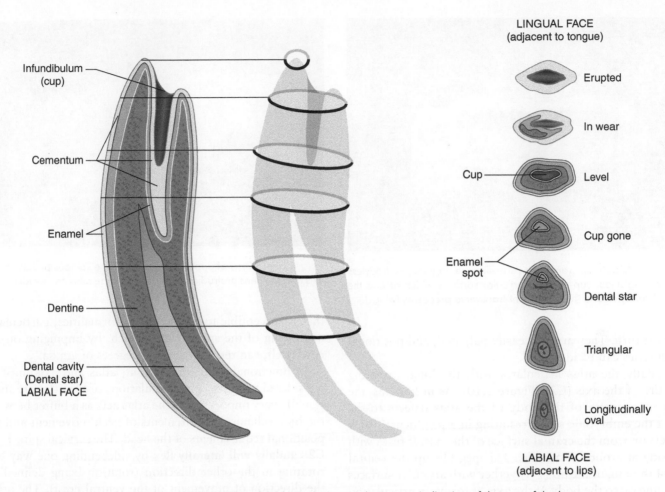

LINGUAL FACE
(adjacent to tongue)

Erupted

In wear

Cup — Level

Cup gone

Enamel
spot

Dental star

Triangular

Longitudinally
oval

LABIAL FACE
(adjacent to lips)

Infundibulum
(cup)

Cementum

Enamel

Dentine

Dental cavity
(Dental star)
LABIAL FACE

Figure 2.8 Dentition: the cross-sectional appearance of the lower incisor teeth gives an indication of the age of the horse.

consequences! Despite all this, many conferences and lectures on back pain will mention that the neck is the most mobile part of the spine and move swiftly on to the intricacies of pelvic lesions and overriding dorsal processes. From the osteopath's point of view it is an area of huge interest. It is accessible, changes are palpable and the effect of treatment on the mechanics of the rest of the spine can be astonishing.

Surface anatomy

Anatomically, the seven bones of the cervical spine adopt an inverted S-shape with the occiput to C3 flexed (convex dorsally) and C3 to the thorax following an extension curve (convex ventrally). This is at variance with the outer contour of the neck and means that, whereas the upper cervical spine is fairly close to the dorsal surface of the neck, the lower cervical vertebrae drop sharply ventral towards the midline of the neck. Therefore, in order to locate the transverse processes, palpation must be much lower down (ventrally) than might be expected from the human equivalent.

The visual and palpatory landmarks are the wings of the atlas, the jugular groove, and the transverse processes of the cervical vertebrae. Muscles that may be identified are the brachiocephalicus and sternocephalicus lying each side of the jugular groove, and the trapezius, splenius, and obliquus capitis.

Anatomical components

Occipito-atlanto-axial complex

Starting at the top is the atlas (Figure 2.9). This is essentially a very chunky version of the bodyless, ring-shaped, human atlas. However, the articular surfaces receiving the skull condyles are much deeper than the human equivalent, which one might expect given the weight of the skull hanging from it. These joints allow mainly flexion and extension. A Canadian study on post-mortem horses reported ranges of about 86° flexion/extension, 44° lateral flexion and, with cranio-caudal glide, 27° of rotation was observed.

The atlas also has substantial transverse processes, or wings, which can be observed and palpated. These wings are large to provide an area for the attachment of some powerful neck muscles. They protrude laterally and are very easily seen starting just below the root of each ear. They are useful landmarks when observing the neck movement in

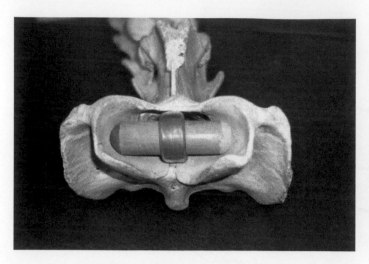

Figure 2.9 Atlas (C1): cranial view showing the ring-shaped bodyless atlas bearing deep, cup-shaped, articular surfaces which receive the occipital condyles and the prominent transverse processes (wings).

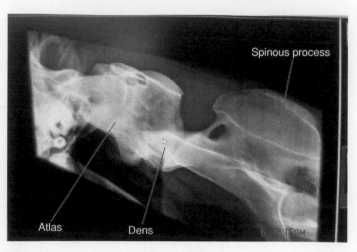

Figure 2.11 X-ray of upper cervical spine: the spinous process of the axis and the dens protruding into the ring of the atlas can be identified.

the short turn. They are also easily palpated, and positional asymmetries can be identified.

Caudally the atlas articulates with the long, imposing structure of the axis (C2) (Figure 2.10). As in humans, the ossification centre of the body of the atlas defects to the axis at the embryonic stage, resulting in a peg (dens) which projects up from the cranial surface of the axis. It fuses with the body at around 7 months. This peg fills up the ventral part of the ring of the atlas. Together with articular surfaces spreading on to the body of the axis, it forms an articulation ideally suited for rotation. In fact, in the post-mortem study, the average neck rotation was 108°, which is about 73% of the total rotation in the cervical spine.

The spinous process of the axis dominates X-rays of this region with its crest-like appearance to which is attached the powerful nuchal ligament (Figure 2.11). It is an area

that is susceptible to congenital abnormalities, particularly narrowing of the spinal canal which, by impinging on the cord itself, can result in varying degrees of ataxia.

In functional terms the occiput, atlas and axis must be considered together. The articulations of the atlas are functionally very important, as the atlas acts as a buffer between the biomechanical requirements of neck movement and the positional requirements of the head. The cervical spine from C2 caudally will laterally flex by sidebending one way and rotating in the other direction (rotation being defined by the direction of movement of the ventral crest). The atlas, however, needs to adopt a different pattern. It will laterally flex one way and rotate the same way in order to keep the head facing forwards. If this ability to counteract the rotation tendencies in the lower cervical spine is impaired, the horse will develop all sorts of only partly effective tricks to look around while keeping the eyes level. This is clearly seen in one of the more important tests in a diagnostic routine: the short turn to assess lateral flexion of the neck (Chapter 7).

Cervical spine (C3 to C7)

Caudal to the occipito-atlanto-axial region, the mid- to lower cervical spine (C3 to C7) has vertebrae with a more consistent box-like shape with a well developed ventral crest, but with very poorly developed spinous processes on the dorsal aspect. These vertebrae begin to snake away from the dorsal surface. Their position can be found by locating the plate-like transverse processes, jutting out laterally, which can be palpated through the overlying muscle above the jugular groove.

The bodies differ from the fairly square human form. They have a rounded, knob-like head at the cephalic end which articulates with a deep fossa in the caudal surface of the vertebra above. Between the two surfaces from C2

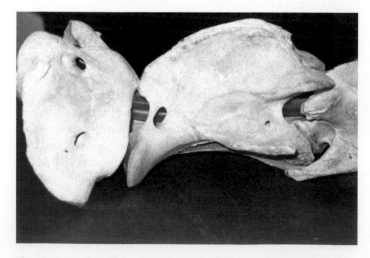

Figure 2.10 Axis (C2): the lateral view shows the large spinous process. Protruding up into the ring of the atlas is the dens.

caudally, intervertebral discs separate the bodies of the vertebrae. These discs are slightly thicker in the cervical region than elsewhere but are, in general, fairly thin, forming only approximately 10% of the length of the horse compared with about 25% in humans. They consist of an outer fibrous annulus and an inner nucleus pulposus, but the boundaries between the two are not distinct and the fibrous quality of the nucleus pulposus reduces the prolapsing tendency of the human structure.

Connecting the vertebral arches, the large, flat, caudal facet joints radiate laterally to articulate with the medially directed cranial facets of the vertebrae below. They are orientated to allow increasing amounts of flexion and extension moving caudally down the cervical column. They also allow lateral flexion from 25 to 45°. Rotation is however limited, which is why optimum function of the atlanto-axial joint in this range is so important.

The vertebral arches and bodies enclose the vertebral canal. The canal varies in width, which can be of clinical significance. The sagittal diameter is greatest at the top of the neck, where most movement occurs. It becomes narrower between the third and fourth cervical vertebrae (C3/4) and then increases towards the lower cervical region. The C3/4 region is a common area for cord compression, which may present as ataxia affecting mainly young thoroughbreds as they start to work; this is sometimes referred to as wobbler syndrome.

Ligamentum nuchae

Dominating the upper border of the neck and confusing unwary osteopaths on the position of the cervical vertebrae is the ligamentum nuchae. This gives the deceptively straight contour of the neck which conceals the serpentine course of the cervical spine below. It supports the head and neck, but is elastic enough to allow the head to drop in order to graze. It is thought to be important in maintaining the normal contours of the back, acting as a bowstring between the poll and withers. As the head is lifted, the bowstring slackens and the supportive traction on the caudal parts of the spine is lost. This is possibly the reason why repositioning the head during exercise can help some cases of back pain, not to mention osteopathic treatment to the neck having beneficial effects more caudally. It has also been proposed that it has a role in the oscillating locomotion pattern of the head and neck in motion by virtue of its elasticity where energy which is stored during stretch can be recovered to lift the head.

The architecture of the ligamentum nuchae is unlike the human version in that it is a paired structure with each of the members of the pair consisting of two distinct parts. One part is the rope-like funicular portion which extends from the nuchal crest on the occipital bone to the spinous processes of the thoracic vertebrae of the withers. It then continues caudally as the supraspinous ligament, becoming increasingly fibrous. At each end, synovial bursae separate the ligament from some of the vertebrae. The first is the nuchal or atlantal bursa which lies over the arch of the atlas, and there is sometimes a second bursa over the spinous process of the second cervical vertebra. The supraspinous bursa separates the ligament from the most prominent part of the withers. Infections of the nuchal and supraspinous bursae are referred to as poll evil and fistulous withers respectively and formerly required extensive surgery to excise the infected, necrotic tissue. In the UK, these conditions have become less common with the control of brucellosis in cattle.

From the underside of this funicular portion of the ligament, the lamellar part fans out to attach on to the dorsal surface of the second to the sixth cervical vertebrae below. This forms an elastic sheet which gives an elasticity to the flexion and extension of the neck, a quality which is apparent in the movement of a relaxed, well functioning horse.

Muscles and movement

The main ligament is the nuchal ligament. Others such as the ventral longitudinal ligament, which is absent until the level of T5, and the dorsal longitudinal ligament are not well developed. Stability and mobility are augmented by the musculature of the region. These muscles also have an important proprioceptive function and bear familiar names such as multifidus and intertranverse muscles. The larger muscles are not as richly innervated and are involved in producing movement (Figure 2.12 and Table 2.2).

There is some distinction between the muscles of the upper cervical spine and the caudal cervical spine, reflecting the fact that functionally the occiput, atlas and axis work very much as a unit.

Upper cervical flexion is produced principally by concentric contraction of the ventral muscles, sternocephalicus, longus capitis and longus colli. Sternocephalicus, also known as sternomandibularis, is obvious from a surface view as it forms the ventral border of the jugular groove.

Extension is produced by bilateral contraction of the erector spinae and dorsal cervical muscles. Lateral flexion and rotation are produced by cranial and caudal oblique and straight muscles of the head, assisted by longus colli, splenius, semispinalis and brachiocephalicus. Of these, brachiocephalicus can be seen as the dorsal margin of the jugular groove. Splenius is also fairly superficial at its cranial end and runs caudal to brachiocephalicus.

The lower cervical and cervicothoracic movement is principally one of flexion, extension and lateral flexion. Flexion is produced by the bilateral action of the scalenes, with the longus colli and sternocephalic muscles. Brachiocephalicus may also be involved, although its principal action is to move the forelimb. Extension follows from erector spinae and dorsal cervical contraction. Lateral flexion is the result of unilateral contraction of ventral muscles such as scalenes

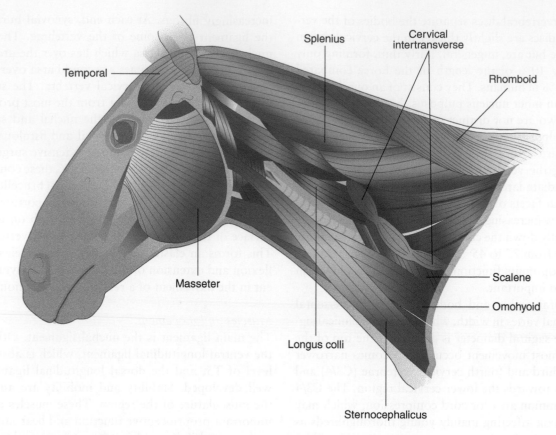

Figure 2.12 Cervical muscles: these provide stability and mobility to the neck.

Table 2.2 Cervical muscles

Muscle	Origin	Insertion	Action
Sternocephalicus (also known as sternomandibularis)	Sternal manubrium	Caudal rim of mandibular ramus	Bilateral contraction – flexion of neck and poll Unilateral contraction – lateral flexion and rotation of head and neck
Longus Capitis	Transverse processes of C3 to C5	Tubercle of occipital bone	Bilateral contraction – flexion of poll Unilateral contraction – lateral flexion and rotation of upper cervical spine
Longus Colli	Vertebral bodies from C2 to T6	Ventral tubercle of C1	Flexion and rotation of cervical and cranial thoracic vertebrae
Splenius	Spinous processes of T2 to T4	Occipital crest, mastoid, wing of atlas, transverse processes of C2 to C5	Bilateral contraction – elevation of head and neck
Brachiocephalicus	Mastoid process	Humeral crest	Protract limb or lateral flexion of head and neck when limb fixed.
Semispinalis	Transverse processes of T1–T7 and articular processes of C spine	Occiput	Extension of head and neck
Scalenes	First rib	Transverse processes of C4–7	Flex the neck
Multifidus	Transverse processes	Spinous processes of 1 to 4 vertebrae above.	Extension and proprioception
Intertransversus	Run from transverse processes of adjacent vertebrae		Lateral flexion of neck

and sternocephalicus, as well as most of the dorsal cervical muscles. The limited amount of rotation in this region is produced by small, deep muscles such as multifidus cervicis.

During normal movement the splenius acts to reduce downward movement of the neck in trot, or to elevate it in walk to allow full protraction of the forelimb by brachiocephalicus. Sternocephalicus has a reciprocal action to control elevation of the neck.

Thoracolumbar Spine

Overview

For some reason, most animal anatomy books deal with the thoracic and the lumbar spine in one breath. It may be because the line of the vertebral bodies forms a straight span referred to as the thoracolumbar bridge. Until about 6 months of age, this forms a gentle curve that is convex dorsally. With maturity the weight of the internal organs slung below this bridge can be supported by drawing the curve down to close-pack the vertebral bodies into a fairly rigid, straight structure. The same principle applies if someone is sitting on top, which is why, from strength and stability considerations, one would not choose to buy a horse with an obvious sway back. It is difficult to evaluate the exact course of the thoracolumbar spine from a surface view because of the varying heights of the dorsal spinous processes (DSPs). Whereas, in the cervical spine, spinous processes seem to have been left out, the thoracic spine makes up for this omission.

The height increases sharply from the first thoracic (T1) spinous process to a maximum height of around 10–15 cm at the fourth and fifth thoracic vertebrae (T4/5), which is the point at which the height of a horse is measured from the ground. From T4/5 caudally, the height tails off to become negligible again in the sacrum.

Orientation

To someone accustomed to the modest number of 12 thoracic vertebrae in the human, a horse's 18, together with same number of ribs, can be disorientating. Although the spinous processes are palpable, it is often difficult to identify each prominence in order to count the individual vertebrae. However, a reasonable guideline may be obtained by taking the high point (T4/5), together with the scapula overlying T1 to T7 to give the humpy shape of the withers. Following the last rib up to the vertebral attachment will give the position of T18, and riders generally sit above T13.

Anatomical components

The basic unit of the thoracic spine is a short vertebral body, large dorsal spinous processes, and stubby transverse processes which bear a facet for articulation with the rib. The six lumbar vertebrae have longer bodies, large, laterally projecting transverse processes, and shorter, cranially-sloping spinous processes. These features vary along the length of the thoracolumbar spine (Figure 2.13).

The varying height of the spinous processes makes it difficult to imagine the position of the vertebral bodies. An

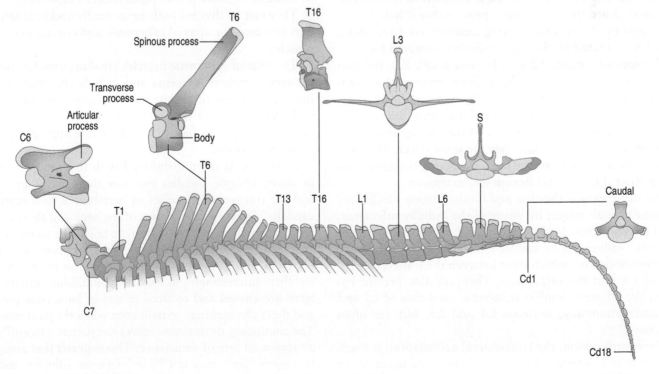

Figure 2.13 Thoracolumbar spine: the vertebrae vary in construction according to region.

added complication is that they also vary in orientation. Those of the upper thoracic spine all slope caudally until T16 (the logically named anticlinal vertebra) which points vertically upwards. Those caudal to T16 as far as L6 are directed cranially. At the sacrum they again point caudally, which means that the distance between the spinous processes at this junction is relatively large and therefore allows a greater range of movement at the lumbosacral joint. Of interest in this region is that post-mortem studies have shown that, not infrequently, the spinous processes do not arise in an exactly perpendicular fashion from the vertebral arches, but instead veer to one side or the other. This suggests that to rely on positional factors alone for identifying areas of spinal dysfunction may not be helpful.

Not only does T16 signal a change in spinous process orientation, but it is also usually the point at which the orientation of the facets changes, for which it also, less logically, attracts the label of the diaphragmatic vertebra. From T2 to T16, the facets are small, tangentially orientated with the cranial articular facet facing dorsally and medially, and the caudal facing ventrally and laterally. At T16, the caudal facets change dramatically to become radial (medial facing) along the lines of the cervical vertebrae. Caudal to T16, the radial orientation allows cranial and caudal facets to interlock.

These variations in structure have implications for movement. Although mobility is relatively restricted compared with the cervical spine, the thoracolumbar spine can be divided into four functional and morphological regions.

The first region of T1 and T2 is adapted to flexion and extension, aided by a T1 spinous process that is half the size of T2 and by the lack of a strong ligamentous attachment. Rotation is limited by the large radially orientated facets.

The second region, T2 to T16, has small, flat and tangentially orientated facets which allow movement in rotation, and lateral flexion ranges mainly between T9 and T14. Above this region, the attachment of the ribs to the sternum limits movement and caudal to T14 the change to radially orientated interlocking facets has the same effect. The large spinous processes with strong interconnecting connective tissues restrict dorsoventral flexion and extension.

The third, caudal thoracic and lumbar region has limited movement in all ranges by virtue of the radially orientated, interlocking facets. In the caudal lumbar spine, movement is further influenced by lateral joints, unique to the horse and the rhinoceros, which form between the transverse process of L6 and the sacral alar. They are also present between the adjacent lumbar transverse processes of L5 and L6, and, commonly, between L4 and L5, but are often ankylosed.

The fourth region, the lumbosacral articulation, is much more mobile as a result of facet orientation and ligamentous structure. Dorsoventral flexion and extension are allowed by the widely spaced spinous processes and the absence of the supraspinous ligament, as well as the laterally facing caudal facets of L6 and the medially orientated sacral facets. The poorly developed intervertebral ligamentous structure makes this joint susceptible to injury. The orientation of the facets limits rotation and lateral flexion.

Most radiographic damage found in the thoracolumbar spine is centred around the midpoint (T13/14) where the interspinous spaces are narrowest. Post-mortem studies show that, if extension of the spine exceeds 4 mm, there will be repeated impingement of the dorsal spinous process summits. This pathological process is described as overriding dorsal spinal processes or 'kissing spines', which are a common cause of back pain in horses and generally affect segments between T12 and L2. It is most often seen in thoroughbreds or thoroughbred crosses, and there is only a low incidence in ponies.

Muscles and movement

The muscles of this region are divided into two categories. The epaxial muscles are those dorsal to the transverse processes and can act as extensors of the spine. The rest of the trunk muscles, ventral to the transverse processes, are hypaxial muscles.

The epaxial muscles

The epaxial muscles are often referred in anatomy texts as being numerous and complicated and of which the details 'are not of clinical significance'. Some description is, however, warranted as they have important contributions to make in the control and production of movement.

They can be divided both functionally and anatomically into two sets, the epaxial cybernetic and epaxial gymnastic muscles.

The *epaxial cybernetic* muscles are short muscles running between vertebral segments and include the interspinales, intertransversarii and rotatores. They are richly innervated with proprioceptors which monitor vertebral position and provide continuous feedback to facilitate appropriate postural adjustments.

Multifidus is often mentioned with this group, running in short, oblique bundles between the spinous processes and the transverse processes of vertebrae 2 to 3 segments caudally. These run the course of the neck and thoracolumbar spine with an extension into the tail as the sacrocaudalis dorsalis. These are tonically active in all movements requiring trunk stabilisation, suggesting a role in intersegmental stability. Interestingly, in humans, multifidus activity patterns are altered and reduced in size in back pain patients and these changes may remain even when the pain resolves. The continuing dysfunction leaves the patient susceptible to an increased rate of recurrence. This suggests that analgesic treatment alone may not be a long-term solution and the role of osteopathy in restoring segmental function may be of significant benefit.

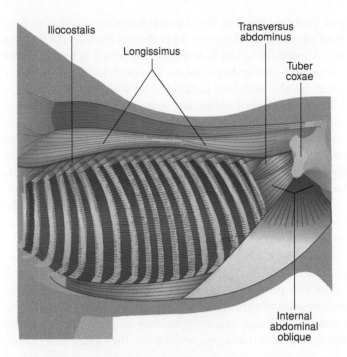

Figure 2.14 Epaxial gymnastic muscles: these run in three columns and are responsible for producing movement.

The *epaxial gymnastic* muscles are the ones that produce movement. They form an unbroken chain of muscle running from the pelvis to occiput, tending to fuse over the loins, fan out in the trunk and split into additional units in the neck. They ascend in three columns (Figure 2.14).

The lateral column, the iliocostalis, runs from the thoracolumbar fascia and ribs 4 to 18 to insert on the transverse process of C7 and caudal border of the ribs to depress the ribs, thereby assisting expiration. The cervical extension runs from the first rib to the transverse processes of C3 to C7 and extends the neck.

The middle column is formed by longissimus, also referred to as longissimus dorsi in the thoracolumbar spine. This is the largest and longest of the epaxial muscles filling in the space between the dorsal spinous processes and the transverse processes. It is involved in stabilising the back and preventing excessive dorsoventral and lateral movements. It is frequently implicated in injuries resulting from direct trauma, fatigue or strains following a fall, and is the site of tender points on palpation. Together with the most medial group, the spinalis thoracis and the juxtavertebral multifidus, these muscles form the bulk of the topline (Figure 2.15). Where these muscles are weak and underdeveloped, the spinous processes jut out prominently, a condition that is often described as loss of topline.

The hypaxial muscles

Ventral to the transverse processes, the hypaxial muscles either complement or oppose the actions of the epaxial muscles. In terms of gross movement, the hypaxial muscles are antagonistic to the epaxial muscles, but with regard to complex movement they work synergistically to create vertebral column stability and controlled, smooth movement. The hypaxial muscles include psoas and quadratus lumborum as well as the abdominal muscles.

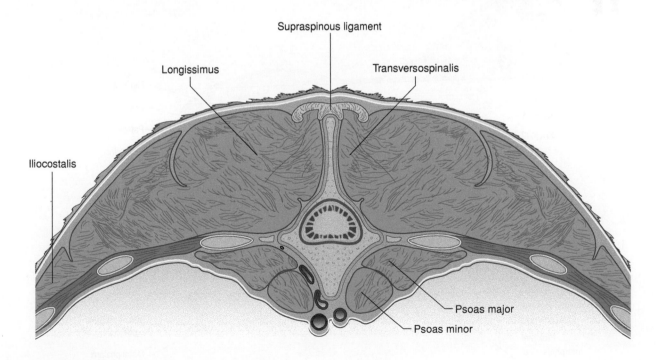

Figure 2.15 Transverse section of spine: this shows the three columns of the iliocostalis, longissimus and transversospinalis (spinalis, rotatores, intertransversarii, multifidi).

Psoas major arises from the transverse processes and bodies of the lumbar vertebrae and combines with iliacus in its descent from the wing and shaft of the ilium to form a common head inserting into the lesser trochanter of the femur. It flexes and externally rotates the hindlimb and contributes to the stability of the lumbar spine. Assisting in this stabilising function is quadratus lumborum, running from the last ribs and lumbar transverse processes to the sacrum.

The abdominal muscles lie on the ventral surface of the trunk. They form a long, not very thick support apparatus for the considerable weight of the viscera and are also involved in respiration and locomotion. They are very like the human structures and even bear the same names. Rectus abdominis, running from the costal cartilages of the fourth to the ninth ribs to the pubic rim, flexes the thoracolumbosacral regions of the spine, or slightly laterally flexes and rotates when working unilaterally. This is complemented by the actions of the external and internal abdominal muscles and the transversus abdominis. In addition to supporting the viscera, they can also lift the floor of the abdomen, compressing its contents to assist in expiration, parturition, urination and defaecation. Their role in expiration is particularly important in older animals with breathing difficulties where the line of the abdominis externus may be seen as a prominent line running from elbow to ilium.

Results from electromyographic and kinematic studies are beginning to show the intricate details of how these muscles and the bony parts of the skeleton function together to produce movement. There are a number of theories, one of the best known being the bow and string which is based on the interaction of the hypaxial and epaxial muscles and their effect on the vertebral column. The stiff core (the bow) is formed by the thoracolumbar spine with the contraction of the epaxial muscles tending to compact the vertebrae. The ventral string is formed by the hypaxial muscles, contraction of which tends to curve the bow. This effect is countered by the weight of the viscera on the ventral string which tends to flatten the bow.

At low speeds such as walk, a fair bit of flexibility in the thoracolumbar spine allows lateral flexion and rotation and, to a lesser extent, flexion and extension. At higher speeds, there are advantages to stabilising the vertebral column so that the 'bow' is straightened. Stiffening the column will allow the propulsive effort generated by the hindlimbs to be transmitted through the spine to produce forward movement. It will also facilitate balance and stability in those inherently unstable asymmetric gaits, the canter and gallop.

THE LIMBS

The legs of the horse can be a little confusing for human osteopaths. The elements making up the limbs of horses and humans are similar but the proportions, orientation and function are quite different (Figure 2.16). In addition, the

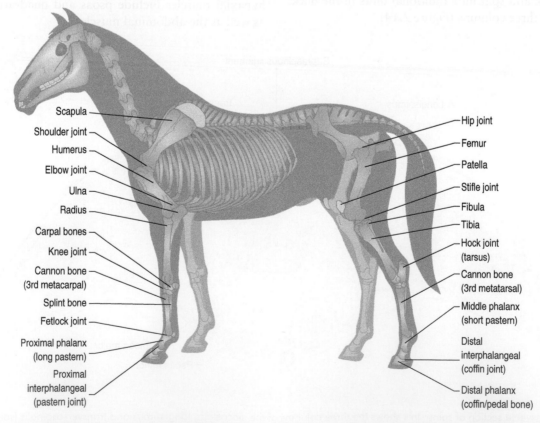

Scapula
Shoulder joint
Humerus
Elbow joint
Ulna
Radius
Carpal bones
Knee joint
Cannon bone
(3rd metacarpal)
Splint bone
Fetlock joint
Proximal phalanx
(long pastern)
Proximal
interphalangeal
(pastern joint)

Hip joint
Femur
Patella
Stifle joint
Fibula
Tibia
Hock joint
(tarsus)
Cannon bone
(3rd metatarsal)
Middle phalanx
(short pastern)
Distal
interphalangeal
(coffin joint)
Distal phalanx
(coffin/pedal bone)

Figure 2.16 Overview of limbs: in human and equine limb anatomy, differences in nomenclature, proportion, orientation and function exist.

horse requires various ligamentous and tendinous apparatuses just to stand upright. Further confusion can arise in the realm of nomenclature as equestrian folk play fast and loose with joint names, and anatomy books over the years have introduced alternative terminology – often without reference to previous incarnations.

Overview

Equine limbs are specifically adapted for speed, and in the process have lost versatility. They have been lengthened, particularly below the carpus and tarsus, by bringing the equivalent of the wrist and heel well off the ground, a posture which is referred to as an unguligrade. This is at variance with the human stance where the heel remains in contact with the ground in what is termed a plantigrade posture (Figure 2.17). Essentially, the horse runs on its third fingernail which takes the form of a hoof. In practical terms, the practitioner must shift the eye proximally to locate the joint which is its human equivalent. For example, in the foreleg, the elbow lies close to the thorax, and the carpals (the equivalent of the human wrist and confusingly referred to as the knee) occupy a central position in the limb. In the hindlimb, the horse equivalent of the knee (termed the stifle) lies well up towards the abdomen.

The limbs are carried by two specialised girdles which are different to reflect their particular functions. The thoracic girdle which bears the forelimbs, having no clavicle, is without a bony connection with the vertebral column and is therefore eminently suitable for a shock-absorbing role. The pelvic girdle is strongly linked with the spine in order that the power generated by the hindlimbs can be transmitted through the spine to produce forward propulsion.

Much of the muscle bulk is located in the girdle and proximal limb region. Distal to the carpals the propulsive mechanism is largely tendinous as the energy acquired by the fibres when these tendons are stretched is released as they are allowed to recoil.

Features unfamiliar to the human anatomist include the equine version of digital pads and the arrangement making up the hoof.

The following description of the limb will review the basic structures and some surface anatomy which may be useful to the practitioner. Details of origins and insertions and exact anatomical relationships can be found in textbooks devoted to the subject.

The section will be divided into the girdles and the proximal limbs, both thoracic and pelvic, followed by the distal limbs which are similar in both fore- and hindlegs. An overview of the ligamentous support mechanisms will also be given.

THORACIC GIRDLE AND PROXIMAL FORELIMB

Overview

The thoracic girdle and forelegs are adapted for movement, mainly in flexion and extension ranges, as well as support, with 60% of the weight of the horse going through the forelimbs. They also fulfil a shock-absorbing requirement (Figures 2.18–2.21) and are therefore susceptible to a number of pathologies (Figure 2.22). The girdle is formed from a system of muscular attachments linking the scapulae with the thorax.

The proximal forelimb extends from the shoulder region to the carpals. It is composed of the scapula and humerus, making up the shoulder joint, with the distal end of the humerus and the proximal radius and ulna forming the elbow joint. The carpal joint or knee is made up of seven main bones and often a pea-like first carpal bone. The fourth carpal bone has a tubercle on its caudal surface which may be the equivalent of the fifth carpal in other species.

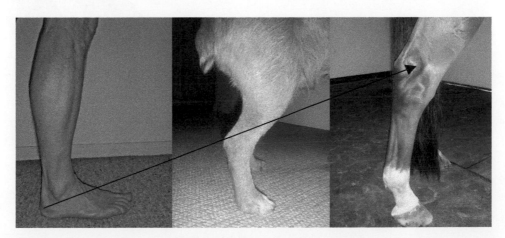

Figure 2.17 Plantigrade to unguligrade posture: human posture (left) is plantigrade with the heel in contact with the ground whereas that of the dog (centre) is digitigrade with just digits in contact with the ground. The equestrian limb (right) has been lengthened below the carpus and tarsus by bringing the equivalent of the wrist and heel well off the ground with only the 'fingernail' (hoof) touching the surface in an unguligrade stance.

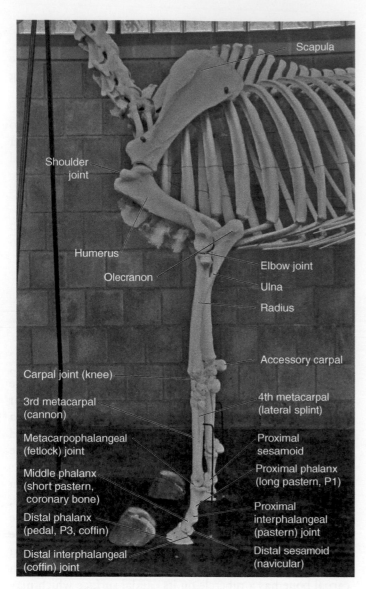

Figure 2.18 Skeleton of the forelimb.

Scapula

Shoulder
joint

Humerus

Olecranon

Elbow joint

Ulna

Radius

Accessory carpal

Carpal joint (knee)

3rd metacarpal
(cannon)

4th metacarpal
(lateral splint)

Metacarpophalangeal
(fetlock) joint

Proximal
sesamoid

Middle phalanx
(short pastern,
coronary bone)

Proximal phalanx
(long pastern, P1)

Distal phalanx
(pedal, P3, coffin)

Proximal
interphalangeal
(pastern) joint

Distal interphalangeal
(coffin) joint

Distal sesamoid
(navicular)

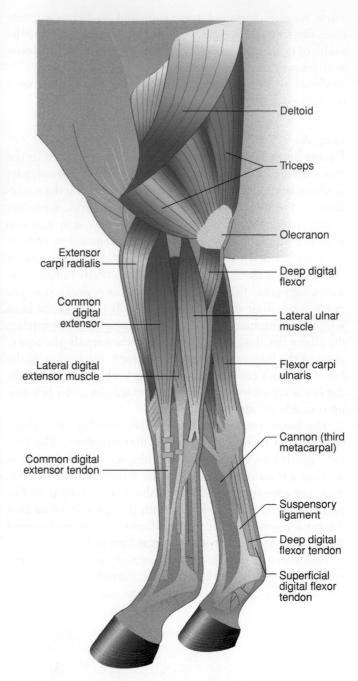

Figure 2.19 Superficial muscles of the forelimb.

Deltoid

Triceps

Olecranon

Deep digital
flexor

Extensor
carpi radialis

Lateral ulnar
muscle

Common
digital
extensor

Flexor carpi
ulnaris

Lateral digital
extensor muscle

Cannon (third
metacarpal)

Common digital
extensor tendon

Suspensory
ligament

Deep digital
flexor tendon

Superficial
digital flexor
tendon

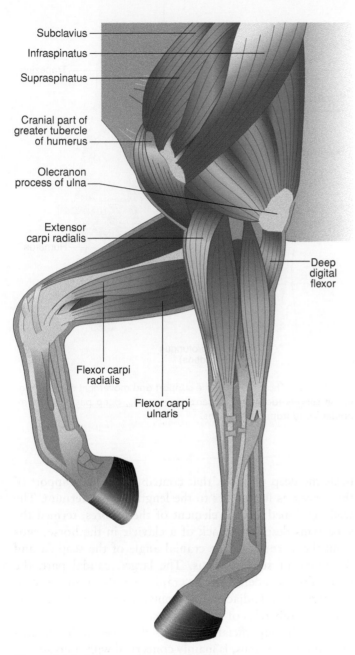

Subclavius

Infraspinatus

Supraspinatus

Cranial part of
greater tubercle
of humerus

Olecranon
process of ulna

Extensor
carpi radialis

Deep
digital
flexor

Flexor carpi
radialis

Flexor carpi
ulnaris

Figure 2.20 Deep muscles of the forelimb.

Thoracic Girdle

This is composed of the scapular region and its connections to the thoracic and cervical spine.

Functional anatomy

The forelimbs have no actual bony link with the thorax as there is no clavicle. The connection is through a synsarcosis (syn = connection with; sarcosis = of flesh) and takes the form of a muscular sling, suspended between the struts of the forelimbs, which cradles the thorax. This muscular link

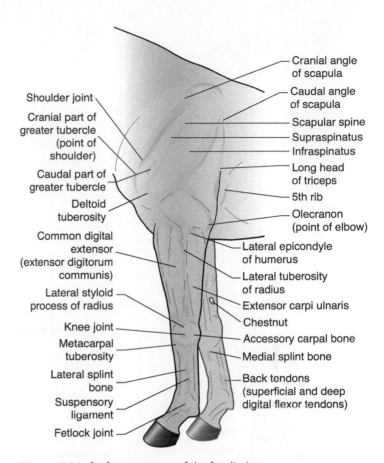

Shoulder joint

Cranial part of
greater tubercle
(point of
shoulder)

Caudal part of
greater tubercle

Deltoid
tuberosity

Common digital
extensor
(extensor digitorum
communis)

Lateral styloid
process of radius

Knee joint

Metacarpal
tuberosity

Lateral splint
bone

Suspensory
ligament

Fetlock joint

Cranial angle
of scapula

Caudal angle
of scapula

Scapular spine

Supraspinatus

Infraspinatus

Long head
of triceps

5th rib

Olecranon
(point of elbow)

Lateral epicondyle
of humerus

Lateral tuberosity
of radius

Extensor carpi ulnaris

Chestnut

Accessory carpal bone

Medial splint bone

Back tendons
(superficial and deep
digital flexor tendons)

Figure 2.21 Surface anatomy of the forelimb.

facilitates the shock-absorbing function of the forelimb. It is the rotation of the thorax in the sling that allows much of the lateral movement evident in dressage manoeuvres or fast turns in polo. In addition, the contraction of serratus and pectoral muscles lifts the thorax in relation to the forelimbs to change the centre of gravity.

The focus for this union is the scapula which is important both in support and movement. It provides an area of attachment for the sling muscles. It also rotates about a pivot point as well as sliding over the thorax ventrally and cranially during limb protraction, and dorsally and caudally during limb retraction, thereby making a key contribution to the range of forelimb movement.

Anatomical components

The scapula is a triangular bone which slopes caudally on the thoracic cage from the point of the shoulder. It has palpable cranial and caudal angles. Between the angles, the dorsal border is extended by a non-bony extension, the scapular cartilage, to which serratus ventralis is attached.

The external surface is divided by the sloping ridge of the scapular spine which separates the infraspinatus and supraspinatus muscles. It is palpable in the body of the scapula but diminishes distally and does not form an acromium as is the case in humans.

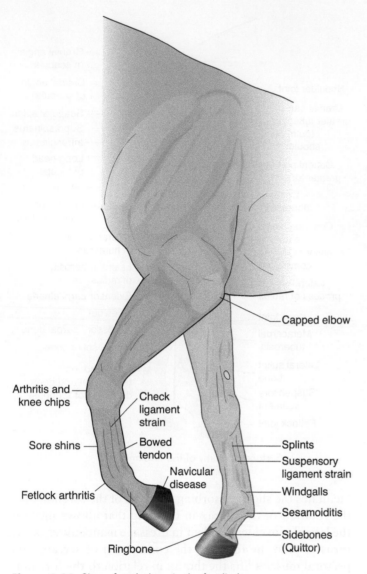

Figure 2.22 Sites of pathology in the forelimb.

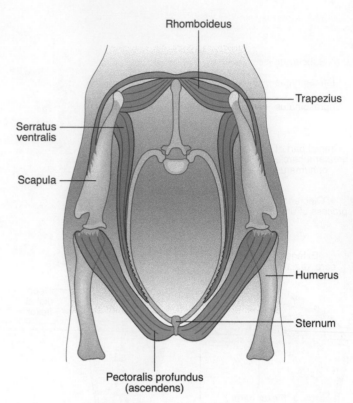

Figure 2.23 Thoracic sling: the support and movement of the thorax in the sling is facilitated by serratus ventralis, deep pectoral, rhomboideus and trapezius muscles.

It is the arrangement of the muscles associated with the scapula that contribute to support and locomotion functions. The support and movement of the thorax in the sling is facilitated by serratus ventralis, deep pectoral, rhomboideus and trapezius muscles (Figure 2.23). The deepest structure of the sling is the serratus ventralis. This is a bulky, extensive muscle with fleshy fingers converging on to the scapular cartilage from an origin stretching from the fourth cervical vertebra to the tenth rib. Its principal function is to support the thorax. In addition, activity of the cervical part rotates the scapula to retract the limb, while the thoracic part produces protraction.

Assisting the serratus ventralis are elements of the pectoral muscles. These lie in two layers, superficial and deep (Figure 2.24). It is the pectoralis profundus, also referred

to as the deep pectoral, that contributes to the support of the thorax as it attaches to the length of the sternum. The well developed cranial element of these fibres, termed the subclavius despite the lack of a clavicle in the horse, runs from the sternum to the cranial angle of the scapula and the fascia of supraspinatus. The larger, caudal part, the pectoralis ascendens, passes craniolaterally from the caudal sternum and adjacent abdominal floor up to the greater and lesser tubercles of the humerus.

Pectoralis superficialis, composed of pectoralis descendens and transversus, is mainly concerned with limb adduction. Both parts arise from the cranial section of the sternum. The cranially situated pectoralis descendens runs down to the crest of the humerus. Caudal to this on the sternum, the pectoralis transversus passes laterally to the medial fascia of the forelimb.

The dorsal component of the thoracic sling is formed by trapezius and rhomboideus. The scapular spine provides an attachment for trapezius as it descends from the supraspinous ligaments almost from the poll to beyond the withers. The cervical part acts on the forelimb to bring it forward, while the thoracic part retracts the limb. Acting together, they lift the scapula.

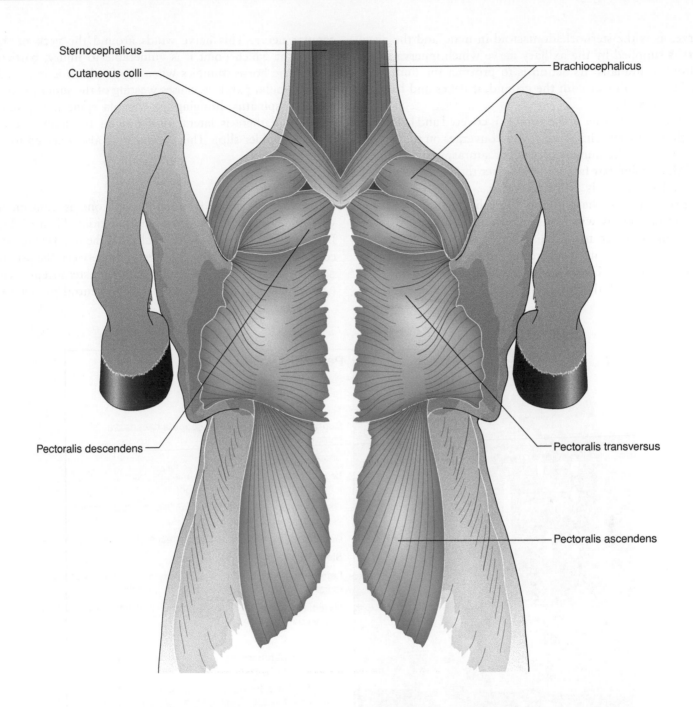

Sternocephalicus

Cutaneous colli

Brachiocephalicus

Pectoralis descendens

Pectoralis transversus

Pectoralis ascendens

Figure 2.24 Pectoral muscles: elements of these contribute to the thoracic sling. Pectoralis profundus is formed from the subclavius and pectoralis ascendens, and pectoralis superficialis is composed of pectoralis descendens and transversus.

Lying deep to trapezius, the rhomboideus runs from the supraspinous and nuchal ligaments of C2 to C7 to insert on to the medial surface of the scapular cartilage. This also raises the scapula.

Girdle muscles associated with the scapula but more involved with neck and limb movement are the brachiocephalicus and latissimus dorsi.

The brachiocephalicus runs from the temporal bone and nuchal crest and combines in the shoulder region with fibres running from the transverse processes of the cervical spine to attach to the humeral crest and associated fascia. It is divided by a fibrous band which is the remnant of the clavicle. Its nerve supply reflects its human equivalent. The proximal part of the brachiocephalicus is supplied by the accessory nerve, as is the sternocleidomastoid in man, and the distal part is supplied by the axillary nerve which innervates the deltoid in humans. Its action is to protract the limb or, if the leg is in contact with the ground, it flexes and laterally bends the neck.

The caudal border of the scapula is covered and held on to the thorax by latissimus dorsi as it converges on to the teres tuberosity of the humerus from the supraspinous ligament and thoracolumbar fascia of the lower thoracic and lumbar spine. This muscle is a limb retractor.

Either side of the scapular spine lie the supraspinatus and infraspinatus which insert on to the tubercles of the humerus and act to stabilise the shoulder. The tendon of the infraspinatus is protected from bone by a bursa which, if inflamed, may cause the horse to stand with the leg abducted. Both muscles are supplied by the supras-

capular nerve. This nerve winds around the neck of the scapula at which point it is vulnerable to injury, particularly if the horse stumbles when the forelimb is retracted. Suprascapular paralysis causes wasting of the supraspinatus and infraspinatus, bringing the scapula spine into prominence, and there is lateral deviation of the limb at each stride (shoulder slip). This condition is also referred to as 'sweeney'.

Surface anatomy

Observing the horse from the front, one is confronted with a landscape of grooves and undulations (Figure 2.25). Descending from the neck on each side, the jugular grooves containing the external jugular veins lie between the prominent brachiocephalic dorsally and the sternocephalicus (sternomandibularis) muscle ventrally. A central line denotes

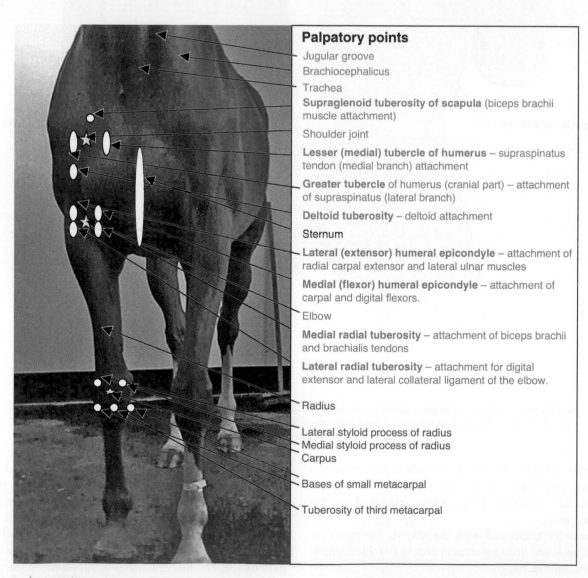

Palpatory points

Jugular groove

Brachiocephalicus

Trachea

Supraglenoid tuberosity of scapula (biceps brachii muscle attachment)

Shoulder joint

Lesser (medial) tubercle of humerus – supraspinatus tendon (medial branch) attachment

Greater tubercle of humerus (cranial part) – attachment of supraspinatus (lateral branch)

Deltoid tuberosity – deltoid attachment

Sternum

Lateral (extensor) humeral epicondyle – attachment of radial carpal extensor and lateral ulnar muscles

Medial (flexor) humeral epicondyle – attachment of carpal and digital flexors.

Elbow

Medial radial tuberosity – attachment of biceps brachii and brachialis tendons

Lateral radial tuberosity – attachment for digital extensor and lateral collateral ligament of the elbow.

Radius

Lateral styloid process of radius
Medial styloid process of radius
Carpus

Bases of small metacarpal

Tuberosity of third metacarpal

Figure 2.25 Surface anatomy of the forelimb.

the position of the trachea covered by the sternothyro-hyoid muscle. Between the bulging descending pectoral muscles is the median pectoral groove overlying the sternum. Laterally, the pectoral muscles are separated from the brachiocephalicus by a shallow lateral pectoral groove, which widens above into the jugular fossa. This is sometimes referred to as the supraclavicular fossa, despite the absence of a clavicle.

From the side a number of features can be identified (Figure 2.21). A shallow line of indentation sloping upwards and backwards towards the withers gives the position of the spine of the scapula. Palpation along this line gives a good idea of the orientation of the scapula (or slope of the shoulder), which should ideally be around 45° to the horizontal. Either side of this indentation are the muscles of supraspinatus and the less easily identified infraspinatus, leading down to the point of the shoulder, a bony prominence formed by the cranial part of the greater tubercle of the humerus. The caudal part of the greater tubercle is also palpable. Overlying much of infraspinatus, the deltoid muscle can be seen passing down to attach to the palpable deltoid tubercle lying at the distal end of the prominent crest which descends from the greater tubercles on the lateral surface of the humerus.

Proximal Forelimb

Overview

The humerus extends from the shoulder to the elbow joint where it connects with the ulna and radius. Below this, the structure causes limb orientation to diverge from the human arrangement. The firm connection of the short ulna to the proximal radius prevents supination and pronation movements which contribute to manual dexterity in man. This also prevents the adoption of the somewhat unnatural position of palms facing forwards, which is the starting point for all human anatomical descriptions. So from here down there is a departure from the familiar. In contrast to the human, the distal limb extensors, although originating from the lateral epicondyle of the humerus, will then run on the dorsal surface of the limb while the flexors, mainly from the medial epicondyle, are found on the caudal or palmar surface of the limb.

The carpus, made up of two rows of carpal bones and three synovial joint spaces, is referred to as the knee. Over these, a series of synovial sheaths and canals transmit the tendons of muscles acting on the digits.

Anatomical components

Compared with the elegant, willowy, human humerus (described by a vet as 'pathetically thin'), that of the horse is a thick, squat structure, allowing it to withstand the great forces passing through it. Even so, it is very occasionally

shattered by unsynchronised muscle movement at the gallop. From its articulation with the glenoid cavity of the scapula at the shoulder, the spheroidal nature of the shoulder joint suggests the ability to move in a number of planes. In practice, however, movement is limited to flexion and extension by the closely knit tendons of infraspinatus and, to a degree, supraspinatus laterally and subscapularis medially.

Also laterally, running from the caudal border and spine of the scapula to the deltoid tubercle on the humerus, is the deltoid muscle whose action is to flex the shoulder. A major contributor in this activity on the medial side is the teres major from the caudal scapula which inserts, with the latissimus dorsi, on to the teres tubercle of the humerus.

The humerus runs distally and caudally, ideally at about 50°, to the easily seen point of the elbow formed by the olecranon process of the ulna, lying tucked into the thorax at the level of the fifth rib.

The elbow, like other joints in the limb, is mainly designed for flexion and extension. Unlike other joints, its resting position is midway between full flexion and extension braced by collateral ligaments and the antagonistic action of flexors and extensors. The humerus forms an angle preferably of around 145° with the ulna and radius. Flexion through the joint is not straight, but slightly outward rotating. When this rotation is exaggerated, particularly in trot, the outward swing is more pronounced and it can contribute to an action where the horse is said to 'dish', although this comes more from the distal limb and poor farriery.

From the point of the elbow, the extensor muscles, principally the triceps, form a rounded muscle mass cranial to the elbow joint. The largest section, the long head of triceps, crosses two joints to insert on to the caudal border of the scapula and acts to flex the shoulder while extending the elbow. The lateral and medial heads act only to extend the elbow as they originate from the shaft of the humerus. A bursa lies between the triceps insertion and the olecranon. An acquired bursa may also be found between the olecranon and the skin which, if bruised, may result in a cold, painless swelling known as capped elbow.

Flexion of the elbow is produced by biceps and brachioradialis. Biceps is not only the most important flexor of the elbow, but also has a function in passive stabilisation of the limb as part of the stay mechanism. It has a single origin from the supraglenoid tubercle and runs down the intertubercular groove but separated from the bone by a bursa. The bicipital bursa may become inflamed, resulting in shoulder lameness. The biceps inserts mainly on the radial tuberosity. An important characteristic is that it has an internal fibrous band within the belly of the muscle which splits away distally to blend with the extensor carpi radialis. This band, known as the lacertus fibrosus, crosses the flexor aspect of the elbow and is taut in the standing animal which helps to maintain carpal joint extension.

If the humerus seems unfamiliar to the human anatomist, the forelimb, made up of the ulna and radius, is also different. These differences have implications for ranges of movement and orientation of the limb.

The main anatomical difference is in the ulna. The ulna is referred to as a 'reduced long bone' in that it finishes in a union (fibrous in many animals) on the caudal surface of the radius, ending just proximal to the centre of the radius. There is often a fibrous cord distally which represents the distal ulna. This lack of separation between the radius and ulna does not allow for the movements of supination and pronation.

The radius forms a 145° angle with the humerus and should drop vertically from the elbow joint to the carpus. With the ulna terminating proximally, the radius itself widens distally to articulate with the carpus at what is referred to as the knee but which is, in fact, the equivalent of the human wrist. Here the radius is grooved on its cranial surface to accommodate the extensor tendons. It has medial and lateral styloid processes for the attachment of collateral ligaments.

The carpal bones are a collection of seven or eight bones and are arranged in proximal and distal rows between the radius and the third metacarpal bone (Figure 2.26). They are named for their position, although this gives the impression that the ulna extends to the carpus which it does not. Also at variance with human descriptions, the radial side is found medially and the ulnar side is situated laterally.

Bearing these vagaries in mind, the proximal group from medial to lateral comprises the radial carpal, intermediate carpal and ulnar carpal, and these have a weight-bearing function. Projecting from the palmar surface to articulate with the lateral styloid process of the radius and the ulnar carpal, but not bearing any weight, is the accessory carpal

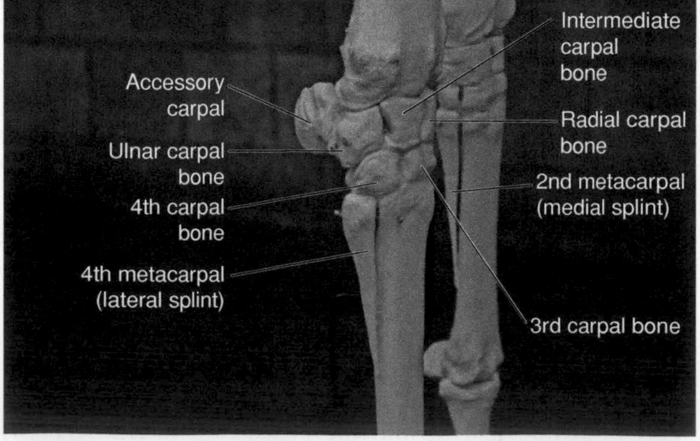

Figure 2.26 Carpal bones: this collection of seven or eight bones are arranged in two rows.

bone which equates to the human pisiform. It is a sesamoid bone acting as a pulley block for the tendons of flexor carpi ulnaris and ulnaris lateralis.

The distal row has three bones which are, from medial to lateral, the second, third and fourth carpal bones. There is often a pea-sized first carpal superimposed over the second carpal and embedded in the palmar carpal ligament. On X-ray it may be mistaken for a chip fracture. A fifth carpal is occasionally seen.

The carpal joint is fully extended when standing and flexes about 95° through the radiocarpal joint and 45° at the midcarpal level. There is little movement at the carpometacarpal junction.

Surface anatomy

The rounded aspect of the shoulder is formed by the brachiocephalicus. The cranial part of the greater tubercle of the humerus (point of shoulder) is palpable through this muscle. Caudal to this is the caudal part of the greater tubercle and running distally is the humeral crest ending in the deltoid tuberosity (Figure 2.21).

Distally, the main palpatory points are the prominent olecranon process forming the point of the elbow, as well as the lateral epicondyle of the humerus and the lateral radial tuberosity which identify the position of the elbow joint itself. These latter two landmarks may be located by palpating up the lateral shaft of the radius between the swelling muscle bodies of the extensor digitorum communis in front and the extensor carpi ulnaris behind until a vertical band of tissue, the lateral collateral ligament, can be felt joining humerus to radius.

At the distal end of the radius, the medial and lateral styloid processes are palpable, and of the carpal bones the accessory carpal bone can be felt projecting caudally.

PELVIS AND PROXIMAL HINDLIMB

Overview

The hindlimbs take only 40% of the weight of the horse but generate 85% of the power for forward propulsion. To facilitate this, there are firm connections between the legs, pelvis and lumbar spine in contrast to the synsarcosis of the thoracic girdle and forelimb relationship. The limbs also have a mechanism involving the stifle and hock which provides a rigid strut through which force can be transmitted from the ground into the spine.

The hindlimb is composed of bones and joints which, in part, resemble the human form although some of the terminology is different (Figures 2.27–2.31). The hip joint, formed from the pelvis and femur, compares well with its human counterpart. However, distally, the femur meets the tibia at the stifle joint which, complete with its patella, is the equivalent of the human knee joint although it is sited well

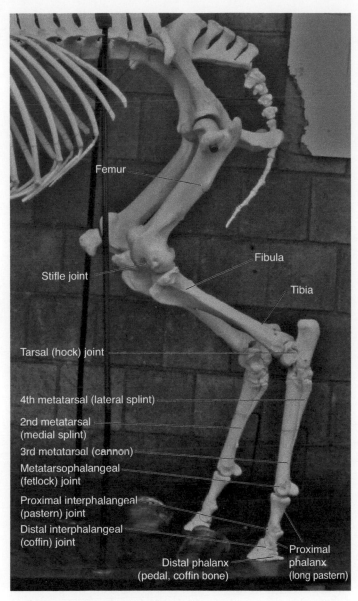

Figure 2.27 Skeleton of hindlimb.

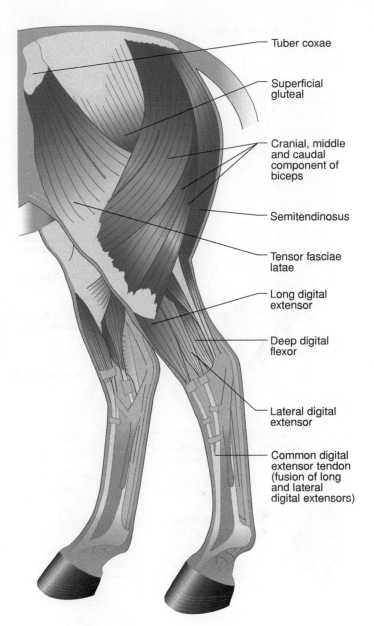

Figure 2.28 Superficial muscles of hindlimb.

up towards the abdomen. This may cause some confusion as it is the carpal joint in the foreleg which is referred to as the horse's knee. An *aide-mémoire* for the name and site of this articulation is the catch phrase 'a knee in the groin stifles all comment'! The stifle has a locking mechanism providing support when the horse shifts much of the weight on to one leg. The tibia runs down to the talus which, together with the calcaneus and the tarsals, forms the hock or tarsus. The calcaneus is the largest bone of this joint and it protrudes caudally to form the point of the hock which is the equivalent of the human heel.

Anatomical components

The pelvis is composed of the pelvic bones and the sacrum. The sacrum is the familiar triangular shape made up of five

fused vertebrae. It lies slightly tipped between the two pelvic bones with its caudal end higher. This orientation is not immediately evident, as the eye is inevitably drawn to the dorsally protruding tuber sacrale of the ilium and the downward slope backwards towards the tail, which, one might be forgiven for assuming, is the line of the sacrum. In fact, the body of the sacrum lies deep to the tuber sacrale.

The sacrum is connected to the ilium by sock-shaped flat surfaces inclined about 30° to the horizontal. This connection combines a synovial articulation with an extensive fibrous union with associated strong ligaments. There is the usual discussion about whether these joints move, which is familiar territory to those who remember the human medics' intransigent position based on post-mortem

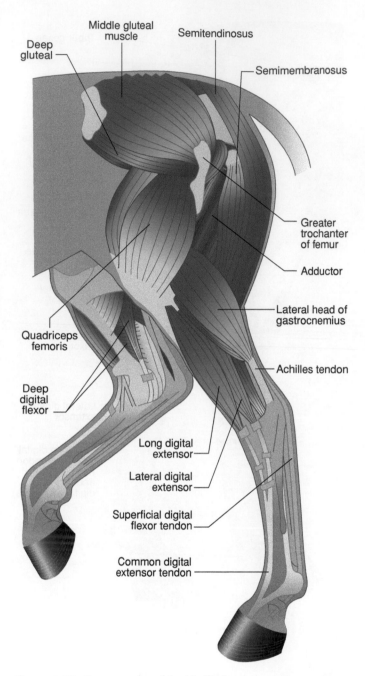

Figure 2.29 Deep muscles of the hindlimb.

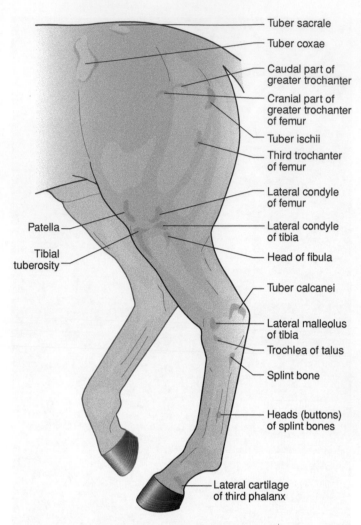

Figure 2.30 Surface anatomy of hindlimb.

dissections. However, there is some consensus that they can be a source of pain as the ligaments are subjected to great stress as a result of the forces transmitted through them into the trunk from the hindleg via the hip. One of the findings commonly reported in these cases is 'asymmetry of the hindquarters'. This introduces the subject of pelvic structure and landmarks.

The pelvis, particularly the ilium, does not form the comfortable bowl shape familiar in human anatomy (Figure 2.32). It is a much more elongated structure providing an area of attachment for large, powerful muscles required to

manoeuvre the hindlimb. The ilium rises from the pubis and ischium by a strong shaft which then broadens at the end into a blade with two palpable prominences at either end. One is the more cranially situated tuber coxae or pin bone which protrudes in front of the quarters and is the equivalent of the human anterior superior iliac spine. It may be fractured by, for example, walking into a gatepost. It is quite a broad projection and so the highest point is used to assess pelvic levels. Not too far distant is the expansion on the other side of the blade. This is the tuber sacrale which is the posterior superior iliac spine in human terms. The tubera sacrale of the two sides come together over the lumbosacral junction to form the points of the croup. This may be referred to as the 'jumper's bump', if they appear more prominent as a result of epaxial muscle atrophy. At the other end of the ilium, the shaft contributes to the acetabulum along with the ischium and pubis.

The ischium projects out backwards to end at the tuber ischii, or tuber ischiadicum which is the equivalent of the

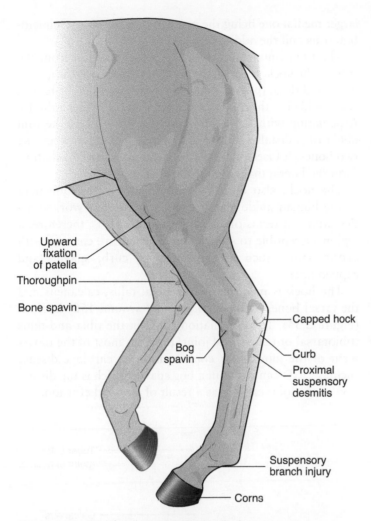

Upward
fixation
of patella

Thoroughpin

Bone spavin

Capped hock

Bog
spavin

Curb

Proximal
suspensory
desmitis

Suspensory
branch injury

Corns

Figure 2.31 Site of pathology in the hindlimb.

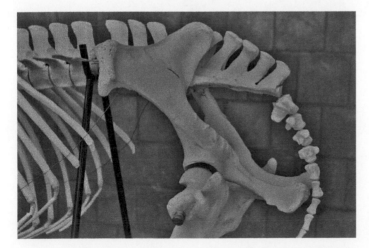

Figure 2.32 Pelvis: lateral view of this elongated structure which provides an area of attachment for the large, powerful muscles required to move the hindlimb.

bony bits that humans sit on (bursitis of which is termed 'rider's bottom'!). The L-shaped pubic bones come together ventrally at the pubic symphysis, running parallel with the ground, and osteopathic evaluation may identify dysfunction of this region, particularly postpartum.

Projecting behind the pelvis and attached to the sacrum is the tail. This is formed by approximately 18 caudal vertebrae which, after the first three, start to lose shape and articulations to form simple rods joined with cartilaginous discs. Cranially, the space between the first and second caudal vertebrae is located by moving the tail up and down and can be used for 'low' epidural anaesthesia such as is used in assisted delivery or profuse distal limb pain. The alternative site for epidural anaesthesia, at the lumbosacral level, is convenient because the spinous processes diverge here to provide a large gap for access to the spinal cord. However, the target is some way from the skin (over 8 cm) and may be missed. The muscles of the tail, particularly the sacrocaudalis dorsalis, link with the multifidus muscles of the lumbar spine and sacrum, which have an important role in the segmental stabilisation of the spine. As these muscles have been shown to be implicated in recurrent back pain, the tail is a useful 'handle' on these structures.

The acetabulum of the pelvis receives the heavy and strong femur to form the hip joint which lies several centimetres below the palpable greater trochanter. Despite the ball-and-socket arrangement, the teres (or round) and accessory ligaments, running from the acetabulum and pubis respectively and inserting into the head of the femur, effectively restrict movement to flexion and extension. The accessory ligament, unique to the horse family, limits abduction and is said to prevent cow-kicking! Overlying the hip, the gluteal muscles form the bulk of the quarters and insert into the greater and third trochanter of the femur. The trochanteric bursa, lying between gluteus medius and the greater trochanter, may become inflamed, causing the horse to stand with the limb adducted and to swing the leg in an arc during movement. The lesser trochanter, lying medially, forms the insertion of iliopsoas.

The cranial, medial and lateral parts of the shaft are dominated by the attachment of the quadriceps muscles. Caudally, biceps femoris and the adductor muscles are inserted.

From the hip, which is located some way cranially from the ischial tuber, the femur runs at a surprisingly straight angle downwards, rather than from the point of the buttock to which the eye may be drawn. It ends in the stifle joint which lies almost within the skin of the abdomen. The stifle joint is composed of three separate compartments: the femoropatellar and the medial and lateral femorotibial joints. There is often communication between the femoropatellar and medial femorotibial joint. On the cranial surface, the diamond-shaped patella articulates with the trochlea formed from a V-shaped groove in the femur lying

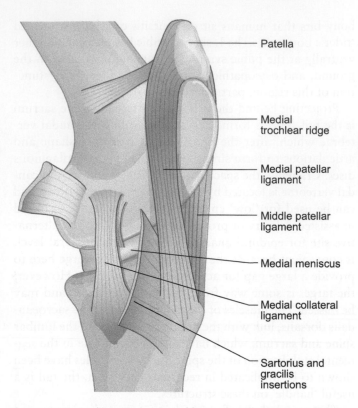

Figure 2.33 Locking mechanism of femoropatellar joint: medial view of left stifle joint showing the medial patellar ligament hooked over the medial trochlear ridge.

between a large medial ridge and a smaller lateral ridge. Above this articular surface is a small shelf facing dorsally called the resting surface, which only comes into contact with the patella at full extension during movement and at rest. The medial, middle and lateral patellar ligaments ascend from the tibial tuberosity and diverge with gaps between them as they attach to the patella. As the stifle is fully extended, the medial patellar ligament is hooked over the medial trochlear ridge, thus locking the limb and allowing it to remain in this position at very little energy cost (Figure 2.33). It has been suggested that the patella locks as a result of a slight medial rotation of the tibia and unlocks with slight lateral rotation. Upward fixation of the patella is a disorder which may occur when the horse is temporarily unable to unlock the stifle and the leg is held in extension. The locked leg tends to be dragged with partial flexion of the distal limb joints.

The caudal surface of the femur ends in lateral and medial condyles which connect with the slightly concave surface of the tibia to form the femorotibial articulation. This includes familiar features from the human knee such as menisci and cruciate ligaments, although these appear to be less troublesome in terms of pathology. Above the condyles, the medial and lateral supracondylar crests give origin to the gastrocnemius. Projecting from the sides are the epicondyles, the

larger medial one being the point of insertion for semimembranosus and the adductor muscles.

The tibia runs obliquely in a caudal direction from the stifle to the hock, forming the region referred to as the gaskin or second thigh (possibly because the 'first' thigh, or femur, is embedded in the quarters and does not look like a thigh). Articulating with the lateral condyle of the tibia, the thin fibula runs distally with an interosseous space between the two bones. It fuses with the lower third of the tibial shaft to form the lateral malleolus at the hock joint.

The hock, also known as the tarsus, is the equivalent of the human ankle and is one of the hardest worked articulations in terms of shock absorbance. It is, therefore, a region susceptible to strains and degenerative changes with exotic names such as thoroughpins, curb, spavins and capped hocks.

The hock is made up of the tibia, talus, calcaneus and the tarsal bones to form an angle of around 150° in front (Figure 2.34). The articulation between the tibia and talus (tibiotarsal or tarsocrural joint) provides most of the movement of the joint. Poor conformation or cartilage disease such as OCD can result in a bog spavin which is the distension of the joint capsule as a result of synovial effusion.

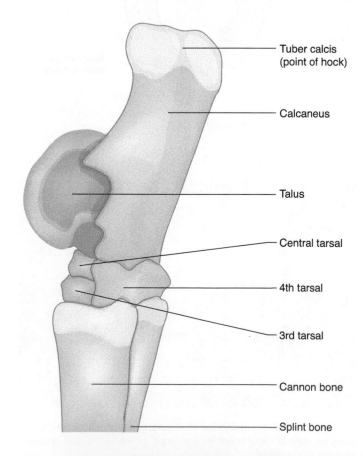

Figure 2.34 Hock: lateral view of the right hock made up of the tibia, talus, calcaneus and tarsal bones. Note that the hock joint is situated at some distance from the point of the hock.

The calcaneus has a projection, the tuber calcis, which is termed the point of hock and is the equivalent of the human heel. Gastrocnemius and the tarsal tendon of the biceps femoris and semitendinosus are attached here. The point of the hock may acquire a subcutaneous bursa in response to trauma, and a cold, painless swelling of this structure is referred to as a capped hock.

The tarsal bones themselves are in three rows and have mainly a shock-absorbing role as well as providing insertions for the hock flexors such as tibialis cranialis (tibialis anterior) and peroneus tertius. The proximal row, made up of the tarsus and calcaneus, articulates with the middle row composed of the central tarsal bone. This in turn articulates with the distal row formed of the fused first and second tarsals as well as the third tarsal. Below the calcaneus, the fourth tarsal spans the middle and distal rows. The distal joints have a relatively small degree of movement and are subject to degenerative changes, termed bone spavin, causing hock pain, swelling and a gradual onset of lameness.

The three main ligaments are the two collateral ligaments and the plantar ligament which runs from the calcaneus to the fourth tarsal and head of the lateral splint bone. Strain of the plantar ligament results in 'curb' which refers to a swelling at the back of the leg below the point of the hock.

Along the tibial shaft is the cranial tibial muscle which flexes the hock. Between this and the digital extensor tendon, the cord-like peroneus tertius extends from the distal femur and ends by bifurcating into the fourth tarsal bone and the third metatarsal. This forms part of the reciprocal apparatus which ensures that, as the hock flexes, so does the stifle (Figure 2.38).

Below the hock is the distal limb comprising the metatarsals and phalanges which are similar in both fore- and hindlegs.

Surface anatomy

The main visible points of the pelvis are the tuber sacrale, the tuber coxae and the tuber ischii, which have already been described (Figure 2.30). The greater (major) trochanter of the femur is covered with muscle but is palpable and marks the position of the hip. It is divided into two separate points, with the caudal part being higher than the cranial part. Distal to this is the third trochanter. The femur ends around the palpable lateral epicondyle. These points can be used to establish the orientation of the femur which is surprisingly vertical.

The deep fascia of the quarters and proximal limb is divided into septa which, in the very fit animal, provides visible delineation between the gluteus superficialis, biceps femoris, semitendinosus and semimembranosus (Figure 2.35). The gluteal muscles arising from the ilium and sacroiliac region provide the rounded mass of the cranial part of the quarters and run down to insert on the greater and third trochanters and shaft of the femur. This region also contains the

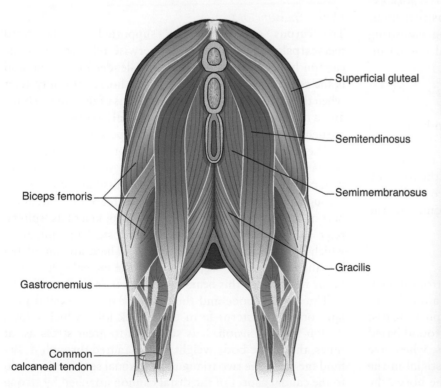
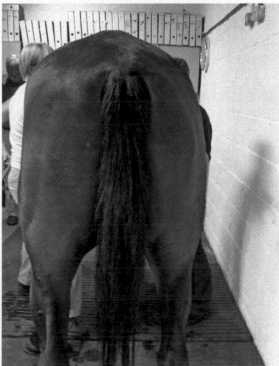

Figure 2.35 Hindquarters: biceps femoris can be felt following a curved course, caudal to which, the semitendinosus forms a distinctive band. The most caudal of this group is the semimembranosus and medially lie the strap muscles of gracilis and sartorius.

tendinous expanse of the tensor fascia lata from the tuber coxae to the patella and tibia. A slight groove may separate the gluteals from the hamstring group. The cranial, middle and caudal components of biceps femoris can be felt following a curved course from the sacrum and ischial tuber over the greater trochanter to an extensive insertion extending from the lateral patellar ligament and the tibial crest down to the fascia of the lower leg and the point of the hock (Figure 2.28).

Caudal to this, the semitendinosus forms a distinctive band passing over the ischial tuber and ending in a tendon which attaches from the tibial crest and leg fascia through to the point of the hock.

The most caudal of this group is the semimembranosus, which is only palpable at the root of the tail as it passes down to the medial femoral condyle.

On the medial surface of the thigh lie the strap muscles of gracilis and sartorius, the most obvious feature being the saphenous vein.

The deep-lying quadriceps inserts on to the patella. The patella is attached to the prominent tibial crest by the medial, middle and lateral ligaments, which are easily palpated.

Running down the cranial aspect of the tibia are the digital extensors and hock flexors. The outline is created by the long digital extensor as it descends to join the lateral extensor tendon below the hock to form the common extensor tendon on its way to insert into the third phalanx.

The caudal aspect of the tibia is made up of the hock extensors, digital flexors and the belly of the gastrocnemius which, together with the tarsal tendon of the hamstring group, form the prominent common calcaneal tendon inserting into the point of the hock (Figure 2.35).

THE DISTAL LIMB

Below the knees and hocks, the distal limbs in both fore- and hindlegs are very similar, with the exception of the shape of the hoof which is rounder and broader in the forefoot. This part of the limb is composed of metacarpals in the forelimb and the metatarsals behind and a column of three phalanges.

Other features unfamiliar to the human anatomist are the equine form of digital pads and the hoof.

Overview

Below the carpals and tarsals, the divergence from human anatomy is even more marked with the loss of a number of elements. Although apes and man retain a manipulating first digit, this has been lost in most land-dwelling, ground-based members of the animal kingdom. Even in dogs, where five metacarpals have been retained, the first is vestigial in the form of a forelimb dewclaw. In the limbs of the horse, the metacarpals and metatarsals have been streamlined down to one principal (third) metacarpal/tarsal or cannon bone and two residual (second and fourth) metacarpals/tarsals

or splint bones. The rest of the limb is continued as three phalanges in a column, ending in the horny hoof in contact with the ground.

Not only is the composition of the distal limb different from the human arrangement but so is the orientation. In the forelimb, the palmar surfaces, rather than facing forward as in the human anatomical position, instead face caudally, thereby affecting the position of the metacarpals or splint bones. The second metacarpal lies medially while the fourth is located laterally. This also means that the digital flexors are found on the caudal surface while the extensors run along the cranial aspect of the limb. This mirrors the arrangement in the hindlimb and the human lower limb.

Functionally, much of the muscle bulk is located in the girdle and proximal limb region. Distal to the carpals and tarsals, the propulsive mechanism is partly powered by releasing the energy stored by stretching the tendons.

Anatomical components

The distal limb is composed of the metacarpals in front and the metatarsals behind which join the phalanges at the fetlock joint. Between the phalanges, which unfortunately are referred to by a number of names, are the pastern and coffin joints. The limb also has several sesamoid bones as well as ergots and chestnuts, which are the equivalent of the digital pads. It also has the hoof.

Metacarpals/metatarsals

The carpus and tarsus are supported on the third metacarpal/metatarsal bones, otherwise referred to as the cannon bones. The cannon bone is slender but strong and is the structure to which those in the horse fraternity refer when they talk of 'bone'. The dimensions of the cannon bone give a measure of the ability of the animal to cope with work, particularly in relation to judging prospective racehorses.

The cannon bone is flanked by the tapering splint bones which are what remains of the second and fourth metacarpals and metatarsals. They dissipate concussion through the carpus and tarsus and reinforce the caudal aspect of the cannon. What is commonly spoken of as 'splints' refer to exostoses resulting from periosteal inflammation which may occur in younger horses. These are found below the carpus or tarsus, mainly on the medial splint bone of the forelimb as this bears more load than the lateral side.

The cannon bone and the first phalanx (proximal phalanx or long pastern) form the fetlock joint which allows flexion and extension. It is subjected to great stress as, at times, the whole body weight is transmitted through it. Behind the joint, the two triangular proximal sesamoids mould to the caudal aspect of the distal cannon attached by strong ligaments to each other and to the cannon and first phalanx. Running between the two sesamoids are the flexor tendons. Depending on the type and use of the horse, the proximal sesamoids are the most frequent fracture sites in the fore-limb, followed by the metacarpal and carpal bones. These are referred to as 'the big three' in racing as serious fracture is likely to lead to euthanasia given the expense involved in repair procedures.

Phalanges and interphalangeal joints
Below the fetlock, the phalanges extend down in a sloping column to the hoof (Figure 2.36a). Each has a number of names related to their position or, less obviously, to their linguistic derivation. The joints are subjected to considerable concussive forces, and the tendons and ligaments have a significant supporting role. These structures are therefore susceptible to injury and are influenced by the biomechanics of limb flight and footfall, so providing an opportunity for farriers and osteopaths to work together to develop a combined therapeutic programme.

The first (P1) or proximal phalanx, though not remarkable in length, is technically a long bone as it has a medullary cavity. Although regarded by vets as an archaic term, owners may refer to it as the long pastern, derived from the Middle English term for the tether or hobble of a horse at pasture. On the dorsal proximal border there is an attachment of the common digital extensor tendon, while on the palmar surface is found the insertion of the superficial flexor tendon and a major insertion of the middle distal sesamoidean ligament. At its distal end, it articulates with the second phalanx at the proximal interphalangeal or pastern joint, which is the least mobile of the phalangeal joints.

The second (P2) or middle phalanx, also known as the short pastern or the more antiquated term, coronary bone, is a short solid structure which runs down into the hoof. It bears a high load over a small surface area and is subject to degenerative osseous changes referred to as ringbone. As for the first phalanx, there are attachments for the common digital extensor and superficial flexor tendons. The second phalanx articulates with the third phalanx and the navicular bone at the relatively mobile distal interphalangeal or coffin joint. At rest the joint is in almost full extension, overextension being prevented by the suspensory apparatus and the deep flexor tendon.

The third (P3) or distal phalanx may also be referred to as the coffin bone, derived from the Latin for basket, or the pedal bone for more obvious reasons. It is shaped very much like a hoof but considerably reduced. On the most proximal point of the dorsal surface is the extensor process. This forms the terminal insertion of the common digital extensor tendon, which is responsible for advancing the foot and extending the knee and fetlock joints. The part of the bone facing towards the ground is composed of a crescent-shaped area and the flexor surface. These areas are divided by the semilunar crest to which the deep digital flexor tendon is attached. The space between the palmar or plantar surface of the third phalanx and the deep digital flexor tendon (DDFT) is occupied by the distal sesamoid or navicular bone, a small, boat-shaped structure contributing to the coffin joint. Between the deep digital flexor tendon and the navicular lies a bursa. The navicular bone is subjected to significant stresses, and degenerative disease of this area, more common in the front feet, causes changes in gait and lameness of insidious onset.

Attached to either side of the third phalanx are the hoof cartilages, sometimes called lateral cartilages, of the foot which have a shock-absorbing function. These project above the hoof and are palpable above the coronary band towards the back of the foot. They are usually slightly springy, but may become hard in 'sidebone', which is a process of slow, progressive ossification of the cartilages. Infection or inflammation of the cartilages is termed 'quittor' from the Middle English for cooking!

Digital pads
Digital pads are well developed in plantigrade animals such as the bear and consist of carpal/tarsal pads, metacarpal/metatarsal pads and digital pads which are all in contact with the ground. Digitigrades such as dogs have raised the heel off the ground leaving only the metacarpal/metatarsal and digital pads in contact with the ground. In horses the only digital pad used for weight bearing is the digital cushion, whose apex lies deep to the horny frog with the base extending caudally to form the bulbs of the heels (Figure 2.36a). The vestigial carpal and tarsal pads appear as chestnuts. Similarly the metacarpal and metatarsal pads, termed ergots, are rudimentary.

The foot
The foot consists of the hoof and those structures contained within it. The hoof is the equivalent of the third fingernail in the human. However, rather than being a partial covering, it encapsulates the distal (third) phalanx and is composed of the wall, the sole and the frog.

The wall is divided into the toe, quarters and heels covering the front and sides of the third phalanx. Caudally, the borders reflect inwards to form the bars, between which lies the frog (Figure 2.36b).

The wall is made up of horn. This is produced by a bulging circle in the epidermis, termed the coronary band, at a rate of around 4 to 8 mm per month depending on the time of year, being fastest in June and July and slowest in February and March. It takes around 9 to 12 months to grow a completely new hoof. Horizontal rings may indicate disease and changes in nutrition. It is composed of horny tubules tied together with intertubular horn which gives it strength to withstand compressive forces. It is not as comfortable with shear or torque forces, and the state of the horn may give an indication of abnormal limb flight which may be corrected by osteopathic treatment. In fact, farriers may comment on the improved state of the feet after osteopathy.

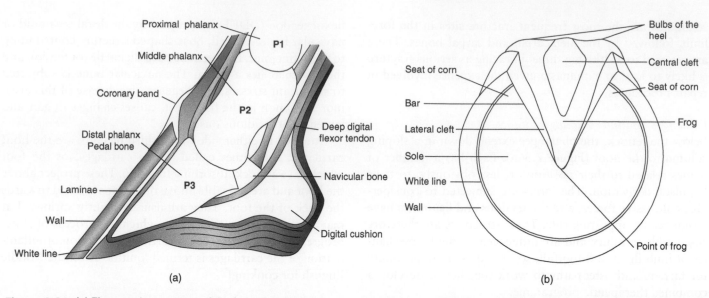

Figure 2.36 (a) The complex structure of the foot allows it to act as a shock absorber. (b) Hoof: this encapsulates the distal (third) phalanx and is composed of the wall, sole and frog.

The wall supports the horse, and expands to absorb shock. It is attached to the pedal bone (P3) by about 600 laminae. Insensitive laminae from the internal surface of the hoof wall project at 90° and interleave with the highly sensitive and vascular laminae emanating from the covering of the pedal bone. Where this arrangement is disrupted, as in laminitis, the feet become painful. This may progress to where the pedal bone, no longer bound sufficiently to the hoof wall, begins to rotate through the sole.

The sole is the concave underside of the foot between the wall and frog. The junction of the sole and wall is the zona alba or white line. The caudal parts between the wall and the bars are known as the angles of the sole and are the seat of corns, the bruised areas resulting from trauma to the underlying dermis.

The triangular frog projects into the centre of the hoof and is made of softer, more elastic horn. Caudally, its base fills the space between the heels.

The complex structure of the foot allows it to act as a shock absorber (Figure 2.36a). As the horse bears weight, downward pressure is exerted on the pedal bone (P3) which moves within the hoof. Force is transmitted from P3 via the interdigitating laminae into the wall which bears most of the weight. It distorts somewhat under the pressure and the heels spread. These mechanical changes help to absorb concussive forces. They also result in changes in blood flow to the area which, acting as a hydrostatic dampener, further dissipates the shock of footfall.

Surface anatomy

The bones, tendons and joints of the distal limb are easily palpable. At the distal end of the radius, the medial and lateral styloid processes can be located, below which, facing

cranially, the tuberosity of the main (third) metacarpal, or cannon bone, is palpable. The cannon bone dominates the front and sides of the limb, and about three-quarters of the way down on either side the nodular distal ends of the two splint bones can be felt, as can any exostoses between these bones and the cannon. In front of the cannon and phalanges, the common digital extensor tendon runs down to the distal phalanx (P3) inside the hoof capsule (Figures 2.29 and 2.30).

Along the back of the cannon, the deep digital flexor tendons overlaid by the superficial flexor tendon are prominent. Deep to this lies the suspensory ligament occupying the channel between the back of the cannon and the splint bones. These structures are easier to identify if the foot is lifted and the fetlock, pastern and coffin joints are slightly flexed.

The position of the proximal sesamoids, encased in a network of well defined ligaments, can be located caudal to the fetlock joint and under the ergot, over which lies a tuft of hair. The upper end of the proximal phalanx is marked by two lateral tubercles receiving the collateral ligaments of the fetlock.

Moving down to the foot, the two lateral cartilages, protruding up above the hoof from their attachment on the distal phalanx, can be palpated above and towards the back of the foot.

STABILISING STRUCTURES OF THE FORE- AND HINDLIMB

Overview

An arrangement of ligaments and tendons provides support for a bony column which is not straight. It is a low-energy system which enables horses to stand for longer than other domestic species. Part of this is the 'stay apparatus', which is present in all legs, with the added feature of a reciprocal system in the hindlimb. Below the knee and hock, the mechanism is similar in both fore- and hindlimbs, with the 'suspensory apparatus' being a major component of the stay apparatus here. Other components are the check ligaments and the annular ligaments.

Forelimb

In the forelimb, the centre of gravity passes caudal to the shoulder, through the elbow, slightly cranial to the carpals and cranial to the fetlock and pastern. Without support, the shoulder and elbow joints would flex, the carpals would be unstable and overextension of the fetlock and pastern joints would occur.

At each point of potential collapse, the stay apparatus stabilises the column.

Proximal forelimb stay apparatus

The shoulder is prevented from flexing by the biceps tendon running from the scapula to the radius. Biceps tendon tension is transferred by its internal tendon, the lacertus fibrosus, which splits away from the main muscle to blend with the extensor carpi radialis and prevents the carpals from buckling forwards and collapsing the knee. Overextension is limited by the tightly packed structure of the carpals as well as the palmar ligament caudally (Figure 2.37).

Hindlimb

Here the centre of gravity drops in a line descending from the head of the femur, running caudal to the stifle and cranial to the hock, fetlock and interphalangeal joints before passing through the hoof. In the unsupported limb, the column would collapse by flexion of the stifle and hock and overextension of the fetlock and interphalangeal joints.

Proximal hindlimb stay apparatus

Stabilisation of the proximal hindlimb joints relies on a locking mechanism for the stifle and a reciprocal apparatus which governs the activity of the stifle in relation to the hock (Figure 2.38). The stifle is locked into full extension when straight as the medial patellar ligament hooks over the medial trochlear ridge of the femur (Figure 2.33).

The action of the stifle is linked to that of the hock through the reciprocal apparatus. Body weight will flex the stifle. This is prevented by peroneus tertius which runs from the cranial surface of the femur to the third metatarsal, but whose action will also flex the hock. This latter effect is countered by gastrocnemius activity assisted by the tendinous superficial digital flexor as it runs from the caudal aspect of the femur attaching to the point of hock on its way down to the second phalanx. This creates passive, antagonistic activity between peroneus tertius and the superficial

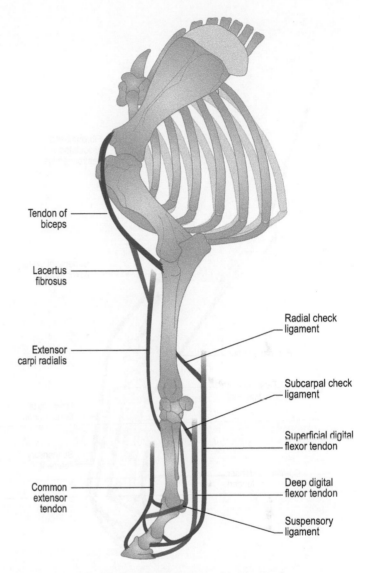

Figure 2.37 Forelimb stay apparatus: this chain of structures stabilises the column at each point of potential collapse.

digital flexor and gastrocnemius to synchronise the action of the two joints.

Distal limb stay apparatus

Below the knee and hock, stabilising structures are very similar in both fore- and hindlimbs (Figures 2.37 and 2.38).

Suspensory apparatus

The fetlock is put under great stress by the downward pressure of the weight of the body. It is prevented from overextension by the suspensory apparatus. This is formed from a number of ligaments whose names reflect their relationship to the proximal sesamoid bones. The principal structure is the suspensory ligament which is also known as the interosseous muscle or the proximal sesamoidean ligament (Figure 2.39). The support is augmented by

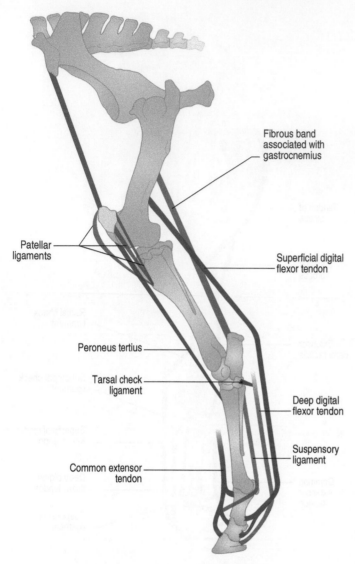

Fibrous band associated with gastrocnemius

Patellar ligaments

Superficial digital flexor tendon

Peroneus tertius

Tarsal check ligament

Deep digital flexor tendon

Suspensory ligament

Common extensor tendon

Figure 2.38 Hindlimb stay apparatus: at each point of potential collapse the stay apparatus stabilises the column.

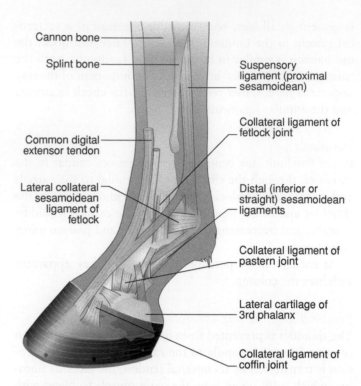

Cannon bone

Splint bone

Suspensory ligament (proximal sesamoidean)

Common digital extensor tendon

Collateral ligament of fetlock joint

Lateral collateral sesamoidean ligament of fetlock

Distal (inferior or straight) sesamoidean ligaments

Collateral ligament of pastern joint

Lateral cartilage of 3rd phalanx

Collateral ligament of coffin joint

Figure 2.39 Suspensory apparatus, lateral view: the principal structure is the suspensory ligament (interosseous muscle or proximal sesmoidean ligament), augmented by the intersesmoidean and distal sesamoid ligaments.

the intersesamoidean and distal sesamoid ligaments with contributions from the accessory ligaments, also known as check ligaments, and the superficial and deep flexor tendons.

The interosseous 'muscle' or suspensory ligament loses the fleshy muscle fibres present in the foal to become entirely collagenous as the animal becomes heavier. It runs from the distal row of carpals and proximal metacarpal in the forelimb or distal tarsal row and plantar ligament in the hindlimb and passes down the caudal surface of the cannon between the two splint bones. Just above the fetlock, it divides into two substantial and easily palpable branches. These lateral and medial branches each attach to a proximal sesamoid bone before passing forwards around the proximal phalanx to join the common extensor tendon

at the level of the pastern joint. At various sites along the structure, mainly in the forelimb, this ligament is subject to inflammation termed desmitis, derived from the Greek *desmos* meaning bond or chain.

Other ligaments having a support role are the deep, cruciate, middle (oblique) and superficial (straight) sesamoidean ligaments. These are functional extensions of the suspensory ligament extending from the proximal sesamoids to the first and second phalanges.

The coffin joint has a similar ligamentous apparatus involving the distal sesamoid or navicular bone, which is held in position by both the suspensory navicular ligaments from the proximal phalanx and the distal navicular ligament running down to the third phalanx.

Check (accessory) ligaments
Under weight-bearing, the fetlock sinks towards the ground and the suspensory ligament comes under tension. This is followed by tension on the superficial and deep digital flexor tendons or 'back tendons' which pass down the rear of the knee or hock and cannon on the way down to the phalanges. Although these tendons have a normal tendinous structure, under conditions of extreme loading they can function more like ligaments by virtue of check, or accessory, ligaments

running from tendon to bone. The superior, or radial, check ligament is a strong, fibrous band which fuses with the superficial digital flexor tendon proximal to the carpus. The equivalent in the hindlimb arises from the tibia and fuses with the flexor tendon above the hock.

The inferior check ligament is also known as the subcarpal/subtarsal ligament. The subcarpal ligament runs from the joint capsule of the knee to join the deep digital flexor in the region of the middle third of the cannon. The subtarsal ligament, originating from the plantar ligament, is long, thin and often absent. Desmitis of the inferior check ligament

may occur in older horses, particularly those involved in jumping.

Annular ligaments

The fascia surrounding the muscles assists in easing the constant strain on limb tendons. In the region of the joints, it consolidates to form fibrous bands, termed the annular ligaments. At the fetlock, the back tendons are held in place by the palmar/plantar annular ligaments, and in the digits their position is maintained by the proximal and distal digital annular ligaments.

Neurophysiological Basis of Osteopathic Medicine

Julia Brooks

3

INTRODUCTION

As a student of osteopathy one begins by learning the theoretical basis of osteopathic medicine. This is followed by years of practice, building up a database of presenting symptoms and signs and interpreting them to form a diagnosis and an effective treatment strategy. The experience-gathering exercise, based on observation and practical intervention, builds up its own language and conceptions. This works well in osteopathic circles where there is, by and large, a measure of mutual understanding. However, in the multidisciplinary environment encountered when working with animals, it is helpful to establish channels of communication which are comprehensible to all groups.

This is particularly important when entering a veterinary practice where there may be preconceived ideas as to what osteopathy represents and little knowledge of the underlying principles. An exchange that occurred whilst I was working in a large veterinary group illustrated the way that misconceptions can exist between the professions. At the time I was looking at regional hair-length variations in the horse to see whether this affected infra-red thermography readings. This involved laboriously measuring the length of each hair in clumps taken from different parts of the horse. The stud vet, passing through, asked what I was doing. In a spirit of mischief, I replied that putting the hair sample into a black box and making a differential diagnosis saved the client a trip into the clinic. He concealed his horror admirably, but the episode highlighted the need to share the osteopathic approach using the common language of neurophysiology and to continue research into the effect and effectiveness of the treatment (Colles and Pusey 2003).

The following chapter explores the protective mechanisms initiated by injury and the clinical presentations that occur in response to these changes, and offers some explanation of the effects of osteopathic intervention.

EVOLUTION OF THE OSTEOPATHIC APPROACH

Osteopathy was conceived in the late 1800s by the Kansas doctor, Andrew Taylor Still. Dr Still was dissatisfied with the medical model practised at that time, which was based on the purgative, laxative and bleeding therapies that had changed little from ancient Egyptian and Greek medicine. Instead, he embarked on a journey of discovery through a detailed study of anatomy by observation and dissection, while noting how the structure enabled the body to function. This led him to propose a system of healing which placed chief emphasis on the structural integrity of the body as being essential to its well-being. His anatomical studies led him to believe that disturbances to this well-being were the result of joint subluxations leading to blockage of blood vessels and pressure on nerves.

However, technological advances in imaging showed that patients frequently present with pain, muscle spasm and poor function without any apparent structural disorder of this kind. Another model was required to account for the dysfunction.

As early as the 1800s, the physiologists Magendie, Bernard and, later, Sherrington were developing new ideas about the way the nervous system worked. A concept evolved of the nervous system as an information network constantly changing and adapting in response to sensory information from the body and the environment. This knowledge allowed a move away from early ideas of pressure and subluxation towards a concept of 'somatic dysfunction'. To use a computer analogy, it is more an aberration in the function of the software, rather than a hardware problem presenting as tissue pathology (Williams 1997).

A common enough irritation for those involved in computing is mirrored in biological systems. Somewhere in the course of entering information from the environment and body, processing the information in the central nervous system and then generating a motor response, something has gone wrong. Clinically, a horse may present with a range of problems such as pain, stiffness, loss of performance and poor co-ordination, but no pathological process can be identified.

To extend the computer analogy further, osteopathy may be thought of as a form of reprogramming. Osteopathic treatment is directed at muscles, fascia and joints. By changing the signals from these structures into the neural network, treatment influences processing of sensory information and motor responses.

Using this model, it is possible to combine information from a detailed case history with the findings from physical examination to form a neuromusculoskeletal rather than a pathological diagnosis. It can also be used to establish a set of identifiable physical characteristics of dysfunction which can be employed as benchmarks against which the success of treatment can be measured.

To build up this picture, it may be useful to review some of the neurophysiological changes that occur in response to injury, in both the short and long term. These processes can then be put into a clinical context, looking at common presentations that will make up an osteopath's caseload in animal practice. The mechanisms whereby these changes can be reversed are also explored.

NEUROPHYSIOLOGICAL RESPONSES TO INJURY

The response to trauma, be it a skin laceration, a joint taken beyond its normal range or an event in the viscera, takes place at a number of different levels as described by Descartes in the 17th century. Initially, there is a localised peripheral reaction at the site of injury. The traumatic event is announced to the central nervous system, first at spinal cord and then at brain stem and cortical centres from which an appropriate motor response is generated (Figure 3.1).

It is tempting to think of this pathway as hardwired, where a harmful event will result in a painful sensation of corresponding intensity, which will last for a certain period of time and then disappear without trace. However, the complex way in which neuronal networks function means

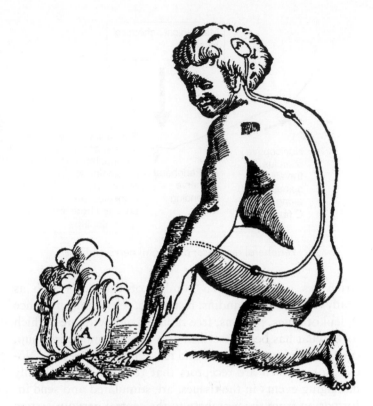

Figure 3.1 Pain pathways: Descartes (1596–1650) described an apparently simple linear depiction of pain pathways. However, he recognised that this could be modified at any level.

that, in reality, the effects of injury cause neurophysiological modifications that may persist long after the clinical signs have disappeared.

On a cellular level, the activity of neurones is determined by the balance of inhibitory and excitatory signals. Those involved in sensing and protecting against potentially damaging events (the nociceptive system) are, under normal circumstances, held in check by the dominance of inhibitory neurone activity. Only when a stimulus is of sufficient intensity will the balance shift in favour of excitation, which sets in motion protective and healing mechanisms. Once healing has occurred, there is a shift back to an inhibitory (pain-free) state. However, far from being a fixed response, the balance point can be moved towards excitation at any point in the network, making the neurones more sensitive to incoming pain signals and therefore more likely to fire at a lower intensity of stimulus. This creates the classic facilitated segment described in the osteopathic texts (Korr 1979).

While appreciating the complexity and interactivity of the network, it may be helpful to look at the response to injury generated at each level of the pathway.

Peripheral Response

The most obvious response to trauma is at the site of injury. Where a horse has fallen, there may be skin abrasions and bruising, joint strains and muscle damage. These

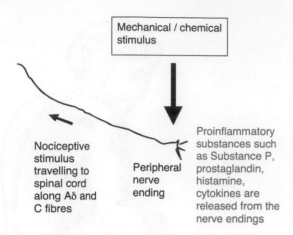

Figure 3.2 Peripheral response: peripheral nerve endings.

structures will produce a number of chemicals such as bradykinin, prostaglandins, histamine, serotonin, substance P, leukotrienes, protons, free radicals and cytokines, which form what has been described as a pro-inflammatory soup, causing local swelling, heat and tenderness (Figure 3.2). Nociceptors, which are receptors that respond to potentially damaging events in the tissues, are stimulated and send information from the periphery to the central nervous system for interpretation. Even at this peripheral level, the sensitivity of the pathway may change as these neurochemicals act on the receptor membrane, lowering the threshold at which it will fire (Raja et al. 1999, p. 31). This creates the hypersensitivity that often follows injury.

Central Response

The central nervous system is informed of trauma to the tissues by signals passing along small-calibre fibres from peripheral nociceptors to the dorsal horn of the spinal cord. Here these fibres arborise, making thousands of connections with other neurones to produce a range of effects (Figure 3.3). There will be communications with tract cells taking information to the brain stem and cortex which, if the stimulus is sufficient, will be interpreted as a painful sensation.

In addition there are connections with the motor neurones of the ventral horn resulting in the muscle spasm that is felt, on palpation, as increased muscle tone and asymmetric function of the joint.

Synapses also exist with the sympathetic neurones of the lateral horn which, when stimulated, cause a shift of blood away from the skin and towards the muscles. This leads to alterations in skin texture that can be detected by palpatory tests such as skin drag, where a local area of increased resistance is detected when the pads of the fingers are run lightly along paravertebral tissues.

Long-term Potentiation and Reverberating Circuits

These peripheral and central reactions form the initial responses to injury. Once the tissues at the injury site have healed, these protective and restorative mechanisms should ideally be switched off. However, changes occur in the spinal cord neurones in response to moderately severe and/or sustained signals from the periphery. These neurones can

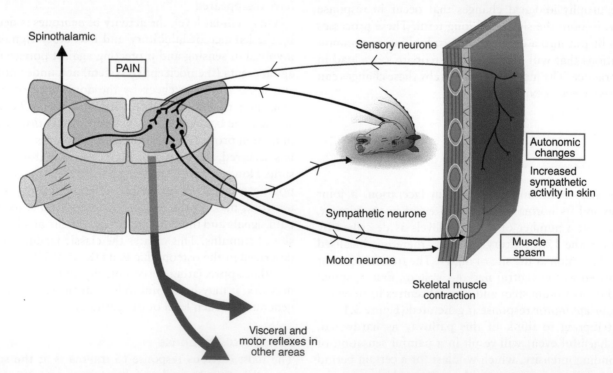

Figure 3.3 Response to injury: pain, muscle spasm and autonomic changes can be used to identify levels of dysfunction and act as benchmarks for monitoring progress.

undergo changes in genetic expression, which make them more sensitive to stimuli in a process known as long-term potentiation or 'wind up' (Bennett et al. 1989). They will produce a pain response at a lower stimulus level and for longer duration than before the initial injury. This is seen frequently in human practice in the patient who can trigger an acute pain reaction with an everyday action such as bending down to put on socks. Similarly, in the horse, recurrent acute back pain for no apparent reason may be a result of the increase in central sensitivity.

In fact a stimulus from the periphery may not actually be needed to drive this pain response. Once spinal neurone sensitisation becomes well established, the interneurones of the pain circuits can continue their activity without any input from the peripheral tissue. This is demonstrated by experiments where ligation of a nerve diminishes sensory signals entering the spinal cord (Jensen and Nikolajsen 1999). Despite this, muscle spasm, autonomic changes and the perception of pain continue, driven by patterns of neuronal activity set up by the initial trauma in what has been described as a reverberating circuit within the spinal cord.

Antidromic Activity

Another aspect of neuronal behaviour that may impact on the clinical picture is the ability of neurones to fire in either direction from the point of stimulus. The traditional view of the way in which a sensory neurone functions is that a signal starts from a receptor in the periphery and travels along the axon towards the dorsal horn of the spinal cord. However, there is actually nothing preventing the neurone from firing at any point along its course as long as there is sufficient stimulus to cause depolarisation. Where the neuronal networks of the dorsal horn have been sensitised, the neurones may fire from the dorsal horn 'backwards' towards the receptors (Raja et al. 1999, p.36). On reaching the periphery, the depolarisation of nerve endings produces an effect mimicking local injury, as they release pro-inflammatory neuropeptides such as histamine, prostaglandins and Substance P (Sluka et al. 1995). This dorsal root reflex may explain those mysterious intermittent and shifting limb swellings and dysfunction for which no pathological cause can be identified.

NEUROPHYSIOLOGICAL RESPONSE TO INJURY IN A CLINICAL SETTING

The obvious difference between human and animal practice is that a verbal description of the site, nature and natural history of the dysfunction is not available. However, using an osteopathic approach, the physiological markers of pain, muscle spasm and autonomic changes in response to an injury can be used to build up a picture of the problem (Figure 3.3).

Pain

Pain sensation is an obvious effect of injury but is difficult to quantify in animals. The horse probably does not perceive pain in human terms. As a herd animal, its survival in the wild depends on being able to keep with the group, as stragglers are vulnerable to predators. In the case of injury, it is in its best interests to make adjustments and carry on moving. This ability to compensate is demonstrated in many horses presenting to osteopathic clinics. Although there may be acute pain in one region, there will often be other areas of longstanding dysfunction, apparent on observation and palpation, with which the horse has coped by making adjustments to the way it moves. The point at which it can no longer make adequate adjustments is where the problem significantly interferes with performance. The process is reflected in a typical history where the owner describes minor asymmetries and imperfections over a long period, leading up to a sudden onset of pain in a particular area without an identifiable cause. Another feature of this type of presentation is that treating the local acute area may be effective in the short term, but problems tend to recur, generally with increasing frequency, intensity and duration.

An example of this process is where a horse presents with recurrent lumbosacral pain with no apparent reason for the onset of each episode. Examination might show upper cervical tenderness and loss of function. Unable to use the momentum generated by the weight of the head to assist forward movement, the horse will compensate by generating the movement with the hindlegs and straining the lumbosacral complex. The neuronal network associated with this region becomes sensitised and a pattern of recurrent pain and dysfunction is established. At this point the owner may recall that it fell on its head at 30 mph while racing as a 2-year-old with no reported ill effects!

Muscle Spasm

Muscle spasm (He et al. 1988) is another common finding on palpation and causes a number of problems. One result is that it will restrict movement, and the owner may report signs ranging from short striding to general stiffness.

A study looking at stride length used computer analysis of video clips of horses moving against a marker board (Woodleigh 2003). The data showed that the stride length in trot of horses presenting to the clinic was significantly shorter (by 17%) when compared with that of controls. After osteopathic treatment this difference no longer existed, the stride length in the clinical group having increased significantly. The ability to extend the limbs in a fluid, symmetric movement is vital in many disciplines, and so improvement in this area will enhance performance.

Movement restriction also occurs in the spine. A small study compared spinal mobility in a control group of horses with that of cases attending an osteopathic clinic

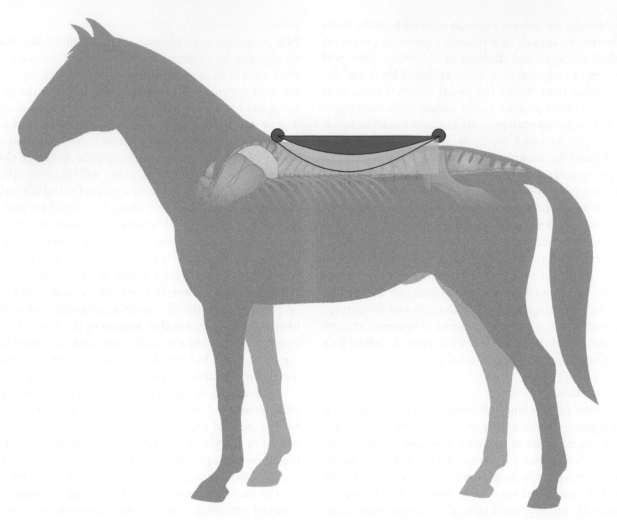

Figure 3.4 Spinal flexibility: the area under the line represents the back position at a particular phase in the stride cycle. Controls: area under line is greater in extension phase (red + yellow areas) than flexion (yellow area). Clinical group: no significant difference in area under line in flexion and extension phases.

(Livingstone 2001). Two markers were placed on the back, with one at the withers and the other at the lumbosacral junction. The horses were videoed in walk and a computer was used to measure the area between the outline of the horse's back and a line drawn between the markers. Readings were taken at two points in the stride cycle, when the spine was flexed and then extended (Figure 3.4). The controls, as expected, showed a significantly larger area when the spine was extended when compared with the flexion phase. In the clinical group, however, there was little difference in area between flexion and extension, which probably reflected the lack of suppleness often reported in cases attending a clinic.

Poor spinal mobility also has implications for paravertebral and gluteal muscle development. An inability to build up these structures resulting in a loss of topline is a frequent complaint of owners (Figure 3.5). Work by Goldspink and co-workers (2002) indicates that it is not stimulation alone

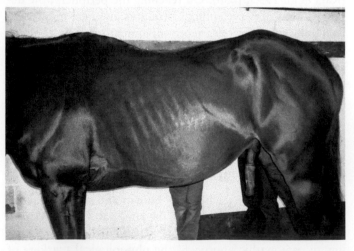

Figure 3.5 Loss of topline: muscle bulk is reduced in the erector spinae and gluteal region.

that increases bulk, but also the action of stretching. Muscle stretch stimulates the local release of hormones allied to the insulin related growth factor. The result is an increase in number and length of the sarcomeres which form the building blocks of muscle fibres. This may well account for owners' remarks that a topline has been re-established following treatment, although the horse is not in training having been allowed time off work for free movement in a field. The ability to move and therefore stretch through the back following treatment stimulates the development of these muscles.

Not only are muscles involved in producing motion, but they also have an important sensory function. Movements are made by a complex interaction of agonist and antagonist muscles. This interaction is largely unconscious and is orchestrated by patterns of neuronal activity originating from within the spinal cord, called central pattern generators (CPGs). However, for optimum function, this neuronal activity needs to be modified to reflect changes in the environment. It is the constant stream of proprioceptive information from muscle spindles and Golgi tendon organs that occurs as joints are moved and muscles change length that provides the central nervous system with detailed knowledge concerning current position and changes in the orientation of the body. In fact, decerebrate cats, where the brain stem has been transected at the midbrain level, and spinal cats, where the transection is at the lower thoracic level, are still able to keep pace with a motorised treadmill on which they are stepping. Under these conditions, the input from proprioceptors maintains balance and co-ordination as well as generating appropriate movement patterns (Pearson and Gordon 2000).

One of the most important areas for providing this type of information is the upper cervical spine. The neurologist Professor Joe Mayhew of the University of Edinburgh describes the case of a horse that presented with unsteadiness following a kick to the poll from a stable mate. Assuming this to be what, in veterinary circles, is descriptively referred to as 'wobbler syndrome', the neck was X-rayed in the expectation of finding some structural damage to the upper cervical vertebrae, with pressure on the spinal cord causing the ataxia. The X-ray was normal. On closer inspection of the neck, there was marked wasting of the suboccipital muscles on one side. It was concluded that the blow to the head had damaged the first cervical nerve, resulting not only in muscle wasting in the area of supply but also, more significantly, in a loss of information on position which is usually generated from these muscles. Although this was an extreme case of information reduction, stiffness in this area will produce some of the same effects because the muscles are unable to change length in response to position changes, and will therefore fail to generate adequate feedback information.

This effect is demonstrated by the following exercise used by a well known professor of neuroanatomy. His students stand supported on both feet by processing information from the eyes, the labyrinth of the ear and the proprioceptors of the musculoskeletal system (Figure 3.6). They are then asked to stand on the non dominant leg (usually the left in right handers) (Figure 3.6a). Wavering in the ranks begins as the point of contact with the floor has been narrowed and the sensory input from the other foot has been lost. The students then close their eyes. Lacking visual cues, the instability becomes much more noticeable as the foot, the limb and the postural spinal muscles make increasingly unrefined

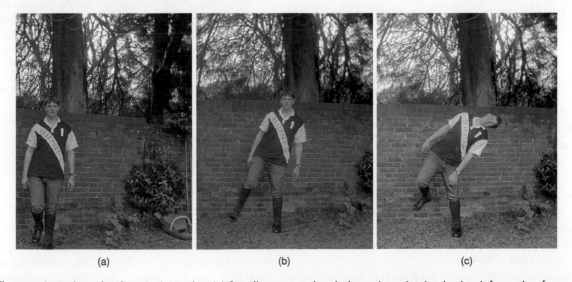

(a)   (b)   (c)

Figure 3.6 The proprioceptive role of cervical muscles. (a) Standing on one leg: balance is maintained using information from eyes, labyrinth and proprioceptors of the joints and muscles of the body. (b) Eyes closed: balance becomes more difficult as information from the eyes is lost. (c) Neck fixed in sidebend: upper cervical muscles are now fixed in length, and proprioceptors which rely on changes in length to monitor orientation no longer provide adequate information on position in space. Balance is difficult with only input from the labyrinth.

adjustments, because of the now incomplete information (Figure 3.6b). Finally, the students are asked to tip the head to one side. This fixes the neck in one position and the all-important proprioceptors in the muscles of the top of the neck are no longer free to monitor position in space from changes in muscle length. Information from the labyrinth alone is insufficient to maintain balance and the students fall (Figure 3.6c). This may explain cases where owners describe their horses as 'pottery', with frequent stumbling and even falls, although extensive diagnostic tests have failed to reveal any pathology.

Autonomic Changes

Alongside pain and muscle spasm, there are also autonomic changes associated with injury (Sato and Schmidt 1973). A painful stimulus results in activation of the sympathetic nervous system. Initially this is a generalised fight/flight response mediated by the brain stem which acts on the vascular walls to drive the blood from the skin to the muscles. In the human subject, this gives rise to the pallor associated with shock. The central response gradually recedes but increased sympathetic activity may persist on a segmental spinal cord level alongside muscle spasm and pain. These segmental disturbances may be palpated in techniques such as skin drag where, by dragging the fingers with light pressure along the paravertebral tissue, changes in tissue texture may be identified.

Infra-red thermography is a diagnostic tool that accords well with this concept of autonomic disturbance as part of a somatic dysfunction. It is a non-invasive means of calculating skin temperature which is, in turn, a measure of surface blood flow and underlying metabolic activity. Therefore, any alterations in autonomic control of blood supply to the surface, or any change in bulk and activity of the underlying muscles, will be reflected in the thermographic image. In practical terms, dysfunction is indicated by a deviation from the normal pattern of the scan rather than absolute temperature, which will vary between individual horses.

In the 'normal' horse, a reproducible thermographic pattern is observed (Turner et al. 1986). This shows some slight regional variation, with surface temperatures over the shoulders and quarters being slightly warmer as a result of the metabolic activity of the bulky muscles of the fore- and hindlimbs. Another area of increased heat is along the line of the erector spinae to form a characteristic dorsal stripe on the thermograms (Figure 3.7). In environmentally controlled conditions, this regional variation is only a matter of ± 0.5°C. Dysfunction is suggested by a difference of more than 1°C (Colles et al. 1994).

Much attention has previously been directed at hot spots to detect local inflammation. However, a facilitated segment will increase sympathetic activity in the lateral horn, which acts on the blood vessel walls to drive blood away from

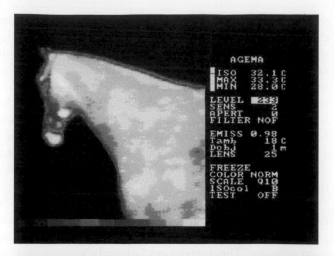

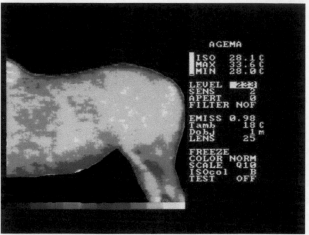

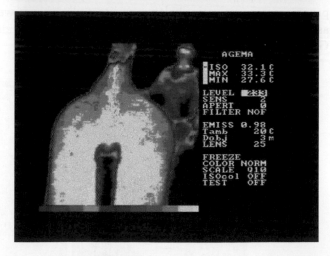

Figure 3.7 Normal infra-red scan: regional variation in surface temperature is ± 0.5°C. The shoulders (top) gluteal region (middle) and erector spinae (bottom) are slightly warmer.

the surface, giving a distinctive segmental strip of cooling that roughly approaches the dermatome distribution (Figure 3.8). An interesting finding in some cases is that, when the feet and lower legs are scanned, the image shows intense cooling of one or both limbs somewhat reminiscent

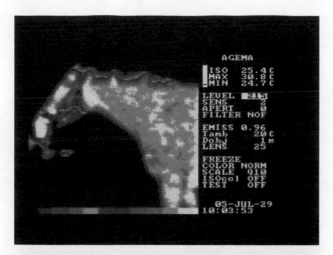

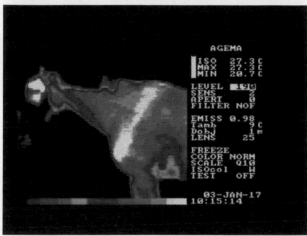

Figure 3.8 Facilitated segment: in a 'normal' neck (above), temperatures vary by ± 0.5°C. Upper cervical dysfunction (bottom) regional variation greater than 1°C indicates increased segmental sympathetic activity. Note: temperature colour scale at bottom of scan runs from left (lower temperatures) to right. Intervals 0.6°C approx.

of human autonomic disorders such as Raynaud's disease and reflex sympathetic dystrophy (Figure 3.9).

The thermographic image can give an overall impression of the longevity of the presenting problem. A centrally mediated, generalised and marked cooling will indicate an acute response to injury (Figure 3.10). In the medium term, where an element of 'wind up' or facilitation in the spinal cord has occurred, the changes will take the form of segmental strips of reduced temperature (Figure 3.8).

Paradoxically, in the very long term cases, the thermographic images appear to be relatively normal on initial inspection. This reflects the damping down of central and segmental autonomic responses and the development of compensatory movement patterns over a prolonged period. However, on more careful viewing, findings such as slight cooling at the top of the neck and abolition of the dorsal stripe are suggestive of compromised spinal function and underlying subtle alteration in segmental autonomic activity.

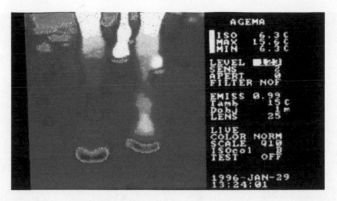

Figure 3.9 Segmental cooling: intense cooling of one or both limbs is reminiscent of human autonomic disorders such as Raynaud's disease.

Reduced heat through the glutei indicates that the hindquarters are no longer generating optimum power to give the horse forward propulsion, which is a common presenting problem. Interestingly, after the first treatment, follow-up scans may show an apparent deterioration with increased regional temperature variation, presumably as compensatory mechanisms are broken down. As clinical signs improve, so the scans approximate the normal pattern.

One study looked at thermographic imaging of horses presenting to a secondary referral veterinary clinic where musculoskeletal problems ranged from general stiffness to idiopathic lameness (Brooks 2003). Scanning was performed at the initial veterinary consultation and prior to every osteopathic intervention. Imaging immediately after treatment was not practical because of the effects of the sedative on the sympathetic nervous system which influences surface blood flow. Given that the established normal for thermographic patterns shows very little regional variation (± 0.5°C), those presenting to the clinic were found to have up to a 3°C discrepancy between different body areas. Following treatment, there was a significant increase in temperatures in the gluteal region and dorsal stripe, which suggested a return to normal sympathetic activity in the area and greater metabolic activity in the muscles (Figure 3.11).

MECHANISMS FOR REVERSING NEUROPHYSIOLOGICAL CHANGES

Treatment procedures all seek to modify the physiological changes occurring as a result of injury. This modification can be made at a number of levels.

Peripheral Modification

The most obvious approach is to dampen down the chemical reaction at the site of injury. This is achieved by administering anti-inflammatory drugs, which form the basis of standard veterinary treatment for musculoskeletal pain

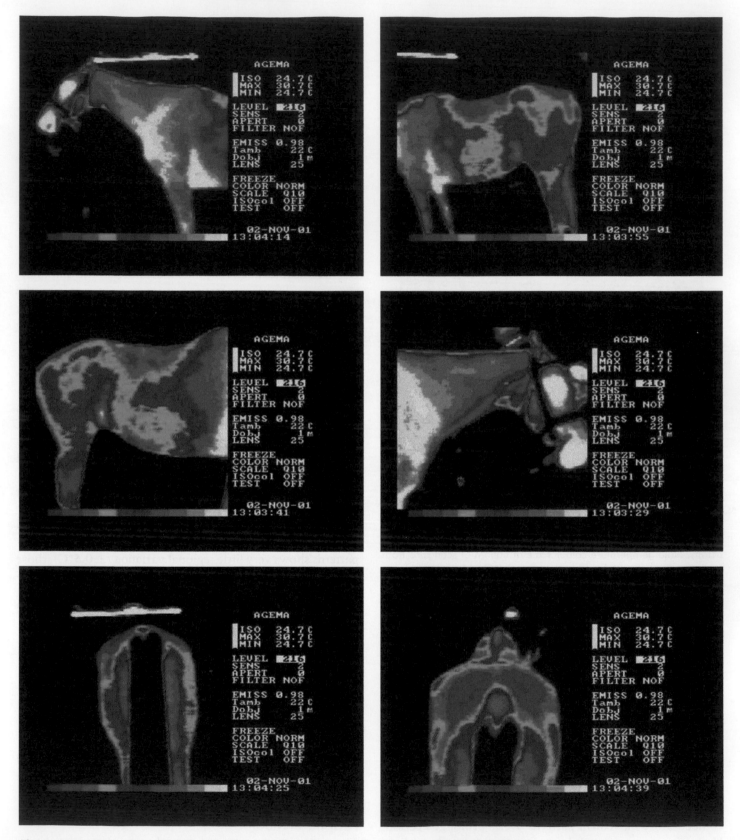

Figure 3.10 Acute injury: generalised cooling over the body is part of a brainstem-mediated autonomic response.

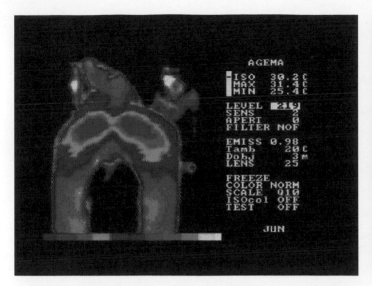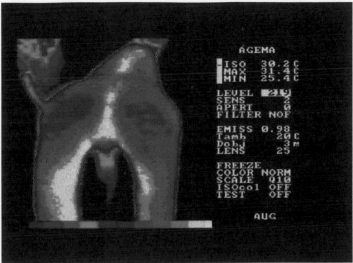

Figure 3.11 Monitoring progress: looking down on to the spine from above and behind the dorsal stripe (erector spinae) and gluteal muscles are evaluated. Pre-treatment scan (left) showed loss of dorsal stripe and low temperatures over gluteal muscle. Follow-up scan (right) demonstrated significant increases in gluteal temperatures and re-establishment of a dorsal stripe.

(Figure 3.12). This reduces local inflammation in the damaged tissue and diminishes the signal traffic from the nociceptors to the dorsal horn of the spinal cord. However, where sensitisation of the dorsal horn neurones has occurred, pain, muscle spasm and autonomic change may persist, driven by this sensitised central neurone pool, even when anti-inflammatory medication has been effective at the periphery. It is these cases that form a large part of osteopathic practice.

Central Modification

Modification at spinal cord level

Fortunately, there are mechanisms which can down-regulate the sensitivity of spinal cord neurones. One of these is the effect of inputs into the spinal cord from large diameter neurones of joint, muscle and skin receptors, which provide information on the position of the body in space and awareness of the external environment. As well as providing sensory information, these inputs are largely inhibitory on the small nociceptive fibres responsible for pain perception. This large fibre traffic can be used therapeutically to modify pain (Melzack and Wall 1965). An everyday example of this occurs when a body part is knocked against a hard object. As the painful sensation is transmitted along small-calibre nerve fibres towards the cord and thence to the brain, the victim can be observed feverishly rubbing the damaged area. It may seem counter-intuitive to apply further physical contact to an injured area. However, the rubbing action stimulates large-fibre input connecting the discriminatory skin receptors to the spinal cord and so inhibits pain pathways (Figure 3.12).

It is by using this route into the spinal cord that physical interventions such as osteopathy can have an effect on pain and therefore muscle spasm and autonomic changes. Treatment is essentially aimed at improving mobility, which increases afferent input from proprioceptors of muscles and joints which act to inhibit or 'gate' pain pathways. This effect is augmented from activity of the discriminatory receptors of the skin, stimulated by the contact with the surface of the body involved in physical therapies.

Treatment may take a number of forms including soft tissue, articulatory, mobilisation and functional techniques, the mechanics of which will be described in subsequent chapters.

Soft tissue and articulatory techniques stretch the skin, fascia and muscles to improve pliability of and nutrition to the periarticular tissues. It also allows the joints to move in a full range.

Mobilisation techniques involve taking a joint with poor mobility to the point of maximum resistance, described as 'the restrictive barrier', and pushing through this barrier with a short-amplitude high-velocity thrust which may be accompanied by a cavitation sound or 'pop'. The resulting mechanoreceptor and associated large-fibre afferent activity into the spinal cord causes an immediate relaxation of the muscles and therefore improved mobility.

A useful approach in longstanding complex cases is functional technique. This uses the idea of 'ease' and 'bind'. A normal joint will reach a point, usually at the middle of its range of movement, where there is minimum tension on the capsular ligaments and overlying muscles, and this is referred to as the point of ease. Any movement away from this point will increase tension or bind. This information

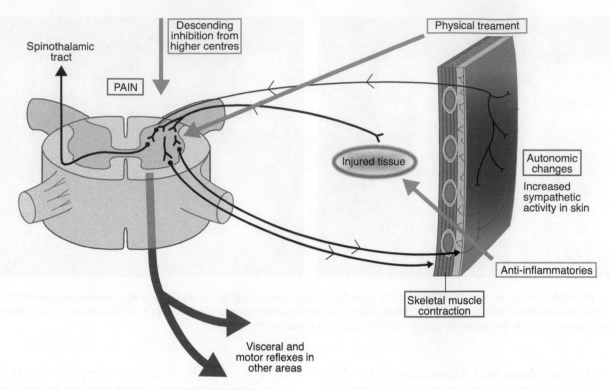

Figure 3.12 Peripheral, central and descending modification of pain pathways: anti-inflammatory medication, physical treatment and centrally acting pharmaceuticals sedation provide a powerful multilevel inhibitory effect on pain.

will be relayed to the central nervous system where it is processed to map joint position and to generate an appropriate pattern of motor activity. Where the normal relationship between the joint structures has been disturbed, this point of ease will be offset and afferent information from that joint will be changed at rest and for any given movement. Difficulties arise with imposing new reference points on well established networks, and the joint is less able to perform appropriately or to co-ordinate movement with other joints.

This new abnormal point may be isolated by testing each range of movement (flexion/extension, sidebending, rotation, translocation from side to side, traction/compression). With the joint held in this position there is minimum tension, and therefore minimum afferent input into the spinal cord. This appears to reduce conflicting information entering the network and allows the old pattern to reassert itself. This pattern is preferred by the system as, over time, neuronal connections have been created that fire more readily to generate a learned response.

Descending modification

Another significant inhibitor of pain circuits is the descending inhibition from centres such as the periaquaductal grey and raphe nuclei of the brain stem (Fields and Basbaum 1999) (Figure 3.12). Increasing the activity of these descending pathways by using specific sedatives, together with large fibre inhibition from physical treatment, can provide a

powerful dual down-regulating effect on the pain pathways (Yaksh 1999).

SUMMARY

This chapter gives an overview of the response of the body to injury in terms of pain sensation, muscle spasm and autonomic activity. It also outlines how these responses may alter the sensitivity of the neuronal network with far-reaching and long-term effects on the neuromusculoskeletal system. It describes how these changes may present in a clinical context and proposes mechanisms for reversing these effects.

In practical terms, in order to develop an effective treatment strategy, it is important to identify all areas that may be involved in dysfunction and quantify the effect on the biomechanics of the body. This process begins with an indepth case history, followed by thorough physical examination of the whole horse.

REFERENCES

Bennett GJ, Kajander KC, Sahara Y, Iadarola MJ, Sugimoto T (1989) Neurochemical and anatomical changes in the dorsal horn of rats with an experimental painful peripheral neuropathy. In: Cervero F, Bennett GJ, Headley PM (eds) *Processing of Sensory Information in the Superficial Dorsal Horn of the Spinal Cord*. Plenum, Amsterdam, pp. 463–471.

Brooks J (2003) Osteopathy in horses using infra-red thermography as a tool to monitor the effect of osteopathic treatment. 4th International Conference on Advances in Osteopathic Research. Royal Society of Medicine, London.

Colles CM, Pusey AG (2003) Osteopathic treatment of the axial skeleton of the horse In: Ross MW, Dyson SJ (eds) *Diagnosis and Management of Lameness in the Horse*. Saunders, London, pp. 819–824.

Colles C, Holah G, Pusey A (1994) Thermal imaging as an aid to the diagnosis of back pain in the horse. Proc. 6th European Congress of Thermography, Bath.

Fields HL, Basbaum AI (1999) Central nervous system mechanisms of pain modulation. In: Wall P, Melzack R (eds) *Textbook of Pain*, 4th edn. Churchill Livingstone, Edinburgh, pp. 309–329.

Goldspink G, Williams F, Simpson H (2002) Gene expression in response to muscle stretch. *Clinical Orthopaedics and Related Research* (403 Suppl), S146–152.

He X, Proske U, Schaible HG, Schmidt RF (1988) Acute inflammation of the knee joint in the cat alters responses of flexor motoneurones to leg movements. *Journal of Neurophysiology* 59, 326–340.

Jensen TS, Nikolajsen L (1999) Phantom limb pain and other phenomena after amputation In: Wall P, Melzack R (eds) *Textbook of Pain*, 4th edn. Churchill Livingstone, Edinburgh, pp. 806–807.

Korr I (1979) The neural basis of osteopathic medicine. In: Peterson B (ed.) *The Collected Papers of Irvin Korr*. American Academy of Osteopathy, Colorado Springs, pp. 120–127.

Livingstone M (2001) PG Diploma Dissertation, Warwickshire College.

Melzack R, Wall PD (1965) Pain mechanisms – a new theory. *Science* 150, 193–207.

Pearson K, Gordon J (2000) Locomotion. In: Kandel J, Schwartz JH, Jessell TM (eds) *Principles of Neural Science*, 4th edn. McGraw-Hill, New York, p. 747.

Raja S, Meyer R, Ringkamp M, Campbell J (1999) Peripheral neural mechanisms of nociception. In: Wall P, Melzack R (eds) *Textbook of Pain*, 4th edn. Churchill Livingstone, Edinburgh, pp. 11–57.

Sato A, Schmidt RF (1973) Somatosympathetic reflexes: afferent fibres, central pathways, discharge characteristics. *Physiological Reviews* 53, 916–947.

Sluka KA, Willis WD, Westlund KN (1995) The role of dorsal root reflexes in neurogenic inflammation. *Pain Forum* 4, 141–149.

Turner TA, Purohit RC, Fessler JF (1986) Thermography: a review in equine medicine. *Compendium on Continuing Education for the Practicing Veterinarian* 8, 855–861.

Williams N (1997) Managing back pain in general practice – is osteopathy the new paradigm? *British Journal of General Practice* 47, 653–655.

Woodleigh M (2003) Can osteopathic treatment under general anaesthetic increase stride length in horses? 4th International Conference on Advances in Osteopathic Research, Royal Society of Medicine, London.

Yaksh TL (1999) Central pharmacology of nociceptive transmission. In: Wall P, Melzack R (eds) *Textbook of Pain*, 4th edn. Churchill Livingstone, Edinburgh, pp. 281–285.

Making a Start in Animal Practice

4

Anthony Pusey and Julia Brooks

Before launching into the field of treating animals, there are a number of factors you may wish to consider. The most effective way of seeing the benefits and the drawbacks of animal practice is to tag along with osteopaths already in the field. They are an enthusiastic group and usually more than willing to share their knowledge and passion for the work. They will have varied interests and experiences, and may help you decide on the direction in which you wish to go. You will also gain invaluable insights into anything from how to approach a wolf in safety to the type of footwear that will protect you from a horse's hoof, without having to go through a painful learning curve yourself. The General Osteopathic Council and the Society of Osteopaths in Animal Practice (SOAP) hold a list of osteopaths working in this area. There are also a number of postgraduate courses on offer, and for new graduates there is always the option of joining a practice with an interest in animals.

There are huge benefits in working with animals, one of which is the development and refinement of a practitioner's osteopathic skills. As information about a problem is from the owner, and is, of necessity, not 'from the horses mouth' and may be incomplete, it is on these skills that we must rely for diagnosis and treatment. This sharpens observation, particularly of the moving body. This is a skill which is under-used in human practice as it is not practical to ask our scantily clad human patients to run up and down in the car park in order to assess the biomechanics of movement. It also hones palpation of tissue state as part of a palpatory archaeological dig to build a picture of past and present dysfunction. The practice of integrating history, observation and palpatory findings into a logical clinical picture on which to base treatment decisions is one of the great challenges.

WHERE TO PRACTICE

There are significant benefits in treating animals. There are also some drawbacks. To begin with, it is expensive in terms of that ever-decreasing commodity, time. When you start to work on your own, you will spend a lot of time on the road to and from stables and clinics. Though it may not be possible at first, developing a centre of operations will improve work efficiency. Ideally, this will be a veterinary clinic. They have the expertise and diagnostic equipment to allow you to concentrate on osteopathy. The other advantage is that, since many horses are insured these days, the vets can process the claim while paying you for the work done. With these advantages in mind, it is well worth contacting your local surgeries. Vets are in private practice and they need to be forward thinking if they are to operate successfully in a competitive market. Owners are often unenthusiastic about long-term pharmaceutical treatment for musculoskeletal problems, particularly in competition horses, and they will value a vet who will take a broad approach. Contacting your local vet may be the first step in establishing a rewarding relationship.

INSURANCE

Time has financial implications but there are other costs such as insurance. An initially comforting thought for those working in a clinic environment is that the osteopath would be covered by the veterinary practice insurance. However, the procedure is that the owner sues the vet and the vet's insurance company sues the osteopath! It is therefore sensible to review your cover. There are various products on the market (e.g. Balens Ltd, Nimrod House, Sandy's Rd, Malvern, Worcs WR14 1JJ; Marketform Ltd 8 Lloyds Avenue, London EC3N 3EL), and the cost will vary depending on the amount of animal work you are doing and the value of the animals involved. Racehorses will often attract a surcharge. As with anything, the maxim 'You get what you pay for' definitely applies here.

The other thing you might like to look at is personal injury cover. Can you afford to pay the mortgage and the school fees while sitting at home with a broken wrist? Most horse vets bear some battle scars, but then they are generally doing nastier things to their patients!

Another reason for insurance company involvement is where the owner wishes to make a claim on a policy. Most companies will cover osteopathic treatment, but there are many different types of policy and the small print may exclude certain conditions.

Payment itself is facilitated by working at a veterinary practice. The client pays the vet and the vet pays the osteopath. If you are working on a referral basis rather than directly with the vet, it may be different. To ensure that payment for treatment does not depend on the vagaries of diverse insurance policies, the onus should be on the owner to establish whether or not fees can be reclaimed. A paragraph on the case sheet along the following lines may be helpful.

If you are claiming treatment costs from an insurance company, it is important that you should contact your particular company to establish whether osteopathy is covered and what conditions apply.

Owners are required to settle all fees on the day of treatment. Where treatment is covered by insurance, it is the responsibility of the owner to reclaim fees directly from the insurance company. It is the owner's responsibility to ensure that their cover is appropriate. Whilst we are always prepared to discuss insurance matters, it is on the basis that we have no special expertise in this field. Our knowledge is based purely on experience of previous claims.

I have read and understood the above.

Signed..... Name (please print name) .... Date ....

SAFETY

Although injuries happen relatively rarely, it is important to reduce the odds as much as possible. You very rarely meet a truly evil horse, but they are herbivores and their survival in the wild over many centuries depended on their ability to react quickly to a perceived danger. Make sure you are not perceived as that danger! There are a number of formal horse handling courses run by the British Horse Society (Stoneleigh Deer Park, Kenilworth, Warwickshire CV8 2XZ), and any of the agricultural colleges now offer a variety of horse-based studies (e.g. Warwickshire College: safety-with-horses@warkscol.ac.uk). If you are not confident around horses, then this is probably the best option. There are also a number of books published on the subject, which will cover the basic rules of safety. Many of these are obvious, such as avoiding an approach to the horse where it does not have a good view of you, i.e. the hindquarters, and, because of the position of the eyes on the side of the head, from directly ahead. The shoulder is about the safest place to stand.

What is perhaps not as obvious is that you may be held responsible for the safety of the owner/handler. A handler should use gloves, protective footwear and a hard hat. The horse will usually be in a headcollar for the examination of active movements. However, in some cases it may be necessary to use a bridle for effective control. A quick look over the tack, checking for frayed stitching and worn leather, will also reduce the possibility of a horse on the loose. Examination and treatment tend to attract quite an audience which should, if possible, be kept on one side of the horse in case it decides to leap sideways (Appendix A).

Preventing unexpected gyrations will be easier in a quiet environment. The noise factor is the disadvantage of treating outside although this may be the only option if you are using certain techniques. A veterinary treatment room will often have a low ceiling with a plasterboard lining. This prevents the horse from rearing up to its full height and either going over backwards or coming down on you.

The safety of the horse is also a consideration. If some of the techniques used involve temporarily unbalancing the horse, as for example when lifting a hindleg, make sure that you are working on a soft surface rather than concrete in case of a fall. Some clinics will provide knee pads for the horse for the same reason.

EQUIPMENT

Another aspect of protection is clothing. The most frequently damaged body part is the foot. Normal shoes will inevitably result in the odd black nail and crushed toe. Boots with steel toe caps are often worn, but there may be a risk of the metal bending and amputating toes. A good pair of walking boots will reduce the chances of injury.

Back protection is also advisable as some techniques involve bending and lifting. Some of the best back supports are easy to put on and off with Velcro fastenings and have extra straps that splint the back without crushing the abdomen.

Other techniques may require resting the weight of the horse's head on your shoulder and neck. There has been at least one reported case of Horner's syndrome as a result of this technique, and many instances of shoulder bruising. One solution is to use the sort of shoulder pads used by rugby forwards, which are integrated into a type of short vest.

Investing in a set of waterproofs will be helpful. Not only does it invariably start to pelt down with rain as soon as you go out to watch a horse moving, but some techniques such as the pelvic lift may leave their mark.

Gloves can be useful for some of the tail traction techniques. Those used in rugby have grip for tails coated in slippery substances designed to make the hair shine, and yet have the fingers cut off to retain the ability to palpate. A lead rope is a useful adjunct to increase pulling power in these techniques if used with a quick release mechanism. Windsurfing harnesses can also be used to reduce the pulling strain.

PROFESSIONAL ETHICS

The 1966 Veterinary Surgeons Act makes it illegal for anyone to diagnose or treat an animal without the input of a vet. Owners may not know this, and when you first start in this area of work it is likely that an owner will make the first approach. It avoids a lot of misunderstandings if the legalities and ethics are explained to the patient at the outset and a referral from the vet is requested. This should be in writing. Referral letters often include a computer printout of the whole veterinary history of an animal, which can be very useful. Expecting a letter is sometimes impractical if treatment is required at short notice, and many osteopathic practitioners have a form which can be sent by fax or e-mail for the vet to sign and return as a confirmation of the referral (Appendix B). A phone call or letter back to the vet to report on your findings is a professional courtesy and helps to keep everyone informed.

INFORMATION SHEETS

There are many myths and misconceptions surrounding physical treatment of horses. Misunderstandings can be avoided by providing a clear, concise information sheet (Appendix D). This will explain to owners some of the underlying principles of osteopathy and outline the procedure involved in the examination and treatment of their horse. It will also be useful to send to vets with whom you are making contact for the first time.

FORMS OF CONSENT

In these days of increasing litigation, you should think about asking the owner to sign a 'consent to treat' form at each consultation. This should also mention sedation if this is to be used (Appendix C).

THE THERAPEUTIC TEAM

There are great advantages to working as a team in this field. The vet/osteopath combination is a powerful one. Two specialists looking at a problem from different angles ensure the best possible care of the animal. The vet makes an assessment to rule out underlying pathology with the expertise of specialist training and access to a battery of diagnostics such as haematology, X-ray and scintigraphy. The osteopath can provide a diagnosis based on knowledge of biomechanics and neurophysiology combined with palpatory skills learned over many years of training and practice. In short, the vet can save the osteopath from any nasty pathological surprises and the osteopath can provide the vet with a specialist skill to tackle biomechanical problems that are common but often difficult for vets to treat.

Alongside the vet, osteopath, physiotherapists and chiropractors, other vital members of the team are the farriers, saddlers and dentists, all of whom have a contribution to make in achieving optimum, pain-free performance from the horse.

5

Case History

Anthony Pusey and Julia Brooks

The case history is often the first point of contact made between the practitioner and those caring for a horse. From it, a picture can begin to be constructed of the horse, its environment and its interaction with the owner/rider.

PRELIMINARIES

It is helpful to have some completed paperwork at this initial stage. There will, of course, be a written request from the vet referring the horse for osteopathic assessment and treatment (Appendix B). It is also sensible to have a consent-to-treat form signed by the owner (Appendix C).

In preparation for this first meeting, a case history sheet can be sent for completion in advance of the consultation. This has the obvious benefit of saving time and allowing the owner a period of reflection in which to crystallise concerns regarding the horse. It also provides written documentation stating their perception of the current problem. This can be used as a baseline measurement against which any future changes in symptoms can be evaluated. Another advantage stems from the fact that a consortium of people are often involved with the care of the horse, ranging from absentee owners to trainers, riders, grooms, family, friends and horse transporters. It is sometimes difficult to establish which of these parties has requested treatment for the horse, and the instigator may in fact not even be present for the consultation. A completed case history in advance avoids the necessity of relying on a sketchy history from the person bringing in the horse.

The format of the case sheet can be varied but certain items of information are essential (Appendix E).

PERSONAL DETAILS

The name and address of the owner should be noted as well as that of the person to whom an invoice should be sent. Contact details of those responsible for the day-to-day care of the horse may also be helpful in order to make or change arrangements for follow-up consultations.

The name of the vet should already be known from the referral note although some owners will use a number of practices for reasons of their own.

A section for details of the horse is included. This may not be as simple as it sounds. Starting with the name, it may have an official designation which is often grand but unwieldy. It is therefore replaced with a more manageable, but usually totally unrelated, stable name. Constantine, the drum horse of the Household Cavalry, was always affectionately referred to as Eric! All possibilities should be recorded.

One way around the identification problem is to make a note of the freeze mark on the shoulder. During a busy clinic in a polo yard or racing stable, one horse begins to look very much like another and the freeze-mark system ensures that the horse matches up with the appropriate case sheet.

At this point, knowing how long a horse has been owned will give some indication as to the scope and accuracy of any subsequent history. Where a horse has been sold on, information may not have been passed in its entirety to the new owner.

DEMOGRAPHICS

The demographic details such as age, sex, height and breed should be recorded.

Age is important as part of a diagnostic and prognostic process. A young horse may present with developmental problems whereas, in an older horse, pathology is more likely to be degenerative in nature. Having excluded pathology, a horse showing mechanical dysfunction early on in life may have suffered some perinatal injury affecting the subsequent neuromuscular pattern development. These cases are often challenging to treat and the prognosis may be more guarded.

The sex of the horse may explain some behaviour patterns and tissue state changes which will vary with hormonal cycles. This is particularly relevant in mares.

Colour is documented for ease of identification. Anecdotal evidence also suggests that response to treatment has been linked to genetically determined tissue type. In the human field, the gene producing red hair, which is the equivalent of the equine chestnut, has been related to lower pain thresholds and increased anaesthetic dose requirement.

Breed will determine attributes such as temperament, conformation and muscle distribution, which in turn predict the type of work that will be suitable.

WORK

Details of the horse's work status are important. If it is not currently in work, the reasons and duration of this layoff should be sought. It should be noted that the length of time off work is not necessarily an indication of how long the problem has existed but of how long it has sufficiently interfered with function to cause underperformance.

Past work regimes are also important as some disciplines carry additional risks. A horse that has spent time in racing may well have had serious falls at speed. Polo ponies will be subjected to frequent sharp stops and turns as well as local soft tissue injuries.

The level of performance achieved in this past work is also helpful. A horse that underachieved or was susceptible to recurrent injury in its original discipline suggests a deep-seated problem resulting from an early injury.

Intended use may give some idea of the owner's expectations. In human practice, I successfully treated a difficult shoulder problem. The patient was delighted and asked if he would now be able to play Chopin on the piano. I replied in the affirmative.

'Good', he replied, 'I've never been able to play it before!'

NATURE OF THE PROBLEM

Presenting problems vary widely in site, severity and aetiology. The complaint may impair performance or it may prevent the horse from carrying out any activity at all. The impact of dysfunction depends on the level and discipline of the work. A minor abnormality in movement will be unremarkable in a leisure hack but significantly affect results in a top-flight dressage horse.

Site

The owner will often have concerns about a specific area. There is also an understandable tendency both in veterinary and human fields to concentrate almost exclusively on a symptomatic region. It is, however, vitally important to probe beyond the immediate problem to reveal any idiosyncrasies in behaviour or movement which co-exist or pre-date the current problem. These might well have been noticed by the owner, but may not have interfered with performance sufficiently to be a cause for alarm. These subtle disturbances may be early warning signals for a future crisis.

A clinical example of this would be a hock joint, which is periodically injected by the vet for recurrent injury. The owner may have noticed a lack of propulsion from behind over a long period. However, no attention has been paid to the poor lumbosacral function that prevents the legs from coming under the body to generate power, but which also subjects the hock to abnormal strain.

Certain problems such as temperament changes, areas of sensitivity in the poll or back, bucking, napping and general stiffness are commonly presenting complaints. In general, upper cervical dysfunction will be reported as a range of signs such as difficulty with collection, forming an outline and unwillingness to accept the bit. Poor cervicothoracic function will affect lateral work, and pelvic problems may be reported as loss of propulsion from behind.

Riders competing in different activities tend to complain of particular problems that affect performance in their specialism. Discussing specific movement issues with them requires knowledge of the language associated with the various disciplines, and it is helpful to review some of the terms in common usage (see Glossary).

Horses involved in jumping may begin to refuse fences, be unable to tackle combinations and be unsuccessful over verticals or oxers. They may take off too early or too late, or trail a hind foot over the jump. Eventers may suffer a loss of propulsive effort from behind or have difficulty negotiating inclines. The dressage element of the discipline may show problems with lateral movements or poorly tolerated collected or extended work. There may be reluctance to accept the bit, or a head tilt.

Onset

The onset and progression of a problem is of diagnostic importance.

Pathological processes can be suggested by the temporal profile. A sudden onset may represent a catastrophic event such as a fracture, while gradual development and inexorable progression of a problem might indicate degenerative disease.

The time scale of the onset is also important when making a biomechanical diagnosis. An acute presentation may result from trauma such as falling in the field or pulling back on a tethered rope, and may be witnessed or surmised by the owner. There are often telltale abrasions and soft tissue injury.

There may, however, be a sudden onset for which no cause can be established. These cases often represent a decompensation process. A horse may have successfully absorbed past trauma sufficiently for adequate, but not optimal, performance. If it is then asked to perform at a higher level or suffers insignificant trauma, the compensatory mechanisms are unable to contend with yet another demand on an already compromised system, and an apparent catastrophe ensues.

A slow, insidious onset is commonly reported. Again, this is often a result of subtle compromise in function over a long period. There may even be radiographic evidence of localised degenerative changes. This does not preclude physical treatment. Identifying ways of reducing abnormal forces through the affected structures will contribute to the management of these cases.

Recurrent dysfunction in the form of a 'boom—bust' syndrome is not uncommon. The horse is treated for a local problem and rested for a while. It appears to recover and is brought back into work. As the intensity of work increases, the injury resurfaces and the cycle begins again. This suggests that the causative factors are not being addressed by treatment. These cases require careful biomechanical examination to identify factors that may be contributing to the problem.

SPECIFIC QUESTIONS

To augment the information already gathered, it may be helpful to ask a few specific questions. Many owners compartmentalise problems, screening out elements of the history which they consider irrelevant. They are often unaware that other aspects of movement and behaviour may be related to the presenting condition. For this reason asking questions about day-to-day activities may bring to light factors of clinical significance (Appendix F).

One of the first enquiries to be made is whether any changes in temperament have occurred. A horse in pain can appear withdrawn and unresponsive or it may become bad tempered and irritable. Musculoskeletal problems are known to have an effect on mood (Jeffcott 1979). In fact, after the first osteopathic treatment, owners will frequently report that 'it is a different horse'.

Questions about movements that stress the system are also useful. A horse may have adequately adapted its movement patterns to cope with a longstanding musculoskeletal problem. However, a specific action such as lifting the leg for the farrier, which requires limb flexion and thoracic and pelvic girdle rotation, may bring to light dysfunction that had hitherto passed unnoticed.

Certain regular activities may reveal problems. For example, a stiff horse may find it difficult or uncomfortable to get down, roll around and regain its feet to stand. Following treatment, owners will often report a return to rolling.

Similarly, urination requires flexion and extension of the thoracolumbar spine, and if this is uncomfortable there may be changes in urinary pattern.

Some problems are brought on or exaggerated by manoeuvres required by riding. The accuracy of this report will depend on the sensitivity of the rider. This will vary from a total lack of awareness of a problem, through to identifying a specific area of dysfunction.

Sensitivity of spinal areas may also be detected, such as irritability of the poll, often noticed when grooming, or thoracic pain when tightening the girth.

PAST EVENTS

Knowledge of past illnesses and injuries as well as previous investigations and treatment for both medical and biomechanical problems will identify areas of weakness in the horse's physiological makeup. It is also helpful in identifying regions of possible dysfunction that may initially seem unrelated to the presenting complaint. An old injury, apparently resolved, may have left behind some residual mechanical disturbance. Medical problems may initiate viscero-somatic reflexes where activity in the spinal cord segment innervating the affected viscera spills over into activation of neural networks supplying the musculoskeletal system. Thus, a bout of colic may leave muscle tension and tissue texture changes in the thoracolumbar region of the spine.

GENERAL CARE

At this stage it is helpful to know about the conditions in which the horse is kept and the level of maintenance care taken. This information may be important in managing the case.

General considerations such as whether the horse is kept out in the field or stabled are noted. If stabled, the horse may have vices which could be the result of, or contribute to, the presenting problem.

Of importance where the back is concerned is whether the saddle is regularly checked and altered to keep pace with the development and fitness level of the horse. Regularity of teeth inspection has implications for structures such as the temporomandibular joint and upper cervical spine. Hoof care and the willingness of the farrier to look at foot biomechanics are also significant.

CLINICAL OBSERVATIONS

The case card will include observations made from clinical examination including conformation, observation of active movements, palpatory findings and treatment methods. If sedation is being used, the dosage should be recorded as being effective or indeed ineffective.

From this record, a report can be written up for the vet, ensuring that all involved in the care of the horse are kept informed.

CONCLUSIONS

Armed with the information from the case history, it is possible to start formulating an idea of the biomechanical stresses experienced by the horse. It will also have been an opportunity to gauge the attitude, experience and expectations of the owner. Restoring a horse to full fitness is a team effort of which the owner/rider is a vital member. With this in mind, together with the history and clinical findings, a treatment and rehabilitation plan should be developed with the owner that is understandable, acceptable and achievable.

REFERENCE

Jeffcott LB (1979) Back problems in the horse—a method of clinical examination. *Vet. Rec. Suppl. In Pract.* 1, 4–15.

Static Observation

Anthony Pusey and Julia Brooks

STATIC EXAMINATION

The case history is followed by examination of the horse itself. This next phase should be embarked upon without preconceived ideas. Discussion with the owner will have suggested regions that are cause for concern, but it is important to assess the structure and function of the whole animal rather than restricting the inspection to a localised area.

The first stage of the process is to observe the horse while it is standing. This view gives the structural blueprint of the horse, comprising its genetic makeup, indications of past trauma and the way it uses its body.

The examination begins with the horse standing square on an even surface. The demeanour is observed and an overview of the conformation of the horse is obtained.

DEMEANOUR

At this early stage it is possible to pick up on personality and behavioural traits. These can range from an inquisitive, interactive animal to an uninterested, introverted horse, apparently focussed on some internal matter. It may be bad tempered or anxious, causing handling difficulties. The eyes are a good indicator of mood. The poetically described soft eyes of a friendly horse may be contrasted with a hard appearance, perhaps from the automatic retraction of the eyes in response to pain or threat. The ears are also indicative of mood, ranging from pricked forwards, which suggests alertness, to flat backwards, denoting fear or aggression.

Behavioural changes are frequently associated with musculoskeletal problems. Encouragingly, a remark often made by owners after the first osteopathic treatment is that the horse is 'much happier in itself' and that it has started to roll and play enthusiastically with other horses. The latter can be a mixed blessing and means that recovery may not be uneventful.

STRUCTURE

The basic structure is modelled on an ancestor adapted for grazing, reproducing, and frustrating predators. Its modern descendant has been modified to develop many different qualities such as speed for racing, power for jumping, flexibility for dressage, agility for polo and the ability to carry a variable amount of weight on its back. These requirements will all have a different structural 'wish list'. The literature describing the most desirable conformation for each discipline is extensive.

Conformation is often considered to be a fixed, unchangeable entity. With respect to bone length, this is true. However, the angles at which these bones meet at joints are determined by the anatomy of the joint, the activity of the overlying muscles and the relationship with adjacent structures. These factors can be influenced by physical treatment.

An examination of skeletal components and the effect of muscular development in response to activity and injury begins with obtaining an overall impression of structure, followed by a more detailed regional assessment. It is performed by observing the horse from the side, from the front and from behind.

Overview

An overview of structure is obtained from the side view. A snapshot impression should give a sense of proportion and

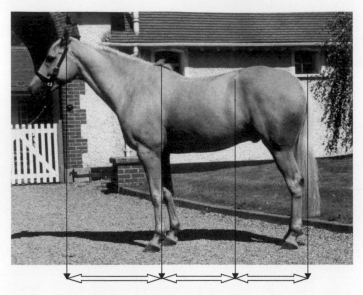

Figure 6.1 Proportions: the body can be divided into thirds to assess the balance and proportions of the horse.

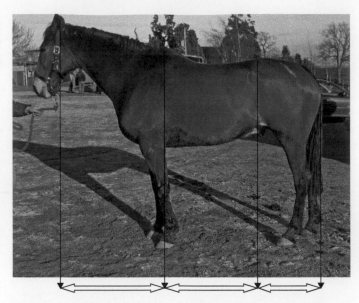

Figure 6.2 Proportions: weak hindquarters transfer power generation to the forelimbs and the thoracic girdle becomes overdeveloped.

balance. This can be confirmed using a number of different systems of which the most practical is probably the rule of thirds. A well balanced horse can be divided into three equal parts (Figure 6.1).

Cranial third: from just behind the poll to the scapula.
Middle third: from the scapula to the point of the hip (tuber coxae).
Caudal third: from the point of hip to the point of the buttocks (tuber ischii).

However, in a phrase borrowed from the car industry, the horse may be a 'cut and shut' job. It can appear to be made up of a number of different horses welded together to form a poorly balanced end product. This may affect the weight distribution through the limbs. Ideally, about 60% of the weight is taken through the forelegs. This gives a centre of mass at around the 13th rib on a line running from the point of the shoulder to the point of the buttock.

The skeletal proportions of a horse may be unalterable. In fact, some variations may be desirable as in the case of short-coupled polo ponies, where the distance between the lower ribs and the pelvic brim is less than the theoretical optimum. This confers strength to the back and the ability to turn at speed but may predispose to overriding dorsal processes. Some horses, such as Arabs, may only have five rather than six lumbar vertebrae.

Muscle mass, which develops in response to functional demands, also plays an important part in the sense of proportion. For example, a horse that is weak in the hindquarters may transfer power generation to the forelimbs. This

results in overdevelopment of the thoracic girdle musculature, which creates an unbalanced appearance (Figure 6.2). In contrast, poor neck function will impair the contribution of the head and neck in forward propulsion and results in increased bulk of the hindquarters.

The structure of one side should be compared with that of the other. It may seem as though the two sides belong to quite different horses. This effect can be caused by a scoliosis, which is identified by looking down on to the spine from above and checking for asymmetry in the ribs. It may also be created by unequal muscle development from musculoskeletal dysfunction.

While looking at the gross outline of the horse, note should be made of scars, swellings and localised muscle atrophy which may be the consequence of injury.

Regional Structures
Once a general impression of proportion, symmetry and muscle development has been obtained, regional assessments can then be made. The factors mentioned here are not exhaustive and emphasis is placed on aspects that may be of interest to the osteopath.

Head and neck
Symmetry is looked for in the eyes, ears, nostrils and frontal region. Changes in fascial tension or rotational asymmetry in the neck due to injury or dysfunction will result in changes in resting position and muscle bulk of the head and neck.

The mandible hangs in a relaxed fashion below the cranium and face. A distance of around 10 cm, roughly the

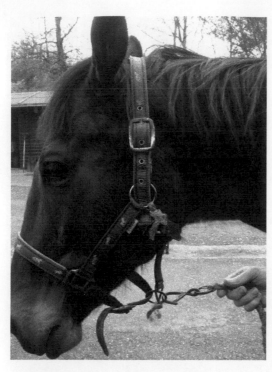

Figure 6.3 Ventral cervical muscles: increased muscle tone here gives a tense appearance to the suboccipital and temporomandibular region.

breadth of a closed fist, separates the mandibular rami and provides adequate space to facilitate airflow. Suprahyoid, infrahyoid and ventral cervical muscle tension give a narrow, tense appearance to the floor of the mandible and the temporomandibular joint (Figure 6.3).

The connection between the head and neck should have a soft, mobile look. Dysfunction in the suboccipital region often gives the impression that the neck has been bolted on to the head to resemble a T-square.

A space of two fingers' breadth separates the temporomandibular joint and the atlas which, together with a long poll, aids flexion. Suboccipital muscle tightness gives a cramped, full appearance to the region between the mandibular rami and the wing of the atlas. This may be different on one side when compared with the other.

The neck itself should show a balance between the dorsal and ventral structures. The neck is held up by the dorsal muscles such as splenius and semispinalis. A neck injury that causes these components to become relatively inactive results in the overdevelopment of the ventral muscles such as the brachiocephalicus to give an 'upside down' neck (Figure 6.4).

Withers

The shape of the withers is determined by the size of the thoracic spinous processes and the bulk of the epaxial muscles.

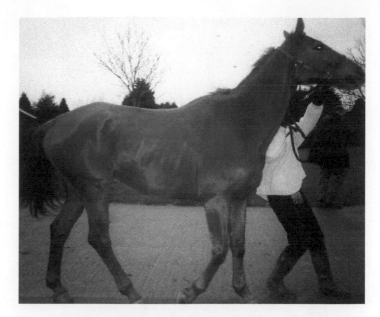

Figure 6.4 Ventral muscles: overdevelopment of muscles such as the brachiocephalicus give the appearance of an 'upside down' neck.

The spinous processes should be of moderate height to provide a large area for muscle attachment and to keep the saddle in place. It is difficult to anchor the saddle on low withers but the converse causes saddle-fitting problems. The development of the thoracic sling muscles during training will have the effect of raising the withers, necessitating saddle alteration.

Dysfunction in the neck and cervicothoracic region results in atrophy of the epaxial muscles giving a characteristic scalloped-out appearance either side of the spinous processes.

Chest

From the front, the forelimbs are separated by about the width of a horse's foot between the two front feet (Figure 6.5). More than this and the horse will tend to have an uncomfortable, rolling gait. If the chest is too narrow, there will be poor lung capacity and the front legs may strike each other during movement.

Lower cervical injuries will result in tightening of the scapular and pectoral muscles, giving a pinched appearance to the chest by drawing the forelimbs together and the scapulae more vertically.

Shoulder

The scapulae are sloped to give expansive forelimb excursion and to absorb concussion. This can be assessed by looking at the point of the shoulder and following the line of the spine of the scapula, dorsally and caudally, towards the withers. Periscapular tightness draws the scapulae into a more upright position, resulting in a short, choppy forelimb action (Figure 6.6).

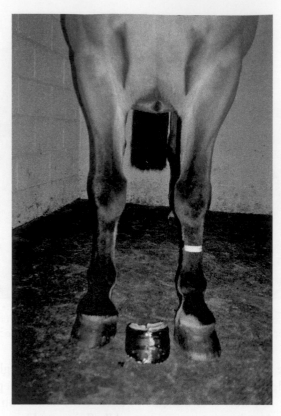

Figure 6.5 Chest and forelegs: the forelimbs are separated by about the width of a horse's foot.

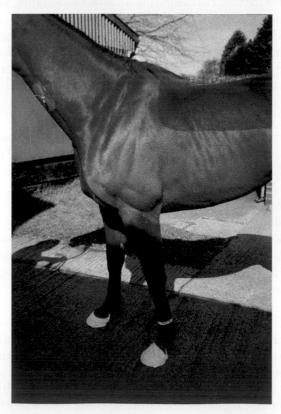

Figure 6.6 Periscapular tightness: the scapulae are drawn vertically and forelimb action is short and choppy.

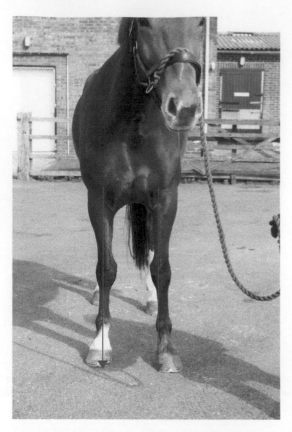

Figure 6.7 Forelimbs: conformational abnormalities, such as splayed feet, will affect gait and predispose to peripheral joint pathology. A plumbline dropped from the point of the shoulder should divide the limb into two equal parts.

The humerus, forming the other part of the shoulder, should slope caudally towards the elbow. A short, horizontally orientated humerus reduces stride scope.

Forelegs

The limbs should hang vertically from the trunk with the weight evenly distributed through both feet. From the front, a plumb line dropped from the point of the shoulder divides the limb into two equal parts. Various conformational abnormalities, such as bow legs (carpus varus), knock knees (carpus valgus), pigeon- or splayed feet, will affect gait and predispose to peripheral joint pathology (Figure 6.7).

From the side, a line descending from the tubercle on the spine of the scapula passes through the centre of the elbow, carpus and fetlock and will touch the ground just behind the heel. The legs should not be held behind this line as stride length is shortened. In navicular disease or laminitis, the forelimb may be positioned in front of the line as a strategy to reduce weight through the front feet.

The back

From above there should be a straight midline from the tail to the poll, with equal muscling on both sides (Figure 6.8). Rotational injuries can disrupt this midline orientation.

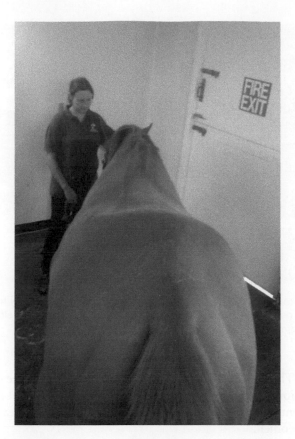

Figure 6.8 The back. The midline should be straight and muscle development symmetric.

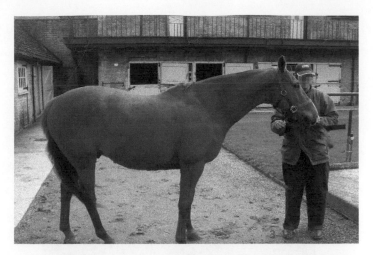

Figure 6.9 The back: should be relatively straight rather than roached, as shown above, or sway backed.

From the side a horizontal line can be drawn between the withers, formed by the spinous processes of the upper thoracic spine, and the croup, made up of five sacral vertebrae. However, dressage riders may prefer an 'uphill' conformation, where the withers are higher than the croup, to enable powerful, upward movements of the front limbs required in this discipline.

The back is relatively straight. It should not be swaybacked, the equivalent of lumbar lordosis in humans, or roached where the lumbar spine is flexed (Figure 6.9). It should also be of moderate length, principally determined by the size of the vertebrae. If the back is too long, it tends to be flexible but weak, whereas a short back is strong but lacks mobility. The thoracolumbar spine must be supported by well toned abdominal muscles which are part of the bow and string mechanism of thoracolumbar support as well as bearing the weight of the viscera (Chapter 2).

Injuries result initially in local asymmetries of intervertebral joint complexes, but later may extend through the spine as compensatory posture and movement patterns are adopted. Seen from the side, the horse often has asymmetry and loss of epaxial muscle development, described by the owner as lack of topline.

Hindquarters

The hindquarters form the powerhouse of the horse, embodying the old adage that a horse should have 'the head of a duchess and the bottom of a cook'. The pelvic skeletal structure is broad, flat and long to provide attachment for muscles.

The croup runs from the eminences of the tubera sacrale back towards the tail, and should be fairly long and slightly downward sloping to the tail to allow lumbosacral flexion and extension. A flat croup restricts the scope of hindlimb movement. This area sometimes appears to slope back from a very prominent tuber sacrale and can be described as a 'jumper's bump' (Figure 6.10). This may be the result of atrophy of the gluteal muscles and affects protraction and retraction of the limb.

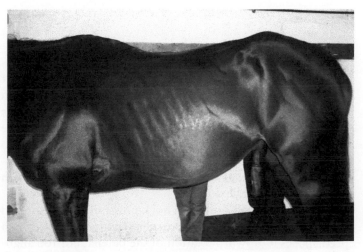

Figure 6.10 The croup: atrophy of pelvic muscles results in prominent tuber sacrale or 'jumpers bump'.

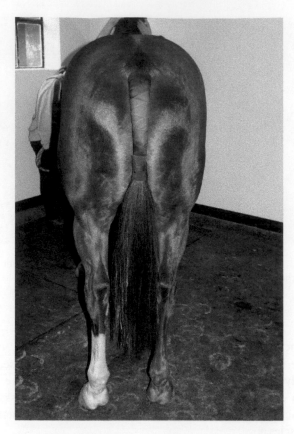

Figure 6.11 From behind: the two tubera sacrale should be level, and pelvic and hindlimb muscles well formed and symmetric.

From behind, the gluteal, quadriceps, hamstring and adductor muscles should be well formed and symmetric (Figure 6.11).

The tail should be relaxed and hang straight. Problems in the lumbar spine and pelvis may result in asymmetric fascial and muscular tension, pulling the tail away from its central position.

Hindlimbs

From the side, a line dropped from the tuber ischii touches the point of the hock, passes down the plantar aspect of the metatarsus and meets the ground about 8 cm behind the heels (Figure 6.12). A limb set forward of this line often causes stride length in the retraction phase to be reduced. Where the limb lies caudal to this line, referred to as camped behind, protraction under the abdomen is compromised and power is lost. This may be associated with poor lumbosacral flexion.

The angles of the stifle and hock joints should be around 155–160° (Figure 6.13). This is neither too straight, which predisposes to upward fixation of the patella, nor too angulated, described as sickle hocked, which may cause plantar ligament strain or 'curb'.

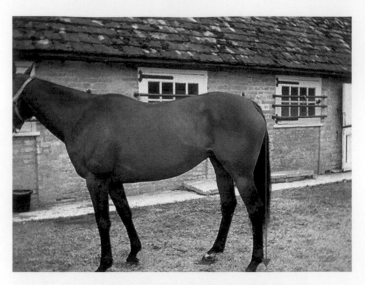

Figure 6.12 Hindlimbs: a line dropped from the tuber ischii touches the point of the hock, passes down the plantar aspect of the metatarsus and meets the ground about 8 cm behind the heels.

The patella is slightly laterally facing following the orientation of the stifle which produces cranial and lateral movement in the protraction phase so that the limb clears the abdomen.

From behind, the tuber sacrale should be level and a line dropped from the tuber ischii divides the limb in two (Figure 6.14). The limbs should be as far apart at the pelvis as at the

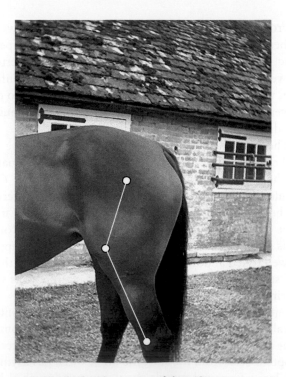

Figure 6.13 Hindlimbs: the angles of the stifle and hock should be around 155–160°.

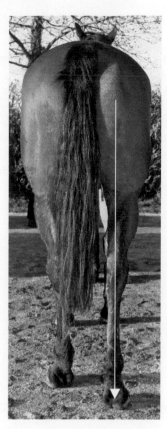

Figure 6.14 Hindquarters: a line dropped from the tuber ischii divides the limb in two.

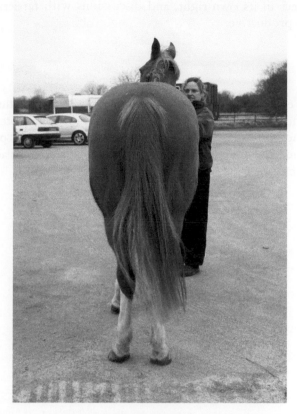

Figure 6.15 Hocks: if the hocks lean towards each other ('cow hocked'), there will be uneven stresses through the carpal joints and this may predispose to degenerative changes.

ground. Feet too far apart or too close together are referred to as 'base wide' or 'base narrow', respectively.

The hocks should be big and without swelling. If the points of the hocks lean towards each other the horse is said to be 'cow hocked' (Figure 6.15). This puts uneven stresses through the carpal joints and may predispose to bone spavin, a degenerative condition of the distal joints of the hock.

Feet

There is a saying, 'No foot, no horse', and this aspect is easiest to assess in the well trimmed foot. The feet should be large and symmetric with medial and lateral hoof walls of equal length. The front hooves are rounder compared with the more oval hind feet.

There are a number of axes used as a guide to foot conformation (Figure 6.16). One of the most important is the hoof/pastern axis formed from a straight line running through the centre of rotation of the coffin, pastern and fetlock joints. Orientation defects of these axes, such as upright or sloping pasterns, low heels with long toes, and medial/lateral imbalances, change the foot flight and may contribute to problems elsewhere.

The foot is the first point of contact with the ground during locomotion, and any dysfunction in the feet will have consequences for the biomechanics of the whole animal. Take note of the type of shoeing. Farriery is a huge

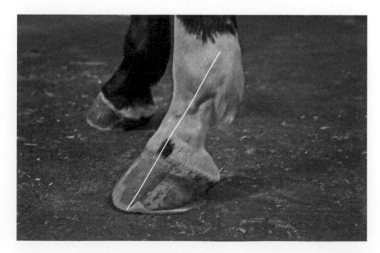

Figure 6.16 Foot: the hoof/pastern axis is formed from a straight line running through the centre of rotation of the coffin, pastern and fetlock joints.

subject in its own right, and discussions with farriers are very productive.

FORM AND FUNCTION

The examination of the skeletal and muscular structure of the horse will give some insight into the functional potential of the horse. This information is taken into the next phase of the assessment which involves the examination of active movements.

BIBLIOGRAPHY

Back W, Clayton H (2001) *Equine Locomotion*. WB Saunders, Edinburgh.

McBane S (2000) *Conformation for the Purpose*. Swan Hill Press, Shrewsbury.

Pasquini C, Pasquini S, Woods P (1995) *Guide to Equine Clinics, Vol. 3, Lameness Diagnosis*. Sudz Publishing, Pilot Point, Texas.

Williams G, Deacon M (1999) *No Foot, No Horse*. Kenilworth Press, Shrewsbury.

7

Observation of Active Movements

Anthony Pusey and Julia Brooks

Observation of the horse as it moves is one of the most important parts of the examination process. It is, after all, usually a failure to perform that brings the horse to the clinic. Alongside investigating the main presenting problem, it is also an opportunity to observe more subtle biomechanical changes that may be compromising the horse's mobility and which may contribute to dysfunction (Appendix G).

As with all forms of examination, it is first helpful to establish a consistent routine in order to build up a mental database of normal and abnormal movement patterns. The routine suggested here is for assessing biomechanical function rather than identifying specific lameness. Lameness resulting from limb pathology requires a veterinary assessment.

Conditions under which the examination takes place will vary but the availability of certain facilities will help in the diagnostic process.

EXAMINATION CONDITIONS

The main part of the examination takes place in a quiet environment on a hard, flat surface extending for about 45 m (Figure 7.1). It should be long enough for the horse to get into its stride and without the added mechanical stress of negotiating slopes. The hard ground allows the sound of hoof beats to be heard. This assists in diagnosis as any musculoskeletal dysfunction will alter the normal, regular rhythm of footfalls. Concrete provides good sound effects but can be treacherous, especially in wet conditions. A dusting of gravel or sand helps to show the direction and force with which the feet contact the ground by noting the orientation of the hoof print and the displacement of loose particles on foot strike.

It may be necessary to use a variety of surfaces. A footsore or unshod horse will move better when on a softer surface. Comparing performances on soft and hard ground and when lungeing is part of a veterinary screen to distinguish between lameness originating from different structures.

An often underrated participant in the examination is the person leading the horse. In an ideal world this person should be proficient and attuned to the osteopath's requirements. Veterinary nurses fulfil this role very successfully. However, in reality the handler may be anyone from a horsebox driver to a non-horsey friend of the owner, and so the principles of the examination procedure should be explained carefully. It must also be appreciated that the safety of persons present is the responsibility of the practitioner.

The horse should wear a headcollar with a lead rope. It is sometimes necessary, for reasons of control, to use a bridle, but this may affect the horse's movements (Cook 1999). The handler is instructed to hold the lead rope or rein at about 45 cm from the horse so that the action of the head and neck can be observed unhampered by external constraints. The pace should be fairly brisk as it is difficult to fully appreciate the flow of movement at a lazy amble. The horse should perform the movements of each phase of the examination several times to get a true appreciation of biomechanical function.

The guiding principles of examination are to look at overall flow of the horse's motion and how movement is transmitted from one area to another. Alongside this is the localisation of regional disturbances in function involving the occipito-atlanto-axial articulations, the mid- to lower cervical spine, the cervicothoracic spine, scapula and forelimbs, thoracolumbar spine, lumbosacral spine, pelvis and hindlimbs.

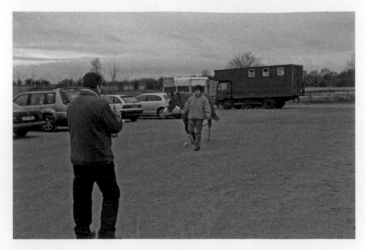

Figure 7.1 Location: a car park provides a large area for observing active movements.

Movement is assessed at walk and trot with particular attention paid to turns and the transitions between these gaits. In order to get a rounded view, movement should be observed from the back, from the front and from the side. Additional information can be obtained by turning the horse in a tight circle and backing up.

OBSERVATION AT WALK

The walk is a four-beat gait, which describes the pattern of footfalls in a stride. In looking at a stride sequence, it is traditional to look first at the left hind as it contacts the ground. This is followed by placement of the left fore, then the right hind and ends with the right fore (Figure 7.2). The amount of time each leg should be in contact with the ground, and the position of each foot in relation to the other, are well documented (Back and Clayton 2001). There is an excellent series of photographs taken by the 19th century photographer, Eadweard Muybridge, showing all phases of the stride (Muybridge 1899). The clinical implication of this sequence is that it gives a distinctive footfall sound pattern, 'clippity clop', with the body moving in a fluid, symmetric, forward progression. Disruption of this normal footfall pattern results from musculoskeletal problems which can be localised

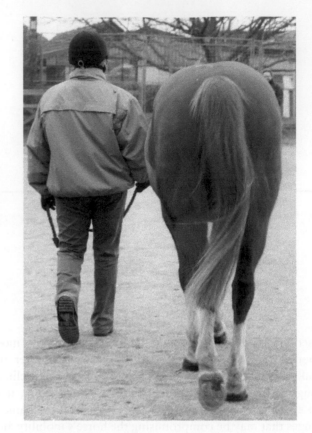

Figure 7.3 Walking from behind: look for vertical movement of the ilia, sacral swing and forward flight of hindlimbs.

from careful observation of the way a horse uses each part of its body.

From Behind
The handler is asked to aim, without deviation, for a fixed point straight ahead. This allows movement to be assessed directly from behind. As the horse walks away from the practitioner a snapshot view is taken to get an overall impression of symmetry and fluidity of the motion. This can then be dissected out to look at the individual elements of limb, pelvic and spinal movement (Figure 7.3).

One of the most striking movements when observing from behind is the way the ilia move up and down like pistons on the sacrum as the leg is lifted and then placed to bear

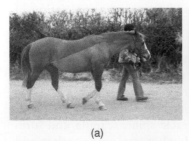
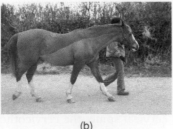
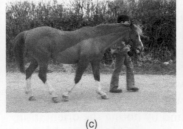
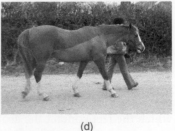

(a)   (b)   (c)   (d)

Figure 7.2 Walk: a four-beat gait sequence, starting with the left hind, left fore, right hind and right fore.

weight. Stiffness in the sacroiliac and lower lumbar regions may suppress this movement unilaterally or bilaterally. The soft tissues often appear bound or tethered over the ilia and sacrum giving a flattened static appearance to the hindquarters, and much of the ventro-dorsal scope is lost.

As the horse moves forwards the hindquarters should show a degree of lateral movement. This is assessed by observing the sacrum swing slightly from left to right across the midline. Pelvic dysfunction may cause this movement to be greater to one side than the other, or indeed it may not shift in one direction at all. The tail may also be held to one side.

The line of flight and elevation of the hindlimb movement should be assessed. As the foot is lifted and brought forwards, it should be possible to see the underside of the hoof. With hindlimb, pelvic and lumbar stiffness the horse is unable to lift the foot up under the body and will instead move it forwards close to the ground such that the undersurface of the hoof is only partly visible. Asymmetry will be reflected in seeing the plantar surface of one hoof more completely than the other.

The hindlimbs should, under normal circumstances, swing freely backwards and forwards with minimal lateral or medial deviation. In cases where the lumbar spine and pelvis are stiff, lateral movement becomes quite exaggerated. The hindlegs swing out and forwards with the feet landing laterally to, rather than under, the body in a motion that has been described as the 'wet nappy' look (Figure 7.4). This re-duces forward propulsion as the energy generated from the leg action is dissipated in sideways movement. The sacrum often appears to be moving in a figure of eight pattern. In contrast to this the hindlimbs may be very close together behind, and this carries the risk of 'interference' when one foot clips the other leg as it is moved forwards.

Long Turn

The horse is brought round to walk back towards the practitioner in a long turn. Usually, the handler stays on the left side and turns the horse away to the right. It may also be helpful to see a turn to the left. This manoeuvre gives an opportunity to assess lateral flexibility in combination with forward propulsion. As the change in direction begins, the neck should be able to sidebend into the turn with the thorax rotating in the thoracic sling followed by spinal and pelvic participation. The lateral flexion is initiated by the front feet which should move sideways into the turn while the back legs cross smoothly behind (Figure 7.5).

Where spinal mobility is poor, the whole horse moves around like a lead pipe with the muzzle thrust forwards, unable to demonstrate the lateral flexibility which characterises axial suppleness. There may be a sense of awkwardness in the foot placement during the turn when the sacrum and sacroiliac joints are stiff. Periscapular muscle tension clamps the scapulae against the chest wall. This interferes with the swing of the thorax in its muscular sling and restricts forelimb excursion. Slight unsteadiness may occur where proprioceptive information is reduced from a poorly functioning upper cervical spine. There are, however, some neurological

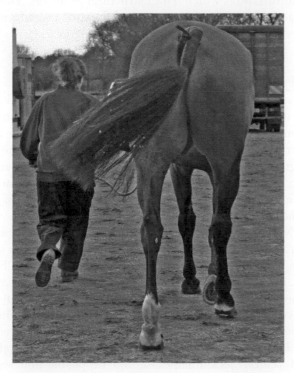

Figure 7.4 Lumbar and pelvic dysfunction: the hind legs show increased lateral movement giving a 'wet nappy' appearance.

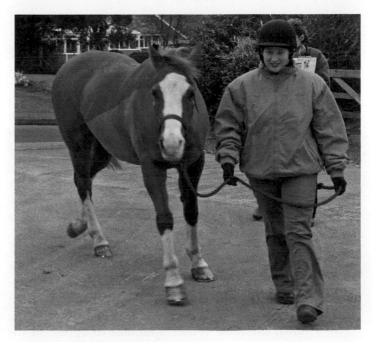

Figure 7.5 Long turn: look for forefoot position, lateral curve of spine and crossing of hindlegs.

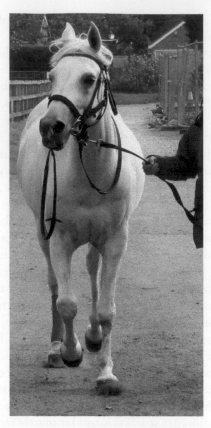

Figure 7.6 From the front: observe the stretching of the ventral neck and pectoral fascia, the space between the legs and the flight of the forelimbs. Photo courtesy of Jonathan Cohen MSc (Ost).

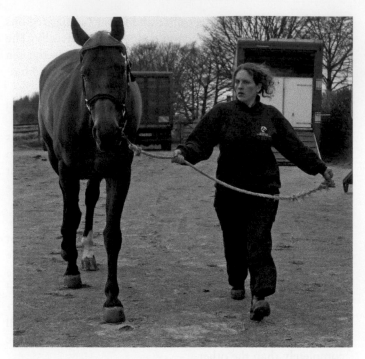

Figure 7.7 Tracking up: spinal dysfunction affects limb placement and a hindfoot appears in the channel of space between the front feet.

conditions that present with ataxic tendencies, and a veterinary opinion may be required.

From the Front

Following the long turn, the horse is walked back directly towards the practitioner. The appearance of the fascia over the face and the set of the ears should be noted alongside the dorso-ventral and lateral excursion of the head as it moves in concert with forelimb footfall. From this view, it is possible to observe the ease, symmetry and orientation of forelimb flight. This movement is influenced by the state of the pectoral and ventral neck muscles and fascia. It should be possible to see a rectangular channel of space between the front legs of around 30 cm in breadth (Figure 7.6). This space extends back between the hindlegs which should follow the line of the forelimbs.

Lower cervical problems often result in a pinched look about the pectorals as the soft tissue is bound down on to the sternum. The forelimbs seem to be drawn together and are close in front. This prevents the forelimbs from striding out and the action is a stilted, rather mincing gait. Dysfunction further down the spine causes a hindleg to appear in the channel of space between the legs as the hindfoot fails to track up directly behind the forefoot (Figure 7.7).

The forward swing of the forelimbs should be straight in flight. Dishing, where the leg swings out laterally, and plaiting, where one foot is placed in front of the other, are both variations which reflect structural problems. This type of action dissipates the energy of forward propulsion and puts uneven strain through the limbs (Figure 7.8).

Side View

By moving to the side and standing about 9 m back from the horse's line of travel, it is possible to follow the sequence of motion from the nose to the tail. This should be a serpentine progression transmitting smoothly through the spine (Figure 7.9). Dysfunction tends to break up the movement into regional patterns which show poor integration with each other. To use a musical analogy it is a series of solos rather than a symphony.

While appreciating the function of the body as a whole, it is also necessary to look at the regional participants in this symphony. Looking at the triangular area enclosed by the eye, ear and wing of the atlas, there should be an appearance of softness and mobility as the head and upper cervical spine function as an integrated unit during movement. The jaw should be relaxed, suspended from the temporal bones like the basket of a hot air balloon. The suprahyoid, infrahyoid and ventral neck muscles should be pliable and seen to be stretching with the swinging motion of the head and neck.

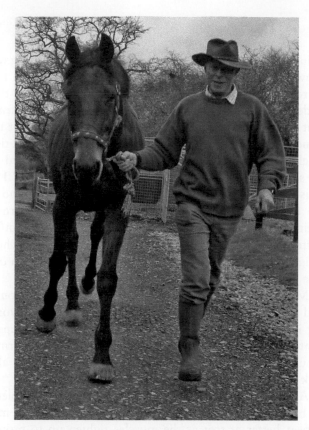

Figure 7.8 Limb flight: dishing, where the leg swings out laterally, reduces forward propulsion and puts uneven strain through the limbs.

A common injury, where the horse falls on to its head, causes the occiput to impact on to the upper cervical spine giving a characteristic pattern of dysfunction. The head appears fixed on the neck like a T-square with none of the normal nodding action, and the muscles of the temporo-mandibular and ventral cervical regions are tense. There

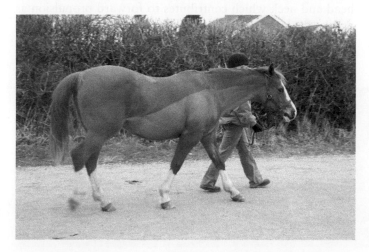

Figure 7.9 From the side: look for the set of the head on the neck, the transmission of movement through the spine and the protraction and retraction of the limbs.

may also be an appearance of increased flexion maintained in the neck below the subocciput in compensation for loss of occipito-atlantal mobility.

After the initial impact there is often a twisting strain through the neck as the horse rotates its body through the air while the head remains a fixed point in relation to the ground. This mid-cervical twist produces a hinge action at the affected level which has been described as a 'fowl neck' movement. The expression arose from a discussion between the osteopath and vet, with one saying that the head and neck movement reminded him of a chicken walking across a farmyard. The other thought that it resembled a turkey. In the spirit of compromise they decided on the generic term of 'fowl' to describe an action where there appears to be a pivot point in the neck from which the head thrusts forwards and backwards. There is often a line of muscle which is more prominent from this pivot point, and the overlying skin puckers on movement.

The flight of the limbs should also be observed, watching for the range and quality of protraction as the limb swings forwards and retraction as it moves backwards. A visual clue to the character of this movement is to look for the 'V' formed from the ipsilateral fore- and hindlimbs, as the fore lifts off just in advance of hind placement (Figure 7.2c).

Extending from the mid-cervical spine to the forelimb, the muscles of the thoracic girdle will stretch out smoothly as the limbs move freely and symmetrically forwards and backwards. A snatching action indicates dysfunction in the region.

Long-term occipito-atlanto-axial dysfunction reduces the forward impulsion derived from the nodding action of the head and causes the shoulder muscles to bulk up to generate the extra movement from the forelimbs. The scapulae become bound down to the chest wall by tense fascia and adopt a more vertical orientation. This restricts the range of protraction and retraction which shortens the stride. To compensate for poor shoulder movement, the distal part of the limb often exhibits a forward flick.

The stretch and recoil of the thoracic spine during movement can be assessed by observing the way the tips of the spinous processes separate and come together again. Where there is sheet muscle tightness through the body, there is an immobile barrel-like appearance to the thorax and forward propulsion is generated principally by the limbs which paddle away underneath.

Lumbar spine and pelvic restriction results in shortened stride. The horse is unable to bring the hindlegs under the body which compromises the forward-propelling mechanism. There is muscle bulking and an appearance of increased effort in the thoracic girdle as the horse transfers activity from hind- to forelimbs to gain impulsion. There may also be excessive neck movement as the horse attempts to overcome inertia by throwing the head forwards.

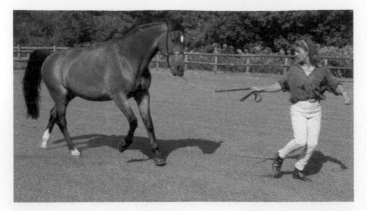

Figure 7.10 Transition from walk to trot: cervicothoracic dysfunction is indicated by a hop and skip action as the horse takes weight-bearing off the front limbs to organise protective splinting of the muscles of the area.

TRANSITION TO TROT

This phase of the examination is important as it follows the musculoskeletal adaptations necessary for the horse to change from the four-beat gait of the walk to a faster, more elevated two-beat trot.

Problems in the cervicothoracic spine are very obvious in this transition. The horse gives a little hop and skip as it throws up its head to take the weight off the front limbs in order to reorganise its muscular support for the more demanding trot. This involves splinting the lower cervical spine protectively and causes the stride to be shortened and muscle tension in the neck to be apparent (Figure 7.10). This usually indicates a long-term well ingrained problem in an area that is difficult to treat because of its position in the heavily muscled sling between the front limbs.

Cervicothoracic stiffness also compromises the bow and string mechanism of movement, affecting lumbar flexion and the ability of the hindlegs to come under the body (Chapter 2). Forward momentum is reduced and it will often appear that the hindlegs are not moving in concert with the forelegs.

OBSERVATION AT TROT

Using the same routines described for the walk, trotting will show up different aspects of a horse's action. Once in trot there should be a co-ordinated, fluid, even movement that is described as a two-beat, symmetrical gait. This means that the hindlimb on one side protracts and retracts at the same time as the opposite forelimb. There is then a period of elevation when all feet are off the ground, followed by the same movement with the other pair of legs (Figure 7.11). This gives the characteristically regular 'clip-clop' sound of the trot. In some horses, such as those used for harness racing in North America and Australia, this diagonal footfall pattern is replaced by the lateral gait of the pace where weight-bearing is taken by the fore- and hindlimbs on one side and then the other.

Musculoskeletal dysfunction interferes with the sound and appearance of this gait. Rather than all four legs working in concert, each limb appears to be working independently to achieve forward propulsion, giving a disharmonious look to the movement. The footfall sounds will also lack regularity.

A general but not incontrovertible rule for acute problems is that movement that looked uncomfortable at walk may appear better at trot as the muscles tighten up to protect the injured area. As the problem becomes more chronic, the horse will find ways of accommodating any dysfunction and the movement will look relatively normal at walk but less efficient with the greater athletic requirement of the trot.

The trot will accentuate problems of the upper cervical spine. This may present with the horse throwing up its chin with the occipito-atlanto-axial and temporomandibular region held fixed. The rest of the neck is stiff and does not appear to participate in the movement of the horse.

As a consequence of the inability to flex and extend the head and neck which contributes to forward propulsion as part of the bow and string mechanism, the horse will have a scurrying action. The spine is held in a straight line, losing much of the graceful serpentine action.

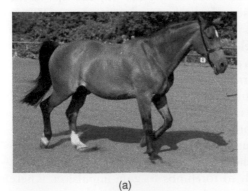
(a)

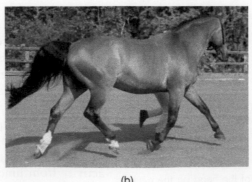
(b)

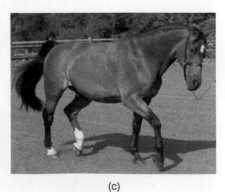
(c)

Figure 7.11 Trot: a two-beat symmetric gait sequence, with diagonal limb pairing and an elevation phase.

Stiffness in the lower cervical and cervicothoracic areas results in short striding, with a stabbing gait as the front hooves are driven into the ground before their full excursion. This may cause blunting of the front of the hooves from increased wear. In addition, the horse often compensates for poor spinal and shoulder mobility by increasing the distal limb movement in a forward flicking action.

SHORT TURN

If there is stiffness and reluctance in lateral movement during the long turn, then the short turn will provide information to localise the dysfunction. The mechanics of this exercise are that as the horse bends its neck into the turn, the thorax rotates in the thoracic sling as the movement reaches the cervicothoracic junction and the horse pivots on its front legs. As the front legs pivot, the hind leg on the outside of the turn moves laterally while the one on the inside crosses under it. This exercise is performed in both directions.

To get the full benefit of this test, additional instructions should be given to the handler and it may even be necessary to demonstrate the manoeuvre. Standing just behind the shoulder with a loose rein, the head is drawn slowly to the side. It is important not to rush this movement, particularly in cases where, over time, a horse has developed trick movements to cope with dysfunction which are easily overlooked during a cursory examination. The horse can then be touched in the flank to encourage the rest of the horse to turn (Figure 7.12).

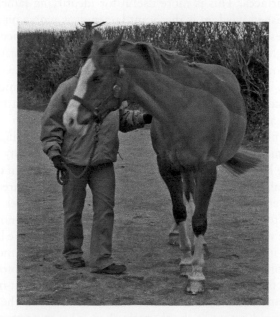

Figure 7.12 Short turn: look at the lateral flexion of the neck, the rotation of the thorax in its muscular sling, the lateral movement of the forelimbs and the crossing of hindlimbs.

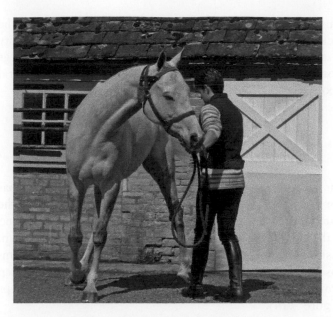

Figure 7.13 Occipito-atlanto-axial dysfunction: the upper cervical spine translocates in a sidebending action and the head rotates on the neck to simulate lateral flexion. The muscles on the convexity do not lengthen.

Levels of restriction in the neck are readily identified. An acute upper cervical problem will present as an immediate movement of the whole body as soon as the head begins to turn as the horse seeks to escape from painful lateral movement through the occipito-atlanto-axial complex. With more chronic dysfunction in this region, the horse develops ways of avoiding discomfort and will tend to translocate in a side-shifting action and rotate the head on the neck to simulate lateral flexion (Figure 7.13). Problems here can also be identified by soft tissue changes. The tissues of the occipito-atlanto-axial articulations on the convexity of the curve may not stretch out, remaining static and tethered as the neck bends sideways. On turning to the other side, there is often a block to movement at this level.

As the horse continues to turn, segments of restricted movement can be identified further down the neck accompanied by puckering of the skin and bunched muscles at the affected level. This is followed by either an immediate shift of the feet as an avoidance behaviour or the involvement of accessory ranges of joint movement as a compensatory mechanism.

Problems in the lumbar spine and pelvis cause the horse to shuffle around placing one hindfoot next to the other rather than the effortless crossing of the legs under the body. Lumbar paravertebral muscles and glutei often show exaggerated activity by bunching up, and the whole manoeuvre appears to require a disproportionate amount of effort. Swishing of the tail is an indication of discomfort.

A scoring system out of 10 is helpful to establish whether improvement has occurred at follow-up consultations. The score reflects the ease with which the neck sidebends and the thorax rotates, and the fluidity of the low back and pelvic movement as the hindlegs cross. Lower scores are an indication of poor lateral flexibility.

REIN BACK

The rein back is a complex movement involving participation from the spine, pelvis and limbs. The handler holds the lead rope close to the headcollar while standing in front and to the side of the horse with a guiding hand on the sternum. Pushing the horse backwards, the neck should flex. The lumbosacral articulation flexes and extends as the hindlegs step straight back fluidly and symmetrically over about five steps (Figure 7.14).

Upper cervical dysfunction may cause the horse to rush backwards in a disorganised fashion as it attempts to avoid flexing the occipito-atlantal articulation. Where the lumbosacral joint is restricted, flexion required for this manoeuvre is transferred further up the spine and there is a characteristic roaching of vertebrae at the thoracolumbar junction and fasciculation of the erector spinae at this level (Figure 7.15). Where the stiffness extends to one or other of the sacroiliac joints, the hindlimbs will not step straight back but will deviate to one side. Tail swishing is a sign of discomfort.

The experience of the horse should be taken into account. In an untrained horse, the movement will appear awkward without this necessarily being a significant sign. A well trained horse will find ways of executing backwards movement despite compromised neck and spinal and pelvic dysfunction.

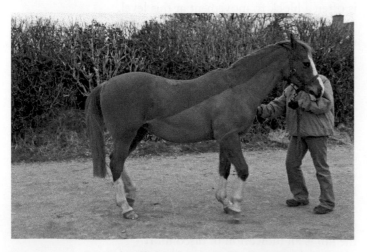

Figure 7.14 Rein back: the neck should flex and the lumbosacral articulation flex and extend as the hindlegs step straight back.

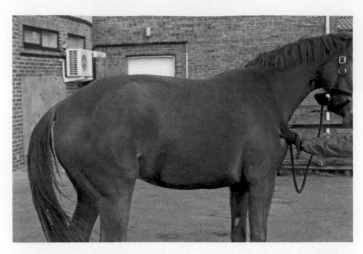

Figure 7.15 Lumbosacral stiffness: lumbosacral flexion, required for backing up, is transferred further up the spine and there is a characteristic roaching and fasciculation of the erector spinae at the thoracolumbar junction.

A scoring system similar to that for the short turn will give indications of progress at follow-up consultations.

FURTHER EXAMINATIONS

It may be helpful to extend the examination to include lungeing and riding under saddle.

Lunge

The horse may be examined on the lunge on both hard and soft surfaces. This is more useful for identifying lameness. Established wisdom is that joint lameness is worse on hard surfaces because of concussion forces. A soft surface will highlight lameness of soft tissue origin as the more yielding ground stretches these damaged structures (Devereux 2006). This is a subject in its own right and large amounts of space are devoted to the subtleties of the examination in veterinary textbooks (Ross and Dyson 2003). From a biomechanical viewpoint it is an effective way of assessing forward movement in combination with lateral flexibility.

The handler stands in the middle of a 15- to 20-m circle and walks the horse for several circuits, first in one direction and then the other. This is repeated for trot and canter. This will often show up a subtle limb lameness that was not apparent when moving in straight lines, as weight on the limbs on the inside of the circle is increased and the turning motion puts torsion through the limb joints to cause discomfort. It is also possible to look at the lateral curve/movement of the spine and compare both sides. The neck turns and the thorax should rotate in the thoracic sling. This is particularly important for balance at higher speeds where the limbs on the inside of the circle work under the horse while those on the outside function laterally to the body. This will confirm findings derived from the long and short turns.

Ridden Under Saddle

Having looked at the freely moving horse it may be useful, if practical, to look at the horse under saddle. This will give a chance to sneak a look at the way the horse is tacked up. A tight bridle will affect head movement and a girth set too far forward will interfere with scapular movement. It will also show how the rider interacts mechanically with the horse and highlight any asymmetries in riding posture to which the horse may be subjected. It may be a case of treating the rider as well as the horse!

REFERENCES

Back W, Clayton H (2001) *Equine Locomotion.* WB Saunders, London.

Cook RW (1999) Pathophysiology of bit control in the horse. *Journal of Equine Veterinary Science* **19**, 196–203.

Devereux S (2006) Examination of the lame or poor performance horse. In *The Veterinary Care of the Horse.* JA Allen, London, p. 96.

Muybridge E (1899) *Animals in Motion.* Dover Publications, New York.

Ross MW, Dyson SJ (2003) (eds) *Diagnosis and Management of Lameness in the Horse.* WB Saunders, London.

Palpatory Examination of the Unsedated Horse

Annabel Jenks

8

Following static and active observation, allow the horse to familiarise itself and settle quietly in a stable before any examination begins.

As described in Appendix A which looks at the safety aspects of treating horses, the examination and treatment must take place within appropriate surroundings and with a competent handler holding the horse.

To palpate means 'to feel, examine, and explore by touch'. This is a unique skill, highly developed by the osteopath, that allows diagnosis, treatment and then re-evaluation of subtle physiological changes within the tissues. It is essential for the practitioner to differentiate between normal and abnormal findings. I advise any osteopath wishing to start equine work to go to their local stables and, with permission, just palpate as many horses as possible, in order to learn to distinguish between normal and abnormal tissue texture and function.

Imagination, intuition and judgement are central to osteopathic palpation (McKone 2007, personal communication). Always listen to the intuitive inner voice and never disregard any thought that immediately arises on observation or examination. This may often be the key to a biomechanical dysfunction or a red flag that must be investigated. If any doubt is raised, the horse must be referred back to the veterinary surgeon for further clinical examination.

It is difficult to separate totally the process of palpation and treatment because the instant an osteopath begins to palpate, changes occur within the tissues and treatment begins! However, an osteopathic assessment and working diagnosis must be made before specific treatment techniques are used.

It is important that the practitioner does not 'pounce' into their palpatory examination but takes time to familiarise and introduce himself or herself to the horse. It is best to begin by talking quietly and approaching from the side towards the shoulder followed by gently stroking the lower neck and withers. Most horses will turn their head, which I always take as a sign that palpatory examination may begin.

With a nervous horse, the practitioner can initially place a hand on the withers and just stand and pause while taking a few long deep breaths. They should concentrate on their own stance and energy while the horse relaxes and becomes more receptive. I was shown this by Eric Laarakker, a Dutch vet who also practises acupuncture and runs a complimentary clinic in The Netherlands. He described this technique as 'earthing' with the horse.

There is no set order to any palpation and treatment but having a framework or pattern to the examination is essential. An initial appraisal of the whole horse will give the practitioner an immediate impression of the tissue integrity. This is followed by an in-depth palpatory and active examination of the neuromusculoskeletal function and dysfunction. Detailed description of tissue sense and anatomical reference points can be found in Chapter 9.

Every practitioner will develop their own unique framework and apply this to each horse as appropriate. The following is just a guide upon which individual procedures can be based.

The practitioner should consider:

- Integrity and quality of the tissue
- Integrity and range of movement of joints
- Crepitations
- Tension
- Tissue texture
- Tone
- Symmetry
- Atrophy
- Overdevelopment

- Scar tissue
- Indentations/old injury sites
- Oedema
- Temperature
- Hydration
- Health of coat
- Sweat patches
- Positive 'athletic feel'

STAGE 1: THE INITIAL APPRAISAL

The initial examination (Figures 8.1.1–8.1.6) is an appraisal of the integrity of the tissues and of any signs of previous or recent pathology and obvious physiological changes within the musculoskeletal structure. It is a procedure that, with practice, will initiate the practitioner into an introductory insight into the horse's vitality and well being. The palms and fingers of both hands are used to enable a large surface area to be palpated.

This initial palpation gives an overall evaluation of the tissues and provides the opportunity to tune into the individual horse before specifically palpating and diagnosing any presenting neuromusculoskeletal dysfunctions. The practitioner should use a caressing motion with the hands, as if stroking a dog or cat. This allows the receptors in the fingers to interpret the underlying tissue subconsciously. Never disregard

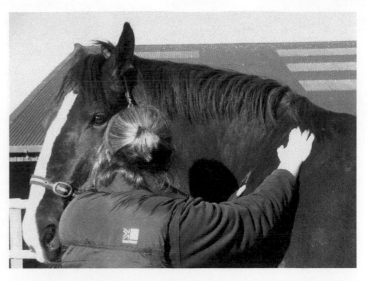

Figure 8.1.2 Progress to the scapula: here the cranial hand moves ventrally and palpates the pectoral muscles and associated tissue as the caudal hand palpates the scapula and shoulder.

any instinctive thoughts at this time and ensure your mind is open to perceptive feedback.

Begin by palpating the upper cervical spine with the hands on either side of the neck, using the whole of the hand, with the fingers relaxed and in contact with the musculoskeletal anatomical contours. Using a stroking and sweeping movement, palpate the cervical transverse processes in a caudal direction (Figure 8.1.1).

Then commence along the scapula and pectoral muscles (Figure 8.1.2). The cranial hand moves ventrally and palpates the pectoral muscles and associated tissues as the caudal hand palpates the scapula and shoulder region. Proceed along the withers and thoracic region (Figure 8.1.3). Run the fingers gently down, either side of the thoracic

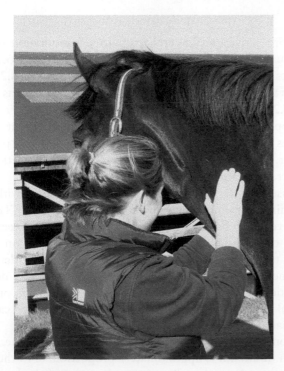

Figure 8.1.1 Begin with both hands stroking the cervical region: utilising the palm and fingers to palpate the cervical transverse processes in a caudal direction.

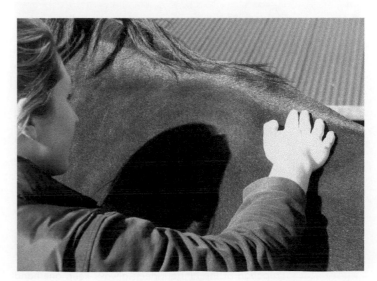

Figure 8.1.3 Palpation of withers and thoracic part of trapezius muscle: use the whole hand to assess the tissue tone.

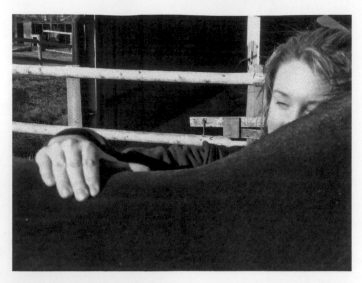

Figure 8.1.4 Palpation of the erector spinae musculature: gently run the fingers and thumb either side of the thoracic and lumbar spinous processes in a caudal direction.

and lumbar spinous processes, along the erector spinae in a caudal direction (Figure 8.1.4). As progression is made towards the hindquarters and caudal muscular tissues, one hand must always remain in contact with the horse (Figure 8.1.5). As with human patients, contact is never broken throughout the examination. Finish this examination with palpation of the hamstring musculature (Figure 8.1.6).

Always palpate both sides of the horse. It is amazing how one side can be relatively supple and free of problems while the other can be quite the opposite.

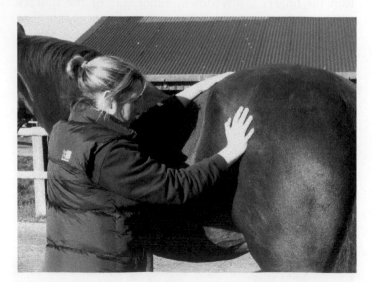

Figure 8.1.5 Palpation of the hindquarters: always keep one hand in contact with the horse as the initial palpation progresses over the hindquarters and associated caudal fascia and musculature.

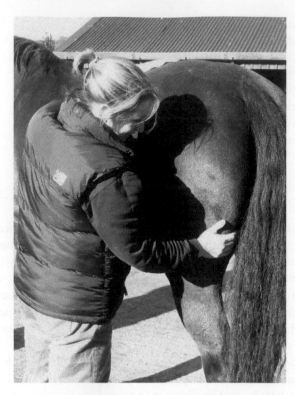

Figure 8.1.6 Finally: finish the initial appraisal with palpation of the hamstring musculature.

STAGE 2: THE ACTIVE IN-DEPTH EXAMINATION

A more active and in-depth palpatory examination of individual joint mobility and the state with the associated tissues follows the initial appraisal (Figures 8.2.1–8.2.38). Begin with an evaluation of the positioning of the atlas (Figure 8.2.1). It is important to gain the horse's confidence and so approach quietly from the side, remembering that some horses may be headshy or initially nervous of the practitioner. The atlas may be held in a dorsal/ventral direction or in a cranial/caudal direction.

Assessing the position of the wing of the atlas with the mandibular ramus allows evaluation of symmetry. This is achieved with fingers being placed in the space between the wing of the atlas and the ramus of the mandible on both sides to compare positioning (Figure 8.2.2). A wider gap on one side indicates that the atlas has rotated in a dorsal direction on the wider side. By placing the fingers on the dorsal aspect of the atlas, cranial/caudal positioning can be evaluated.

Continue with examination of the cervical spine. The width of a hand is approximately proportionate to the size of a cervical vertebra. By placing the palm of the hand on the atlas and moving in a caudal direction along the cervical transverse processes the practitioner can locate and count

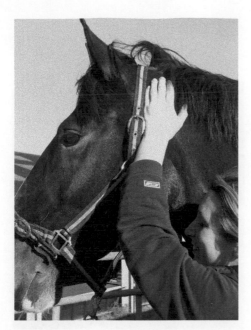

Figure 8.2.1 Begin palpating the atlas position: the atlas may be held in a ventral/dorsal or cranial/caudal direction.

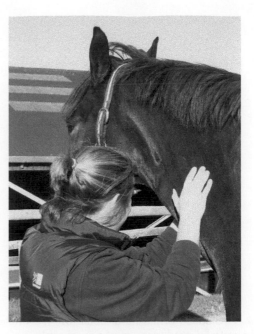

Figure 8.2.3 Continue with palpation of the cervical spine: the width of a hand is approximately proportionate in size to a cervical vertebra. Progress with palpation in a caudal direction.

the vertebrae. Examine and palpate each individual cervical vertebra and assess positioning (Figure 8.2.3).

Having fully gained the horse's confidence, return to the poll region to continue examination of the head and upper cervical spine. The frontal bone is palpated using the palm of the hand (Figure 8.2.4). Continue palpation in a rostral

direction along the nasal bone (Figure 8.2.5) towards the nasal peak (Figure 8.2.6).

Palpate the facial crests and mandibular ramus (Figure 8.2.7), particularly noting the tone and quality of the masseter muscles. Note any facial swellings, evidence of old fractures in the skull and signs and smell of nasal discharge. Look for any soreness or abrasions around the corners of

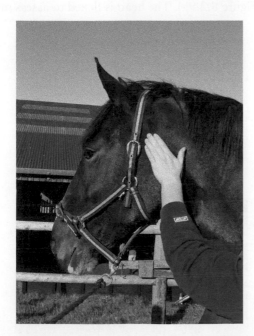

Figure 8.2.2 Assessment of the position of the atlas and mandibular ramus: place the fingers between the wings of the atlas and mandibular ramus and evaluate the positioning. A wider gap between the two indicates that the atlas has rotated in a dorsal direction on that side.

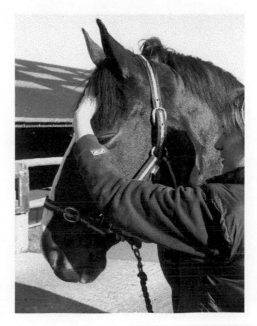

Figure 8.2.4 Cranium examination: begin with palpation of the frontal bone.

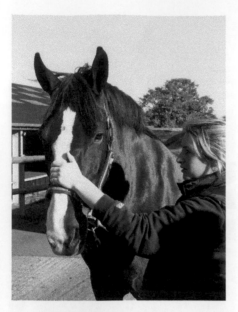

Figure 8.2.5 Palpation of the nasal bone: use the whole hand to palpate in a rostral direction towards the nasal peak.

the mouth and around the face, noting any scarring or irritations caused by tight or badly fitted nosebands, head collars or curb chains. Also, be aware of any tenderness from normal and abnormal teeth eruptions and how the jaw is aligned, e.g. parrot or sow mouth.

Temporomandibular joint mobility is evaluated (Figure 8.2.8). This is followed by assessment of the integrity of the hyoid bone and associated tissues.

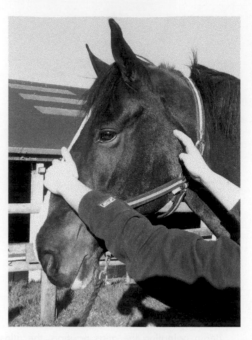

Figure 8.2.7 Palpation of mandibular ramus: note the tone and symmetry of masseter muscles.

Gentle palpation of the ears to include frontal and parietal bones and auricular and scutularis muscles can then be followed by a more active examination of the cervical spine.

Flexing and extending the head achieves an active evaluation of the occipito-atlantal joint function. Flexion of the occipito-atlantal joint is achieved by supporting the poll with the caudal hand while the cranial hand contact is on the nasal region (Figure 8.2.9a). The head is flexed to assess mobility.

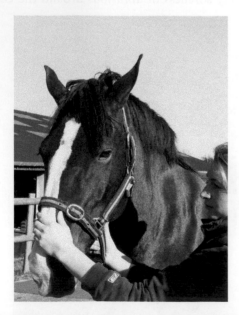

Figure 8.2.6 Gently run your fingers along the nasal peak: note any facial swellings, evidence of old injuries, signs and smell of nasal discharge, soreness or abrasions around the corner of the mouth. Note any scarring or irritation from badly fitting bridles or head collars. Assess the jaw alignment and teeth.

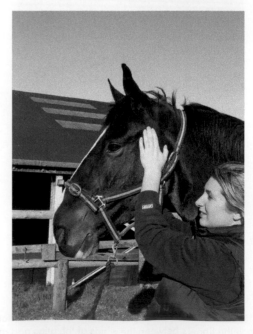

Figure 8.2.8 Palpation of the temporomandibular joints: compare the structure of both temporomandibular joints and associated tissues.

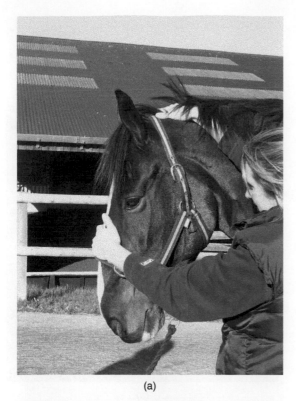

(a)

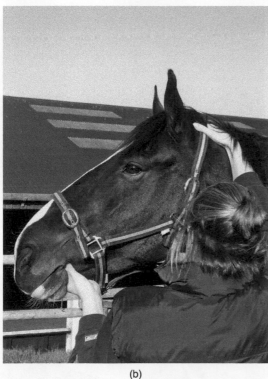

(b)

Figure 8.2.9 (a) Flexion of occipito-atlantal joint: support the poll with the caudal hand. With the cranial hand contact is made on the nasal region and the head is flexed to assess mobility. (b) Extension of occipito-atlantal joint: support the poll with the caudal hand, cup the chin with the cranial hand and extend the head.

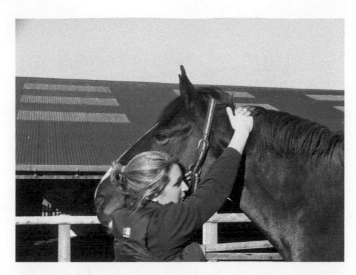

Figure 8.2.10 Springing the axis: interlace the hands and gently spring the axis in a ventral direction.

Extension of the occipito-atlantal joint is achieved by supporting the poll with the caudal hand while the cranial hand cups the chin and extends the head (Figure 8.2.9b).

Springing C2, the axis, can follow this. With the hands interlaced, contact the axis spinous process and gently spring in a ventral direction (Figure 8.2.10).

The remaining cervical vertebrae are then gently laterally flexed by bringing the head round to the horse's side (Figure 8.2.11). This would be done to the left and right. The practitioner must remember that this is just an evaluation

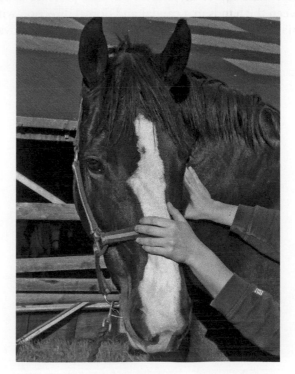

Figure 8.2.11 Lateral flexion of cervical spine: gently flex the lower cervicals laterally to the left and then to the right.

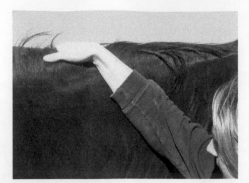

Figure 8.2.12 Examination of nuchal ligament and associated dorsal neck musculature: palpate along the dorsal cervical musculature and nuchal ligament in a caudal direction.

of mobility and the head and neck should not be forced into an uncomfortable position. This is merely a diagnostic examination. Treatment procedures follow later.

All the dorsal and ventral cervical muscles, especially the brachiocephalicus and sternocephalicus, as well as the nuchal ligament from the poll to the withers (Figure 8.2.12), must be examined before proceeding to the pectoral region (Figure 8.2.13). Palpate in a caudal direction along the descending and ascending pectoral musculature.

The mobility of the cervicothoracic junction is then assessed. To perform this, place the palm of the cranial hand on the manubrium of the sternum and associated pectorals, while the palm of the caudal hand is placed on the withers (Figure 8.2.14a). A rhythmical pushing pressure is applied between the hands in a caudal and dorsal direction with the cranial hand, followed by a cranial and ventral movement

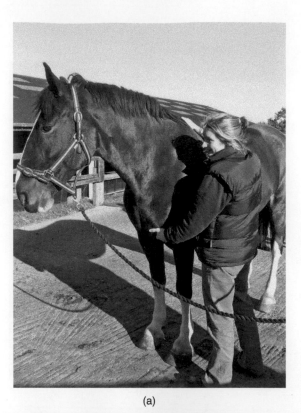

(a)

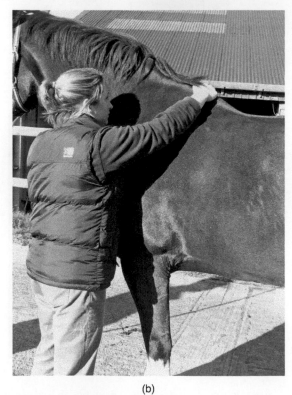

(b)

Figure 8.2.14 (a) Cervicothoracic evaluation: place cranial hand on the manubrium and the caudal hand on the withers. (b) Cervicothoracic mobility: rhythmically push between the hands to evaluate mobility.

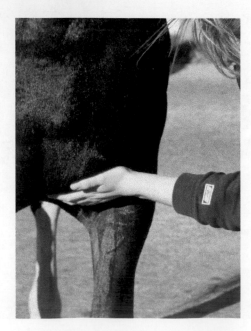

Figure 8.2.13 Palpation of pectoral muscles: palpate in a caudal direction along the descending and ascending pectoral musculature.

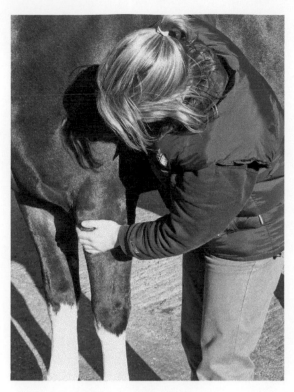

Figure 8.2.15 Palpation of extensor carpi radialis: always compare both sides.

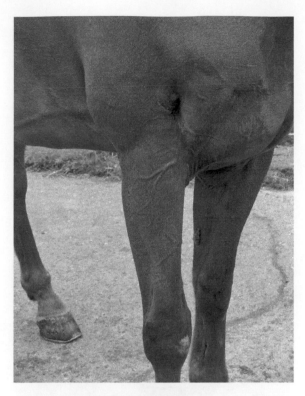

Figure 8.2.16 Note injuries or scars: always record on the case history any anomalies or evidence of injury.

with the caudal hand (Figure 8.2.14b). There should be an impression of fluidity between the hands.

The forelimb is then palpated, noting any atrophy or asymmetry in the extensor carpi radialis muscle (Figure 8.2.15) signifying reduced or over use of the forelimb to 'pull' the horse along. Examine the carpal joints (knee) and fetlock in flexion and extension and also use a rotation and shearing movement for the pastern joint. Always be aware of any degenerative changes and contraindications to fully flexing the carpus with young or older horses.

Observe and record any signs of oedema, heat or scarring from old or recent injuries (Figure 8.2.16). Examine the integrity of the tendons (Figure 8.2.17), again noting evidence of previous pathology. Note the presence of splints on the metacarpal bones, a sign of concussive forces through the limb. If the splint is active, it will be painful on palpation.

If the horse is reluctant to lift the forefoot, the chestnut, which is located on the medial aspect of the forelimb, can be squeezed to encourage it to raise the leg (Figures 8.2.18a and 8.2.18b).

When examining the foot (Figure 8.2.19a), note differences in size, shape, wear and balance between the hooves. The integrity of the hoof can be a good reflection of the horse's general health and management. Wear and balance of the shoes on the shod horse are excellent indicators of how the horse is mechanically moving on each

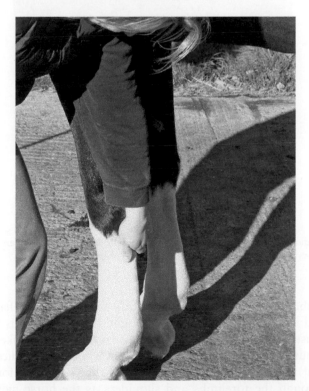

Figure 8.2.17 Examination of the tendons: slide the hand down the palmar aspect of the forelimb. Note any oedema, heat, scarring or signs of old injuries or pathologies. When proceeding to the assessment of the carpal joints, be aware of any degenerative changes or other contraindications to fully flexing the joints.

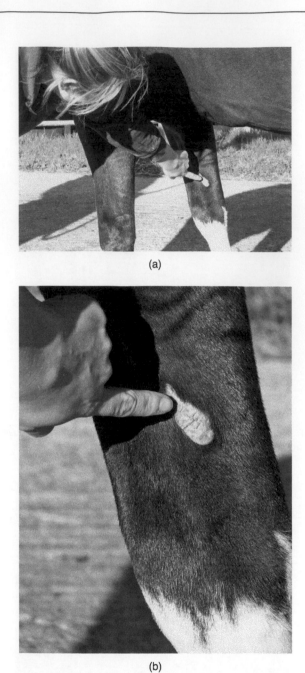

(a)

(b)

Figure 8.2.18 a and 8.2.18b Positioning of chestnut: located on the medial aspect of the forelimb, proximal to the carpals. Squeeze the chestnut to encourage lifting of the leg if necessary.

limb. Feet are often asymmetrical, with one being flatter and the other squarer, more upright and 'boxy'. This will cause unbalanced weight distribution when the feet strike the ground, with more weight on the flatter foot. This indicates that the practitioner should observe the concussive forces through the forelimbs and shoulders as the horse moves, to fully evaluate any dysfunction. If necessary, once again watch the horse walk and trot before progressing with treatment, if this will help consolidate a working osteopathic diagnosis.

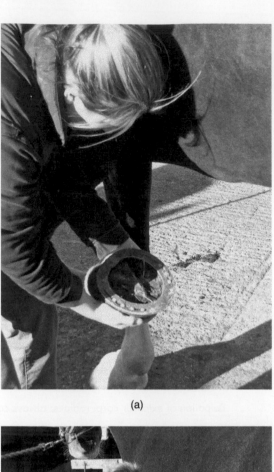

(a)

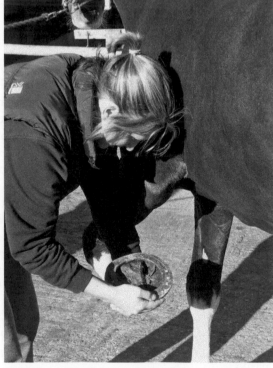

(b)

Figure 8.2.19 (a) Examination of foot and pastern mobility: always support the hoof and leg. (b) Pastern and fetlock mobility: flex, extend and rotate the foot comparing both sides.

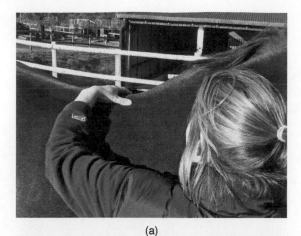

(a)

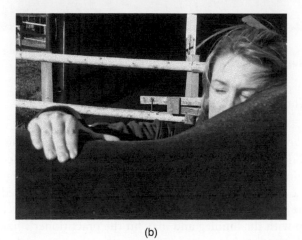

(b)

Figure 8.2.20 (a) Withers and thoracic spine: with the fingers just lateral to the spinous processes, palpate in a caudal direction along the thoracic spine. (b) Deeper palpation of thoracic spine: palpate in a caudal direction the thoracic spine and erector spinae musculature.

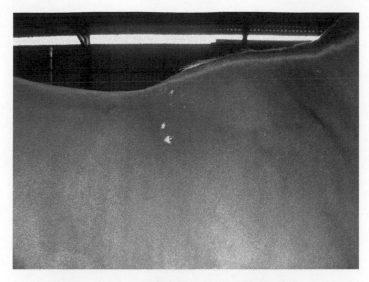

Figure 8.2.21 Areas of white hair: areas of white hair around the saddle region are an indication of saddle pressure points, past or present.

its forehand to pull itself forwards instead of propelling from the hindquarters. Atrophy of the infraspinatus and supraspinatus muscles may occur in conditions such as sweeney where the suprascapular nerve is damaged (Figure 8.2.22).

The mobility of the pastern and fetlock joints is then assessed by flexing, extending and rotating the foot (Figure 8.2.19b).

Palpation then continues from the withers (Figure 8.2.20a) in a caudal direction along the thoracic spine. Follow this with a deeper palpation of the erector spinae musculature (Figure 8.2.20b). Especially examine trapezius and associated muscle and fascial tissue in the saddle region, looking for white hairs (Figure 8.2.21), nodules, hair loss and bald patches caused from the numnah rubbing or saddle pressure points. Be aware of tenderness and soreness over the thoracic spinous processes. Note any inflammation of the supraspinous ligament or any signs of infection, and be aware of fly bites or warble fly larvae in this area.

The scapula musculature is examined, comparing both sides for positioning, angles and muscle bulk. Strong thoracic girdle musculature compared with less developed pelvic girdle musculature may suggest that the horse is using

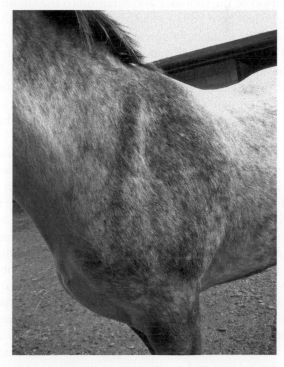

Figure 8.2.22 Sweeney: disuse or neurogenic atrophy of the supraspinatus and infraspinatus muscles. Neurogenic atrophy is due to damage to the suprascapular nerve.

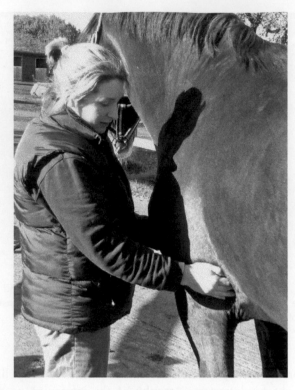

Figure 8.2.23 Palpation of triceps: the muscle should be soft but toned and pliable.

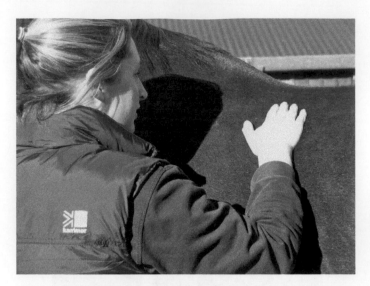

Figure 8.2.24 Palpation along the dorsal third of the ribs: these are often tender due to saddle pressure.

It must be remembered that a muscular sling suspends the thorax. The horse has no clavicles and so there is no bony stabilisation of the shoulder and forelimb to the sternum.

Triceps can be readily palpated and should feel soft and pliable (Figure 8.2.23). Palpate deep into the muscular tissue around and medial to the elbow. The ribs and sternum are common areas for tenderness and tension caused by over-tight girths. Note any abrasions to the skin resulting from an ill-fitting martingale, breastplate, draw reins, girth guards, or girth galls from pinching girths. Horses sometimes hit the sternal region with studs from their front shoes when jumping. Skin lesions may also be caused by inadequate grooming and not thoroughly washing down when muddy or sweaty, especially around the 'armpit' where the skin is very soft and folded. The dorsal third of the ribs can be tender from unbalanced and incorrectly fitted saddles (Figure 8.2.24).

Palpation continues along the thoracolumbar spine for tissue integrity and spinal alignment. A springing technique can be used along the spinous processes to assess mobility. Pain in the thoracics may be due to kissing spines, so it is important to remember common pathologies that may be present in certain regions. Tenderness in the caudal thoracic spine may also be caused by incorrectly fitting saddles. Wear of hair will indicate the positioning of the saddle and give a clue to the balance and positioning of the rider. This is very obvious if the saddle sits over to one side. The symmetry of the back muscles and withers must be observed.

The spinal reflexes can then be tested.

- *Thoracolumbar flexion*: gently run the fingers along the abdomen from the sternum in a caudal direction, encouraging and stimulating the horse to arch its back (Figures 8.2.25a and 8.2.25b). Take great care not to be kicked, as the abdomen is a very sensitive area. A horse tends to kick up with the hindleg and may hit the practitioner's hand.
- *Thoracolumbar extension*: run the fingers gently but firmly either side of the thoracic spinous processes. The horse will hollow its back (Figure 8.2.26).
- *Lateral flexion*: run the fingers along the lateral thoracic region in a cranial to caudal direction. The horse should laterally flex, with the spine becoming concave in the direction of the stimulus.
- *Lumbosacral flexion*: run the fingers gently, but firmly, lateral to the sacrum in a caudal direction. The horse arches its back, flexing the lumbosacral junction (Figure 8.2.27).

Some practitioners use pens or hoof picks to test the reflexes. I personally prefer a more controlled, subtle approach at first, followed if needed by a deeper technique.

Throughout any examination and palpation, the practitioner must continually assess the horse's reactions by observing the ears, eyes, head position and body posture. The horse can strike out with the front legs as quickly and dangerously as the hind legs. As well as biting, the head can be a deadly tool when swinging in any direction and a horse can easily squash both practitioner and handler against the door or walls. Safety of the handler and practitioner is paramount at all times. With practice, minute changes in the muscular tension will help warn the practitioner of imminent sudden movements. However, palpate with caution at all times.

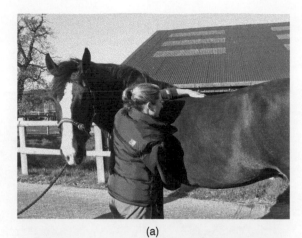

(a)

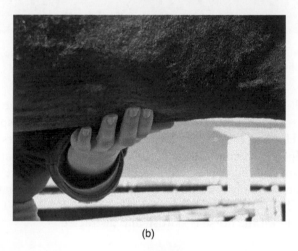

(b)

Figure 8.2.25 (a) Thoracolumbar flexion: the cranial hand is gently positioned on the thoracic spinous processes while the caudal hand is placed on the sternum. (b) Stimulus to produce thoracolumbar flexion: gently run the caudal hand from the sternum in a caudal direction under the abdomen. The horse should arch its back.

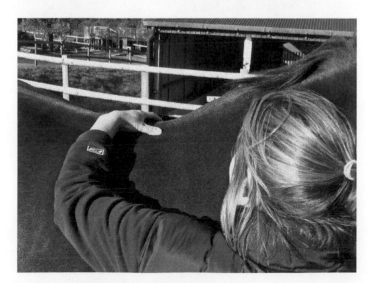

Figure 8.2.26 Thoracolumbar extension: run the fingers gently but firmly either side of the thoracic spinous processes. The horse should hollow its back.

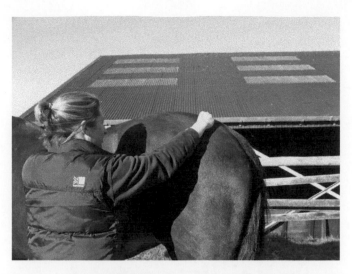

Figure 8.2.27 Lumbosacral flexion: gently but firmly run the fingers lateral to the sacrum along the gluteals in a ventral direction. The horse should arch its back, flexing the lumbosacral junction.

The gluteal, hamstring, quadriceps musculature and associated fascia are palpated (Figure 8.2.28) before evaluation of the pelvic bony landmarks.

The tubera sacrale, tubera coxae and tubera ischii are the bony landmarks to observe and evaluate in order to assess pelvic symmetry.

It is very important that the horse is standing squarely on all four feet with the head and neck straight for an accurate

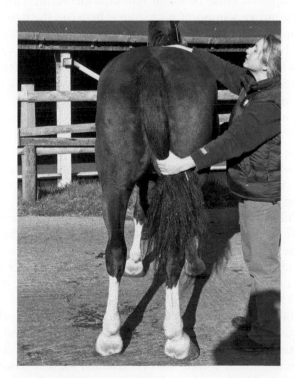

Figure 8.2.28 Safety: always begin any palpation of the pelvis and sacroiliac joints from the side of the horse and assess the risk of standing behind. Never put yourself or the handler at risk.

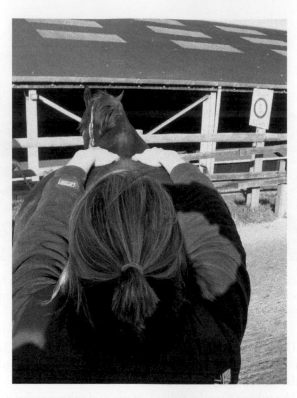

Figure 8.2.29 Evaluation of tubera sacrale symmetry: if it is safe to do so, place the fingers on the tubera sacrale to assess symmetry.

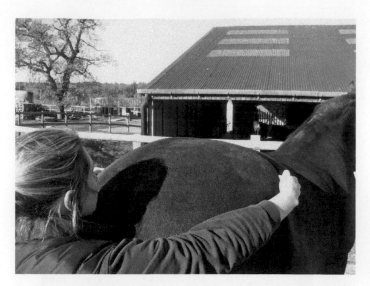

Figure 8.2.30 Evaluation of tubera coxae: if it is safe to do so, place the fingers on the tubera coxae to assess symmetry.

evaluation to be made. Any muscular atrophy or under-development must be taken into consideration. There is a subtle but very important difference between the two and it is important to differentiate between them. To the eye there may be the impression that the tubera sacrale are asymmetric whereas, on palpation of the bony structures, there is symmetry. Pain may be elicited on palpation if there is any spasm or guarding of the soft tissues.

Initially observe and palpate from the side of the horse and then, *only* if it is safe to do so, stand directly behind and assess the symmetry of the pelvic bony landmarks.

Tubera sacrale are the highest points of the hindquarters and can be referred to as the 'jumper's bump' or point of croup (Figure 8.2.29).

Tubera coxae are the prominent bony parts palpated laterally on the hindquarters, sometimes referred to as the point of the hip (Figure 8.2.30).

Tubera ischii are the most caudal points of the pelvis and can be referred to as the point of the buttock (Figure 8.2.31).

Having evaluated any asymmetry in the pelvis, always re-examine the hip region and associated fascia and musculature tissue for tension (Figure 8.2.32). The lumbar spine alignment should also be assessed for any associated scoliosis, which is a lateral curvature of the spine. Examine the sacral positioning and tissue integrity (Figure 8.2.33). Test the sacroiliac movement by springing the joints. There

will be less movement on the side of the sacroiliac joint restriction and the horse may react, showing a pain response.

Holding the tail out laterally will stabilise the horse and help keep its concentration as the hindquarter musculature is examined (Figure 8.2.34a). It must be standing square when examining the hindlimb musculature. Examine and palpate the hamstring and caudal muscles (Figure 8.2.34b). Toggle the tail if the horse is skittish and distracted.

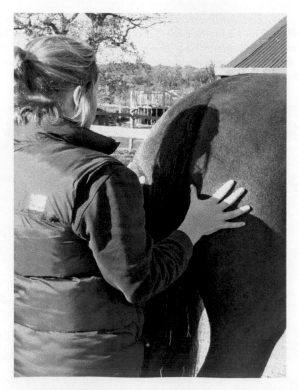

Figure 8.2.31 Evaluation of tubera ischii: if it is safe to do so, place the fingers on the tubera ischii to assess symmetry.

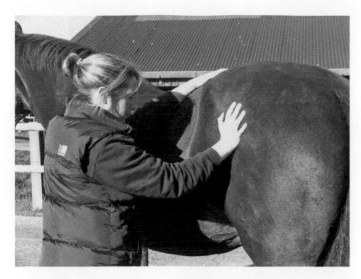

Figure 8.2.32 Palpation of the hip and associated tissue: always have one hand in contact with the spine. Be aware at all times of the horse's reactions to your palpation and examination.

Tail tone and mobility are assessed, standing laterally to the horse (Figure 8.2.35). Gently flex and extend the dock within the horse's tolerance.

Examination of the hindlimb is similar to that of the forelimb but extreme caution should be taken when palpating the stifle as this is another very sensitive region (Figure 8.2.36). The stifle and hock movements are synchronised. The practitioner must have a good understanding of the stay apparatus of the hindlimb, known as the reciprocal system. Always have one hand on the quarters and, with the examining hand, use a stroking movement to examine the distal leg so that the horse is always aware of your touch. Palpate the hock joint for any obvious signs of pathology such as bony enlargements or visible fluid-filled swellings, indicating strain or trauma to the region. On examination

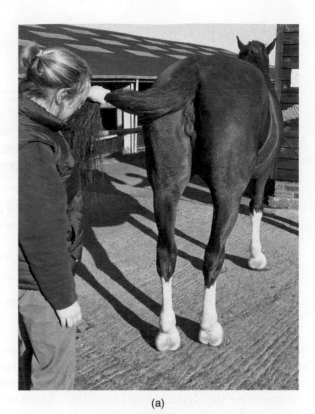

(a)

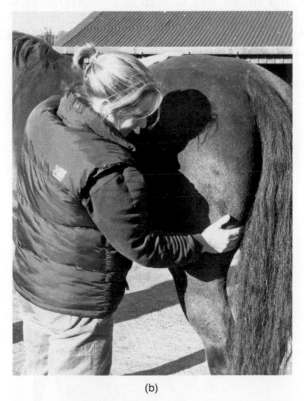

(b)

Figure 8.2.34 (a) Evaluation of hamstrings and caudal musculature: the horse should be standing squarely on all four feet on an even surface. (b) Examination and palpation of the hamstrings: if necessary hold the tail out laterally to keep the horse's concentration.

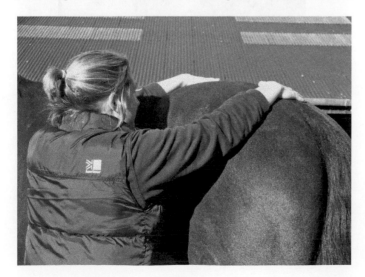

Figure 8.2.33 Examination of the sacrum: palpate the sacrum in a caudal direction.

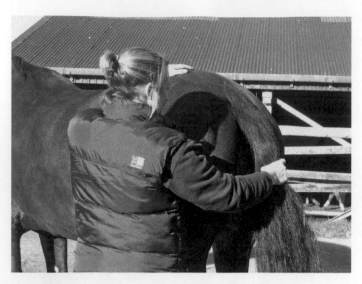

Figure 8.2.35 Examining the tail: stand to the side of the horse and gently palpate the tail to assess flexibility.

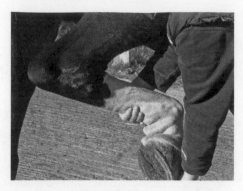

Figure 8.2.37 Examining the hock: be aware of degenerative changes and other contraindications to gross movement of the joints.

of hock flexion (Figure 8.2.37) it is important to be aware of degenerative changes and other contraindications to gross movement of the joints. Remember, the horse may be reluctant to stand on the dysfunctional hindlimb. Examine the foot in a similar way as used in the forelimb by flexing, extending and rotating the hoof (Figure 8.2.38).

After palpation and examination, if there are no contraindications, osteopathic treatment can begin.

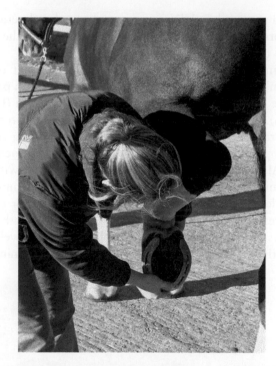

Figure 8.2.38 Examination and evaluation of the hindfoot: flex, extend and rotate the hindfoot comparing both sides.

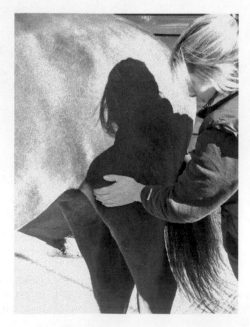

Figure 8.2.36 The stifle examination: always be very cautious when examining the stifle, hold the tail to keep the horse's attention.

Palpatory Examination of the Sedated Horse

9

Anthony Pusey and Julia Brooks

Static examination and observation of active movements will provide some insight into the nature and site of a problem, while further information to localise dysfunction can be obtained using palpation. Under some circumstances, such as when dealing with an anxious horse or examining for deep-seated, longstanding dysfunction, it may be helpful to examine under light sedation (Chapter 12). Ideally, this should be a combination of opioid to reduce sensitivity to pain and an α_2-adrenoceptor agonist to prevent sympathetic flight/fight behaviour. This does not abolish segmental responses to injury but it does make it easier and safer to identify local muscle spasm, joint asymmetry and tissue texture changes.

Initially, it is advisable to follow a routine when examining, which will inevitably become modified with experience. The following is a framework for the systematic palpatory examination of the axial skeleton.

PALPATORY EXAMINATION

Cranium

Horses are susceptible to cranial injuries as a result of falls and minor repeated trauma. Dysfunction may present with a history of temperament change, bitting problems, being headshy and even headshaking.

As a starting point a hand is placed over the frontal bone to feel for the tone and symmetry of the muscles (Figure 9.1). It is often a good indicator of irritability and pain if the muscles overlying the frontal bone are tense and somewhat oedematous to the touch, and the horse may pull away from this contact. A common finding is the presence of two tight muscular bands of temporalis that have a fibrotic feel and give a taut look to the face (Figure 9.2). As a consequence of past head injuries, there may also be an impression of

flattening or scarring of the fascia which feels bound down to the underlying cranium. The ears may seem tethered to the skull rather than relaxed and flexible (Figure 9.3).

It is possible to follow changes in the cranial tissue back into the top of the neck. Resting the fingers just caudal to the occipital bone the tension in the suboccipital muscles can be assessed.

Any asymmetry in the subocciput and cranium will also be reflected into the soft tissues of the nose by virtue of muscular and fascial connections. Moving the hand downwards towards the nostrils, the areas either side of the nasal bones are gently squeezed to give an idea of tissue symmetry and tone (Figure 9.4). Pressure to this area may also have the effect of relaxing the horse, similar perhaps to the way in which a person might obtain endorphin-mediated relief from a headache by pinching the bridge of the nose (Hecker et al. 2001).

Temporomandibular Joint

The cranium and mandible join at the temporomandibular joint. This synovial joint allows opening, closing and lateral shift of the jaw during eating. It should also protract and retract in concert with flexion and extension of the head on the neck such as occurs in locomotion or grazing.

By moving both hands up along the ramus of the mandible to the region behind the ear, the state of the tissue overlying the temporomandibular joint can be assessed (Figure 9.5). Any change in tone and symmetry here will affect the way the mandible hangs from the cranium. This can be further tested by gripping the mandibular rami and exerting gentle pressure downwards and forwards, noting how easily the condyle of the mandible disengages from the fossa in the temporal bone. A little movement should be possible owing to the elasticity of the soft tissues. Where dysfunction exists,

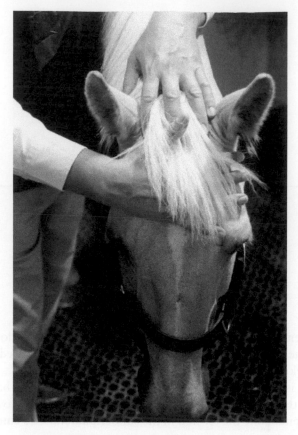

Figure 9.1 Frontal hold: assessing tension and symmetry of temporalis, auricular and suboccipital muscles.

any attempt to distract the mandible will move the whole head. The temporalis and masseter muscles overlying the joint often look and feel flattened and fibrotic.

Moving down from the temporomandibular joint past the angle of the jaw, the fingers are placed medial to each

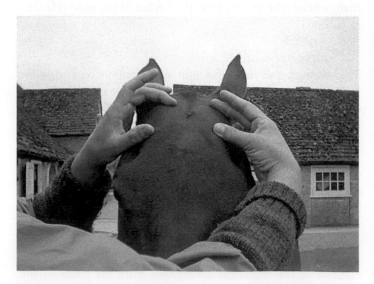

Figure 9.2 Frontal bone: two tense lines of the temporalis muscles have a fibrotic feel on palpation.

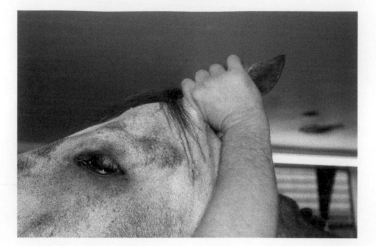

Figure 9.3 Ears: the muscles around the ears should be relaxed and allow flexibility of ear movement.

side of the body of the mandible to palpate the structures of the floor of the mouth such as the geniohyoideus, genioglossus and mylohyoideus muscles (Figure 9.6). Areas of tension in these muscles can reflect back into the hyoid lying deep between the angles of the mandible. Normal tone and symmetry of the suprahyoid and infrahyoid muscles are important in maintaining the optimum patency of the airway.

At this point it might be helpful to reflect on the dental history. Changes in grinding surfaces, presence of hooks, etc., may maintain a problem in this area. Consideration should also be given to the close relationship between the nerve supply to the jaw and the upper cervical spine at spinal cord level which makes the function of these two areas intimately connected (Chapter 2).

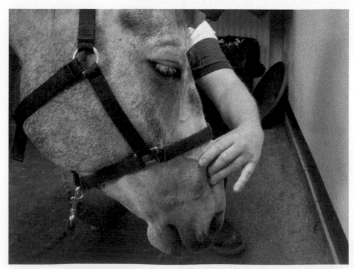

Figure 9.4 Nasal hold : squeezing either side of the nasal bones evaluates symmetry and tone in the tissue.

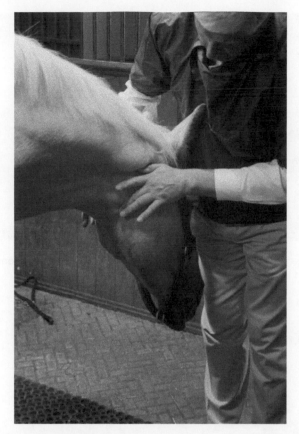

Figure 9.5 Temporomandibular joint: feeling for symmetry and tissue tone over the joint.

Upper Cervical Spine

The occipito-atlanto-axial complex is one of the most mobile parts of the spine executing a large proportion of total neck flexion, extension and rotation. It is also a region of great importance in providing proprioceptive information (see Chapter 3). Dysfunction here can affect the way the whole horse moves, causing a range of problems from

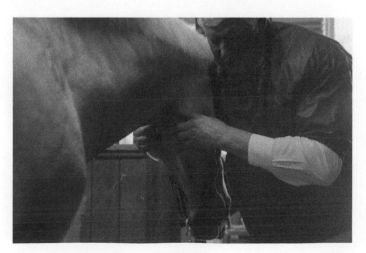

Figure 9.6 Floor of mouth: palpating for symmetry and tone of muscles.

lack of fluidity to uncertainty in foot placement when asked to turn, as balance and coordination are compromised. A thorough examination of the area is therefore essential whatever the presenting problem.

Bringing the hands up caudal to the ears and temporomandibular joint and using the large wing of the atlas as a landmark, the tissues of the occipito-atlantal and atlanto-axial region can be palpated. Tissue texture can give an indication of the chronicity of a problem here, where the gritty feel of a long-term problem can be differentiated from the bunched-up muscle spasm of an acute injury. This can affect the positional orientation of the region which may be palpated as vertebral asymmetry. By bringing the fingers of each hand behind the mandible it should be possible to rest two or three fingers' breadth in the space between the mandibular ramus and the wings of the atlas. Any narrowing of the space or lack of symmetry between the two sides may indicate dysfunction in this area.

Having obtained an overview of soft tissue state, an assessment of joint motion is the logical next step. A general impression of flexion and extension, the principal movement of the occipito-atlantal joint, is gained by placing a hand on the nose near the muzzle and gently pushing to produce a nodding action. This movement should be free and easy. Where there is occipito-atlantal restriction, the head will be resistant to the pressure of the hand and will move *en bloc* without any impression of separation of the atlas from the occiput. This can be verified by placing the hands just behind the ears to palpate the suboccipital region and using the body to push the lower part of the horse's face to produce flexion (Figure 9.7). Keeping one palpating hand in this region and lifting the underside of the muzzle, occipito-atlantal extension can be tested (Figure 9.8).

At the next level down, rotation is the primary movement and atlanto-axial mobility is assessed by holding the lower part of the face in one hand and rotating it upwards while the other hand fixes on to the wing of the atlas and palpates for atlanto-axial excursion (Figure 9.9). This is repeated for rotation in the other direction.

A more accurate impression of individual joint movement can be obtained by lifting the horse's head and resting its mandible on the practitioner's shoulder. This contact acts as a pivot point and so a little time should be spent moving the shoulder up or down the line of the jaw to achieve a point of balance. As the practitioner bends and straightens the knees, range and quality of occipito-atlantal flexion and extension can be palpated in the area behind the ears (Figure 9.10). Moving the hands caudally and locating the wings of the atlas enables palpation of the atlanto-axial joint. A sideways movement of the practitioner with the horse's head still balanced on the shoulder will tilt the head and introduce rotation at this level (Figure 9.11).

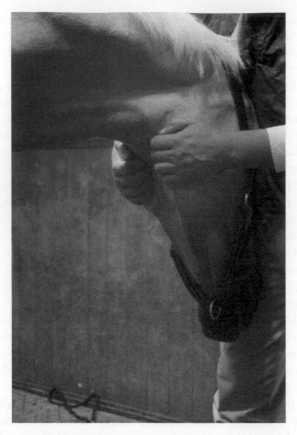

Figure 9.7 Occipito-atlantal flexion: pushing on the horse's nose produces flexion.

Cervical Spine

The cervical spine follows a sinusoidal course and the transverse processes form a ridge running down the neck much more ventrally than in the human equivalent. Much of the dorsal region is occupied by the ligamentum nuchae. Movement of the mid- to lower cervical spine is principally flexion, extension and lateral flexion.

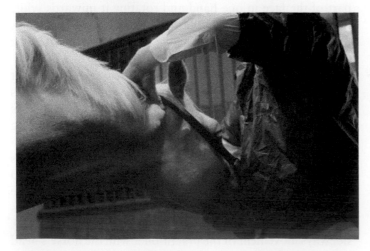

Figure 9.8 Occipito-atlantal extension: lifting the muzzle produces occipito-atlantal extension.

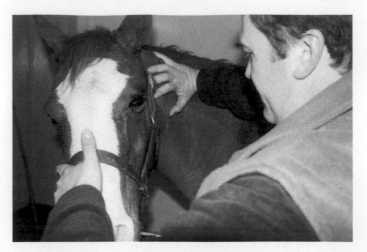

Figure 9.9 Atlanto-axial joint: taking the muzzle round to one side and then the other produces rotation.

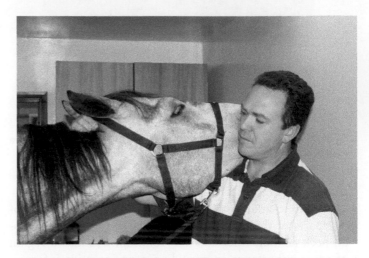

Figure 9.10 Occipito-atlantal joint: flexion and extension can be introduced by the practitioner bending and straightening the knees.

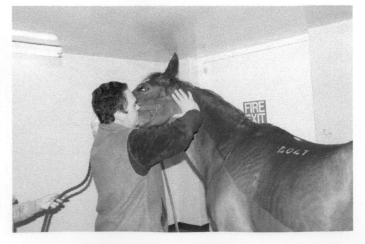

Figure 9.11 Rotation: moving sideways introduces rotation focusing at the atlanto-axial joint.

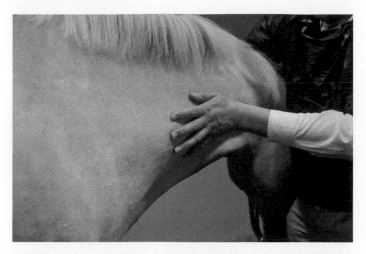

Figure 9.12 Lateral flexion: testing for tissue quality and sidebend in the cervical spine by pushing sideways on the transverse processes.

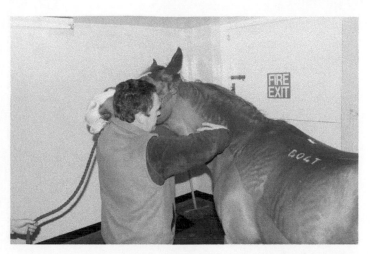

Figure 9.14 Cervical spine: lateral flexion can be tested at each level.

Palpating along the transverse processes, quality of the tissue can be assessed. There may be areas of tissue hypertrophy giving a lumpy feel accompanied by a localised reduction in movement. Lateral movement can be tested by pushing sideways on the transverse processes at each level (Figure 9.12).

Moving to the ventral surface of the neck, a gentle upward impulse from the hand or from the shoulder positioned under the neck will give an impression of local ventro-dorsal shift (Figure 9.13).

Further information about joint movement can be obtained with the horse's head resting on the practitioner's shoulder. Bending and straightening the knees test flexion and extension ranges. Stepping sideways will introduce a degree of lateral flexion, which can be palpated at different levels down the neck (Figure 9.14). By changing body

position and hand hold while testing these ranges, it is also possible to introduce smaller accessory movements such as ventro-dorsal and lateral shifts to form an idea of the composite function of the joint complexes.

Cervicothoracic Spine

Anatomically, the cervicothoracic junction lies deep to the considerable bulk of the thoracic girdle muscles. It is a pivotal point in the coordination of trunk and neck. Mobility here is essential for the fluid movement of the neck, scapula and forelimb. Neurologically it is closely related to the autonomic nervous system as the sympathetic nerves to the head, neck and forelimbs originate from the upper thoracic spinal cord.

Dysfunction here will often be reported as restricted forelimb movement, generalized stiffness and poor performance. There may also be acute pain presentations elsewhere as the horse tries and fails to compensate for deficits in this area.

Cervicothoracic problems may show on thermography as a cold limb, which is perhaps a parallel with Raynaud's phenomenon in humans and suggests increased and inappropriate sympathetic activity (see Chapter 3).

By virtue of its position deep to the surface, it is difficult to palpate movement of individual joint complexes in this region but examination can give an overall impression of suppleness. Standing in front and to one side of the horse with a hand on each shoulder, lateral to medial pressure can be exerted on one shoulder and then the other. There should be an easy transfer of weight-bearing across the midline from one foot to the other (Figure 9.15). A further test of mobility is to place one hand on the prominent spinous processes of the upper thoracic spine and the other on the sternum. The two hands are squeezed towards each other and then released (Figure 9.16). There should be a sensation of 'bounce' as the tissues give under the applied pressure,

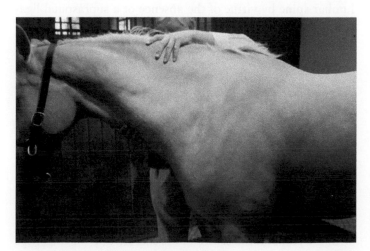

Figure 9.13 Cervical spine: a gentle impulse from the ventral surface upwards towards the nuchal ligament gives an idea of local segmental mobility.

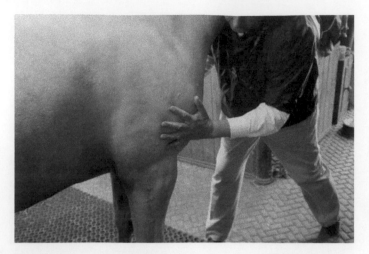

Figure 9.15 Cervicothoracic junction: exerting lateral to medial pressure to the shoulder, there should be an easy transfer of weightbearing from one foot to the other across the midline.

followed by recoil when this is relaxed. Dysfunction at the cervicothoracic region often gives the impression of pushing against concrete. The tissue does not yield to the pressure and there is no recoil.

Thoracolumbar Spine

With the exception of the lumbosacral segment this region is relatively rigid, with movement restricted by the orientation of the facets, the presence of the ribs in the thoracic spine and large transverse processes in the lumbar spine. It provides a strong, resilient scaffold from which the abdomen is slung and from which the limb girdles can act during movement. It also provides somewhere for the rider to sit. Problems here may range from discomfort when saddling, to difficulties

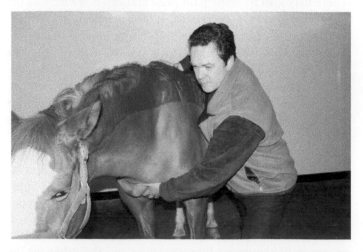

Figure 9.16 Cervicothoracic junction: with one hand on the thoracic spinous processes and the other on the sternum, squeezing the hands towards each other and then releasing should give a sensation of 'bounce' (yield and recoil).

bringing the hindlimbs under the trunk. Points of sensitivity along the back are not uncommon.

Areas of dysfunction may be identified initially by using 'skin drag'. Standing beside the horse, the thumb and fingers are placed lightly on the skin over the paravertebral muscles either side of the spinous processes and are slowly dragged down the spine (Figure 9.17). There may be areas where the hand does not move smoothly over the surface, which indicates altered vascular and sweat gland activity of the skin surface mediated by the autonomic nervous system.

Paravertebral muscle quality and tone can be assessed by standing on one side of the horse and using the thenar eminence to push the erector spinae on the opposite side away from the spinous processes (Figure 9.18). There may be segments of localised muscle hypertonia which have a lumpy feel and are resistant to stretch.

Individual joint mobility from the upper thoracic spine through to the lumbar articulations may be evaluated using dorsal springing. Standing above the horse (it may be necessary to stand on a bale or crate) the fingers of one hand are used to palpate the interspinous space while pushing down and then releasing pressure on the spinous process below with the thenar eminence of the other hand (Figure 9.19). Ideally, the body weight should be dropped through straight arms positioned perpendicular to the spine. There should be a bounce (yield and recoil) in response to the force.

Lack of movement and/or a pain reaction indicates local dysfunction which usually ties in with the findings on skin drag.

Lumbosacral Junction and Pelvis

The lumbosacral joint is worthy of special consideration as it acts as a hinge between the lumbar spine and the solid mass of the sacrum and pelvis. It is the most mobile segment in the lumbar spine by virtue of the absence of a supraspinal ligament and the widely spaced spinous processes. Its principal ranges of movement are flexion and extension. Acute problems here are common, either as a direct result of trauma or as a result of increased loading from dysfunction elsewhere. The mobility of the sacrum between the ilia is also important in pelvic movement where the tubera sacrale should move up and down like pistons on the sacrum when observed from behind.

Running the hands over the lumbosacral area and on to the gluteal muscles, symmetry of muscle development and tone is assessed alongside skin drag (Figure 9.20). The mobility of the sacrum can be tested using sacral springing. Standing to one side of the hindquarters, a hand is placed with the palm on the centre of the sacrum and the fingertips palpating the lumbosacral junction lying deep between the tubera sacrale. Reinforcing this with the other hand, downward pressure is applied to the sacrum and then released.

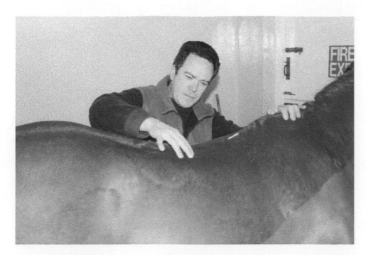

Figure 9.17 Skin drag: fingers and thumb placed lightly on the paravertebral muscles either side of the spinous processes are slowly dragged down the spine, noting areas of resistance to movement ('drag').

There should be a sense of yield and recoil. After testing this in a number of horses, the varying degrees of sacral mobility become apparent, ranging from a healthy bounce to an impression of pushing down on concrete. The sacrum may also be used as a lever for testing lumbosacral movement. Moving the hand caudally below the fulcrum and pushing downwards here will cause the lumbosacral joint to flex (Figure 9.21), while moving the hand onto the sacral base will introduce an element of extension. The direction of pressure exerted by the hand may also be altered to include elements of sidebend and rotation.

The tail is a useful tool in the assessment of the pelvis and lumbosacral spine. Taking the tail 3 cm from the root and

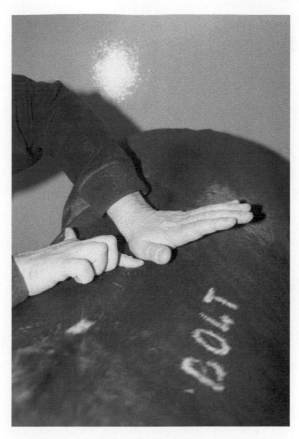

Figure 9.19 Dorsal springing: testing segmental thoracic movement by palpating the interspinous space and pushing down on the spinous process below.

exerting a little traction will give an overall impression of the state of muscle and fascia extending from the tail along the sacrum and into the lumbar spine. If this stretch is uncomfortable, the horse may clamp the tail into the perineum protectively. This is an indication for caution when working

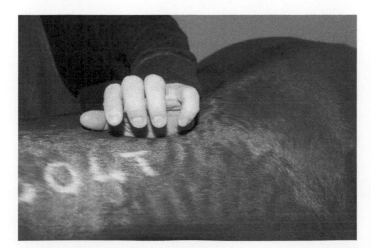

Figure 9.18 Paravertebral muscle tone: using the hyperthenar eminence, the erector spinae are stretched laterally to assess muscle quality and tone.

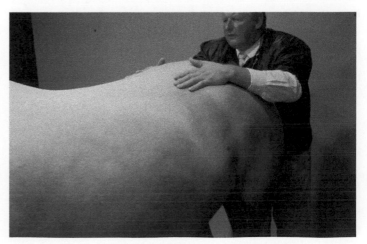

Figure 9.20 Gluteal muscles: quality, symmetry and tone of the gluteal muscles should be assessed.

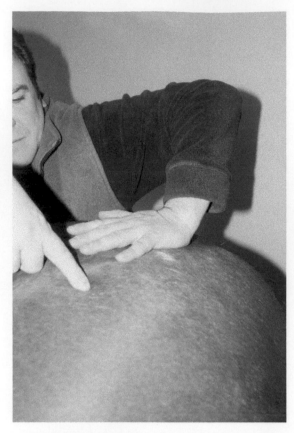

Figure 9.21 Sacral bounce: mobility of the sacrum is established by downward pressure. Pressure caudal to the fulcrum results in lumbosacral flexion.

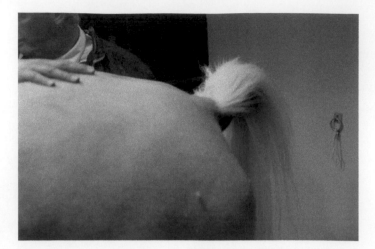

Figure 9.23 Tail: sidebend and rotation of the tail gives a sense of the movement through the sacrum and into the lumbosacral joint.

around the hindquarters until some change in the state of pelvic and lumbosacral tissue has been achieved.

If this contact is tolerated, the root of the tail is taken by one hand while the other is placed on the lumbosacral junction to assess the movement of this articulation. In a normal spine, as the tail is lifted there is a sense that the sacrum dips as it drops ventrally in relation to the lowest lumbar vertebra (Figure 9.22). Moving the tail downwards produces the opposite effect. Sidebending and rotation of the tail will also be reflected through the sacrum into the lumbosacral joint (Figure 9.23).

The soft tissue state of the pelvic region can be evaluated by standing behind the horse and putting the shoulder against the pelvic diaphragm, between the tuber ischii. Pressure is initially applied in the midline pushing directly forwards towards the head (Figure 9.24). The degree of tissue yield will indicate the tension in the pelvic muscles and should also introduce an element of sacral flexion. By gradually changing the direction of push laterally around to 90° to one side and then the other, an impression of spring in the sacroiliac joint should be obtained.

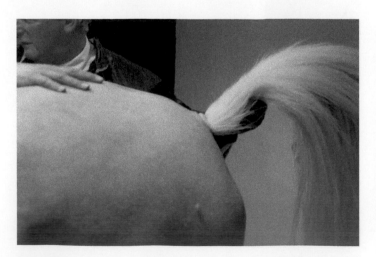

Figure 9.22 Lumbosacral joint: as the tail is lifted the sacrum dips and produces extension at the lumbosacral articulation.

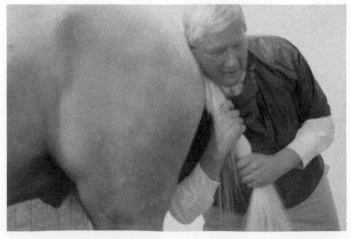

Figure 9.24 Pelvic soft tissue: pushing into the perineum in the midline and then directing pressure laterally in an arc towards the ischial tuberosities will give a sense of pelvic soft tissue state.

Putting it all Together

With this examination of soft tissue and segmental mobility, together with the findings from static and active movement, a treatment plan can be formulated. This should address dysfunction not only in terms of local tissue pathology but also with regard to the way the body functions as a bio-mechanical unit.

REFERENCE

Hecker H, Steveling A, Peuker E, Kastner J, Liebchen K (2001) *Colour Atlas of Acupuncture*. Thieme, Stuttgart, p. 105.

10

Osteopathic Treatment – Overarching Principles

Anthony Pusey and Julia Brooks

This is the point at which the synthesis of case history, active examination and palpation come together in the form of a treatment plan. In almost all cases, this plan should consider the whole biomechanical structure of the horse rather than focusing on the localised area identified as causing the symptoms.

This approach is often a surprise to the owner and sometimes to the vet. I worked with a German vet for a number of years treating horses in the Rhine Valley. At the end of one clinic, he asked me to look at his painful wrist. I examined him, tracing the strain pattern up through the elbow to his shoulder. Asking him to remove his shirt, I examined the thoracic and lumbar spine. To check pelvic function, I asked him to loosen his trousers, at which point he turned to me in some alarm with the words, 'Anthony, if you want to make love to me, just say so.'

This incident illustrates the need to take owners and vets with you when treating a complex problem with involvement at many different levels!

Treatment is not synonymous with technique. Both the philosophy and the mechanics of treatment will depend on the practitioner's morphology, the course of education, working conditions and personal preferences. It will depend on the size, shape and temperament of the horse, and the site, duration and nature of the problem. This may vary during the course of the treatment as the biodynamics change and new aspects of the problem come to light. To be prescriptive about treatment or to be dogmatic about a particular approach is to remove from one's armoury a raft of measures which could be therapeutically effective. It has been said that most approaches will be helpful in 70% of cases, but

it is the recalcitrant 30% that present the challenge. This requires flexible thinking and an ability to listen to advice from many sources, both within and from outside the profession. To use a hunting term, this is 'the thrill of the chase' which ensures that osteopathy remains stimulating and absorbing to the practitioner and invaluable to horse and rider.

Most treatment plans will use techniques that are directed towards restoring movement to the musculoskeletal structures of the body. This allows a normal relaxed standing position and free and easy active movement, and promotes a balanced homeostatic environment to support these functions. Most of the techniques used will be very familiar to osteopaths in human practice although some are adapted specifically for the horse. They take a number of forms including soft tissue stretch, inhibition, articulation, high velocity thrusts, positional release, and functional and cranio-sacral techniques (Ward 1997).

Soft Tissue Techniques

Soft tissue techniques are directed at abnormal muscle and fascial tone resulting from neuromusculoskeletal dysfunction. They aim to improve tone, pliability and nutrition to the muscles and to allow full mobility of the joints.

Soft tissue can be stretched either longitudinally or cross-fibre. A sound knowledge of anatomy and in particular of the origin, insertion and fibre direction of muscles is essential for effective soft tissue stretch of an individual muscle or a group of muscles (Figure 10.1).

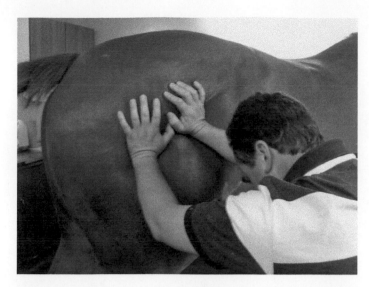

Figure 10.1 Soft tissue stretch: this is an effective way to relax an individual muscle or a group of muscles.

Longitudinal stretch is effected by using the hands to compress the tissue at one end of the muscle and pushing in the direction along which its fibres run towards the other attachment. It is usual to start at the distal attachment and push in a cephalad direction.

In cross-fibre techniques, the belly of the muscle is stretched sideways at an angle of 90° to the direction of the fibres, although this can be varied.

Soft tissue stretch is usually applied rhythmically moving along or across the muscle fibres at a particular rate. It has often been said that each person has his or her own gear or natural harmonic and this applies equally to the horse. The rate should be set to match this rhythm, but may vary according to the desired effect on the tissues. In general a faster rate will stimulate the muscles while a slower rate will relax them.

Inhibition

Inhibitory techniques are natural accompaniments to soft tissue stretching. These techniques are often directed at local areas of altered tissue tone and texture, which may be found within a muscle. In human osteopathy, these areas may be referred to as tender points and in some circumstances as trigger points. Although in the literature there is some distinction between the two, both rely to an extent on subjective feedback from the patient. Tender points are indeed reported as tender by the patient. Trigger points may be sensitive locally but the pain radiates from the point of pressure in distinct patterns, thought to represent a widening field of central sensitisation to noxious afferent input (Bennett 1999). Histological changes have also been identified.

As accurate subjective feedback is not possible in horses, a pragmatic approach will be used in the terminology. The use of trigger points when discussing treatment refers to the

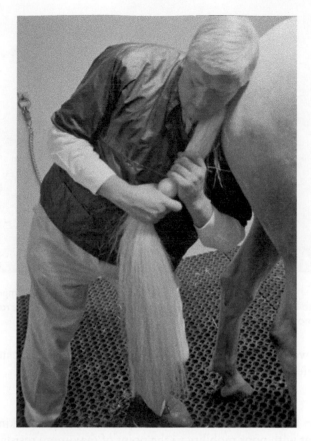

Figure 10.2 Inhibition: pressure is applied to trigger points on the medial side of the ischial tuberosity and pelvic diaphragm to produce muscle relaxation.

point that, when pressure is applied, will 'trigger' a response in the horse.

In practical terms, steady pressure is put on a trigger point until a tissue response is felt. Changes, generally a reduction in tone, will occur locally at the point of contact and spread throughout the muscle as a whole (Figure 10.2). The horse may also lean into the pressure and make postural changes with this point as a fulcrum.

It is important to monitor the tissue response and to release the pressure when relaxation has occurred.

Articulation/Mobilisation

The term 'articulation' will, in this text, be interchangeable with 'mobilisation', and encompasses techniques that improve the pliability of and nutrition to the periarticular tissues and encourage a full range of joint movement. This not only improves the biomechanical performance of the body but, where there is pain, it increases large-fibre afferent input to the central nervous system from the muscles and joint structures which act to inhibit or 'gate' incoming pain signals.

Articulation may be used on one joint or on a number of joints together. This requires not only knowledge of specific joint anatomy, but also an appreciation of the interplay

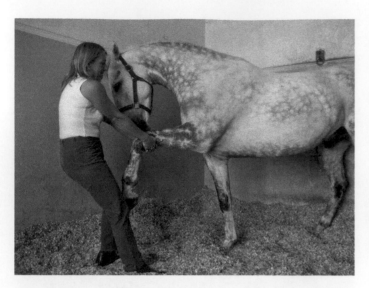

Figure 10.3 Articulation and Mobilisation: these techniques improve pliability of and nutrition to the periarticular tissues and improve range of motion.

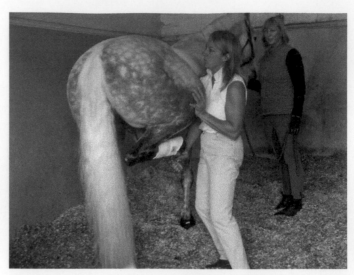

Figure 10.4 High velocity thrust: used in the pelvis, the leg is lifted and pushed sharply upwards and away from the practitioner to mobilise the sacroiliac joint.

between a number of structures and the range that can be achieved (Figure 10.3).

HVT (High Velocity Thrust)

The high velocity thrust or manipulation involves taking a joint with poor mobility to the point of maximum resistance (the restrictive barrier) using knowledge of planes of articular surfaces and joint biomechanics. This barrier is overcome with a short-amplitude, high-velocity thrust which may be accompanied by a cavitation sound or 'pop'. This stimulates a sudden increase in articular mechanoreceptor activity, which changes the pattern of neuronal firing in the central nervous system that is creating abnormal muscle activity. The effect of the thrust is usually immediate with relaxation of muscle tone and improved joint mobility.

The classic example of HVT, often used in chiropractic circles, is where the leg is lifted and pushed sharply upwards and away from the practitioner to mobilise the sacroiliac joint (Figure 10.4). It can also be performed in the neck, peripheral joints and, under general anaesthetic, in the lumbar spine (Figure 10.5).

Indirect Techniques

Almost at the other end of the spectrum from HVT is the family of indirect techniques which include positional release, functional and fascial techniques. They are termed indirect because, rather than pushing directly through a movement restriction, they rely on moving a joint into the position of dysfunction, closely following the forces that created the problem. This approach is particularly useful in chronic, complex cases.

These techniques use the idea of 'ease' and 'bind'. In a normal joint there will be a resting position where there is

minimum tension on the capsular ligaments and the overlying muscles. This is the point of 'ease' and is usually found in the mid-range of joint movement. Any movement away from this point will increase tension or 'bind'. This information is relayed to the central nervous system where it is processed to map joint position and to generate an appropriate pattern of motor activity. Where the normal relationship between the joint structures has been disturbed, the point of ease is offset and afferent mapping information will be changed at rest and during movement. The central nervous system has difficulties in processing this new information within existing well established networks, and the joint is less able to move appropriately or to co-ordinate movement with other joints.

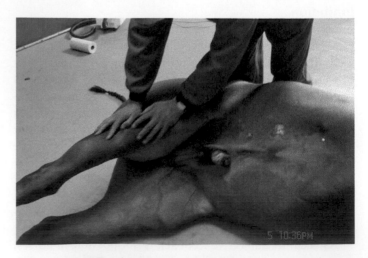

Figure 10.5 HVT: a lumbar roll technique to manipulate the lumbar spine can be performed under general anaesthetic.

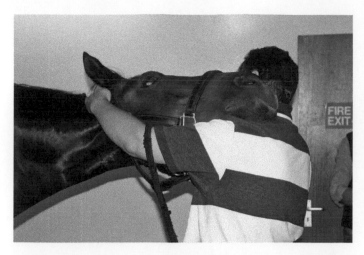

Figure 10.6 Functional techniques: establishing and maintaining a point of 'ease' in the joint complex results in tissue relaxation.

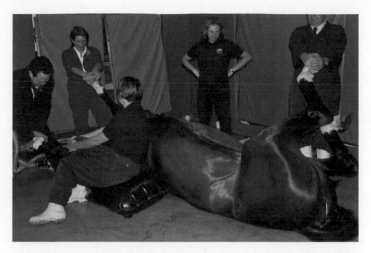

Figure 10.7 Fascial release: whole body fascial release can be achieved by putting the legs and neck in a position of minimum tension, which often reflects the strain pattern of the original injury.

Treatment relies on locating the new abnormal point of minimum tension by testing each plane of movement step by step. Flexion and extension, sidebending to left and right, rotation to left and right, translocation (horizontal or vertical shearing across a midline axis) from side to side and forwards and backwards, traction and compression are tested to establish the point of maximum 'ease'. This position is held until the tissues around the joint relax (Figure 10.6).

At the point of minimum tension, afferent input into the spinal cord is diminished. This appears to reduce conflicting information entering the central nervous system network and allows the normal neurological pattern of activity to reassert itself.

Positional and functional techniques are usually directed at specific joint complexes. Using the same principles of ease and bind, fascial release techniques may be used to produce an 'unwinding' effect on large areas of musculo-fascial dysfunction. A whole body release is possible under general anaesthetic. With the horse supine, each leg is taken by a practitioner and moved to a point of ease which is maintained until a generalised sense of relaxation is felt (Figure 10.7). The body position adopted at this point of minimum tension often reproduces the strains involved in the original injury.

There is much overlap between functional, positional release and fascial release techniques. All are based on manoeuvring the body into the position of least tension. A purist might say that functional techniques test resistance over very small ranges of joint movement whereas in positional techniques the movements are rather more exaggerated. Fascial release takes into consideration regional distortions in movement patterns. In practice, these divisions are somewhat artificial and practitioners will probably use a combination of indirect approaches.

Cranial Osteopathy

Cranial technique requires a highly developed sense of palpation. It is extremely gentle and to the uninformed observer is as exciting as watching paint dry. However, it is remarkably powerful in its effect on horses.

The theory of this effect is based on minute fluctuations occurring in the structures enclosing and supporting the central nervous system as well as the inherent movement of the system itself (Magoun 1951). Optimum function of these components maintains the health of the neural system, which is the prime organiser of the neuromusculoskeletal apparatus. Treatment also has a general de-tuning effect and has been referred to as the 'osteopathic valium'. This perhaps reflects the strong connections between the sensory system of the cranium with the more primitive, emotional parts of the brain, a connection exploited by many mothers as they stroke the face and head to soothe a fractious infant.

The technique hinges around what is termed the primary respiratory mechanism, which describes the constant, rhythmical nature of the movement of the central nervous system and cerebrospinal fluid. The movement, or cranial rhythm impulse (CRI), is generally considered to be around 10 to 14 cycles per minute, but other slower fluctuations may be detected.

The rhythm is in concert with changes in meningeal tension. The dura mater, a continuation of the periosteum which covers the inner surface of the cranial bones, has inwardly directed, sickle-shaped membranous reflections of the falx cerebrum and the tentorium cerebelli. It extends downwards, hanging in the vertebral column like a sheath covering the spinal cord, and attaches to the sacrum caudally. The anatomical unit of the cranial and spinal dura is referred to as the reciprocal tension membrane (RTM). Subtle changes in the dural tensions will influence the functioning of the primary respiratory mechanism.

Associated with the fluid and membrane fluctuations is the biphasic movement of the cranial bones and sacrum. The midline structures such as the sphenoid, occiput, ethmoid, vomer, mandible, hyoid and sacrum will flex and extend, while the paired lateral bones, such as the temporal, parietal and zygomatic bones, rotate externally and internally. Flexion of the key midline structures, the sphenoid and occiput, is accompanied by external rotation of the lateral structures in the first phase of the cycle. The exact opposite occurs in the second phase, with extension of the midline and internal rotation laterally. This internal and external rotation is reflected through fascial planes of the body into the limbs. Integral to this mechanism is the movement of the sacrum by virtue of its dural connections. As the midline cranial structures flex, so the base of the sacrum moves cranially and dorsally, the reverse occurring during the extension phase.

Cranial technique can be performed on a number of levels. The skull is vulnerable to high-impact injuries and some quite firm 'bone-crunching' cranial procedures may be used to 'disengage' the constituent parts of the skull (Figure 10.8). On a more refined level, they may be used to guide and balance membranes of the cranium and spinal column, and influence the fluid circulating within the ventricles and subarachnoid space (Figure 10.9). These techniques usually employ an indirect method by exaggerating the direction of lesion and maintaining this position until a release of tension is felt in the tissues.

In horses, the components of cranial treatment are much the same as in humans although the differences in anatomical

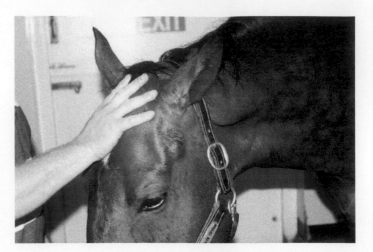

Figure 10.9 Cranial osteopathy: techniques may involve using a quiescent 'listening' hand to monitor and influence the cranial mechanism.

orientation and the smaller cranial scale need to be appreciated (Figure 10.10).

APPLYING THE TECHNIQUES

Techniques employed in the human field are ideally suited, with some modifications, for treating musculoskeletal dysfunction in horses. Those used will depend on the nature of the problem and the preferences of the practitioner. Some consideration must be given to the environment and conditions of treatment. Decisions will have to be made such as whether techniques would be most effective in the enclosed space of a stable or in an open area with room to manoeuvre. Some techniques may be more easily performed when the horse is given a light sedation. Long-standing

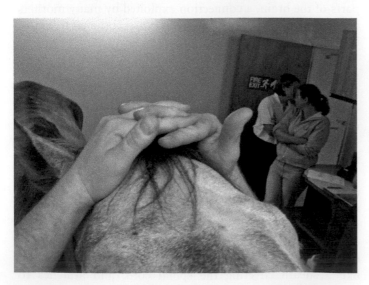

Figure 10.8 Cranial osteopathy: some techniques involve firm pressure applied to the cranium.

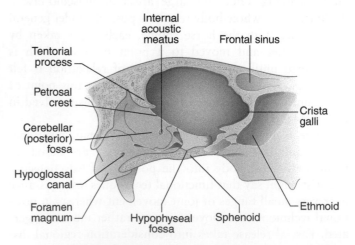

Figure 10.10 Sagittal section of the cranial bones: there are differences in the orientation and size of the cranial structures compared with the human counterpart.

complex problems may be best tackled by using techniques that can only be performed under general anaesthetic.

As far as techniques themselves are concerned, there is no one perfect method for any particular type of presenting problem. The important thing is for the hands to maintain a constant dialogue with the tissues, and to be prepared to change an approach in response to this feedback in order to achieve the desired result of a balanced and fluidly moving horse.

REFERENCES

Bennett RM (1999) Fibromyalgia. In: *Textbook of Pain*, 4th edn, Wall PD, Melzack R (eds). Churchill Livingstone, Edinburgh, pp. 588–589.

Magoun HI (1951) *Osteopathy in the Cranial Field*. Journal Printing Company, Kirksville.

Ward RC (ed.) (1997) *Foundations of Osteopathic Medicine*. Williams & Wilkins, Baltimore.

Osteopathic Treatment Without Sedation

11

Annabel Jenks

'Take the skeleton of a man, tilt the pelvis, shorten the femur, legs and arms, elongate the feet and hands, fuse the phalanges, elongate the jaw while shortening the frontal bone, and finally elongate the spine, and the skeleton will cease to represent the remains of a man and will be the skeleton of the horse.'

Georges-Louis Leclerc, Comte de Buffon (1753)

The procedures described in this chapter are just a few of a number of osteopathic techniques that can be applied. The aim is to provide a base for the osteopath to structure his or her own treatment regime. Each practitioner is an individual, and every patient must be treated as a unique being. Likewise every horse and every presenting problem are unique. Rather than being tied in to a prescribed treatment routine, the approach should be flexible. If the horse does not respond, or responds adversely to a particular technique, there are always alternative methods. If there is no improvement after one or two treatments, the horse must be referred back to the veterinary surgeon for further investigations.

Osteopathic soft tissue techniques precede all mobilisation, stretching and articulation techniques. Reminders of the principles of osteopathy are very relevant at this point.

The underlying principle of osteopathy is that structure governs function, and that disturbances of structure in whatever tissue within the body will lead to disturbances of functioning in that structure and, in turn, of function of the body as a whole. The objective in the osteopathic approach is therefore the complete restoration of the structural integrity in the body (Stoddard 1980, pp. 9–10).

Joint manipulation is the normalisation of position and mobility and the relief of abnormal tensions within the soft tissue structures such as muscles, ligaments and fascia.

Manipulation and mobilisation with soft tissue techniques improve circulation, venous and lymphatic drainage and soft tissue integrity. The aim is to restore and improve the dynamic forces and mechanics within the conformation and limitations of the individual horse, holistically restoring equilibrium throughout the neuromusculoskeletal system.

Once pathology has been excluded, the practitioner can palpate to identify any joint dysfunction such as abnormal tissue changes, hyper- or hypomobility and joint positional changes. As Stoddard (1980, p. 14) constantly reminds the osteopath:

'If the positional relationship of adjacent bones are altered as well as the mobility, then we must note it down and attempt later to restore the normal anatomical relations. If there are altered positional relationships and yet normal mobility, then the position is not of material significance – it is due to anomalous shapes or soft tissue thickenings and we can ignore them.'

This is especially important to remember when examining and palpating the horse's pelvis for apparent positional changes.

Stoddard (1980, p. 22) also emphasises the importance of tissue-tension sense, which he describes as 'the appreciation of the amount of stretch there is in moving tissue, an interpretation of such tension during the process of movement in a limb, joint or muscle. It is dynamic rather than static.'

It is this tissue-tension sense that enables the practitioner to achieve success in manipulation by being able to choose the precise moment a thrust should be made. This, along with the rhythm and timing of a technique, is only achieved with practice and experience.

On all occasions, veterinary permission must have been received. Before commencing, it is good practice to discuss with the owner the expected outcomes and your proposed osteopathic treatment programme.

By removing compensatory factors, the dynamics of the horse change, in some cases revealing underlying pathology. This may result in some unlevel strides when it is trotted up post-treatment. The owner must be warned of this outcome and understand that often the veterinary surgeon wants these secondary compensations to be addressed so that they can then investigate the primary factor. It is common reasoning that sometimes the horse is just not lame enough for a full lameness workup to be performed. When the compensatory factors are removed, the lameness may become more evident and a full clinical examination by the veterinary surgeon can proceed.

On the other side of the coin, the practitioner should leave alone any compensatory factors if the horse is performing well and no symptoms are presenting. *Do not* open up a Pandora's box: you will not be popular with the owner!

Note: Occasionally, especially in the autumn and spring when the horse is changing its coat, slight swellings are seen on the areas that the practitioner has worked on. Lines along the tissues are observed and can concern the owner. It is therefore important to explain that this may happen and is a result of the blood vessels dilating and histamine being released (see Chapter 3). This has no detrimental effect at all on the horse and is part of the natural physiological response associated with soft tissue treatments. The practitioner must, however, communicate this to the owner, explaining the phenomenon before commencement of treatment.

After a full palpatory examination the following techniques can be used, in no specific order. Remember that these should be thought of as examples of osteopathic techniques giving the practitioner a guideline and springboard from which they can expand and form their own treatment programme. This will reflect their personal preferences and the suitability of each procedure for the individual horse receiving treatment.

Osteopathic considerations to contemplate during treatment comprise:

- Neurophysiology
- Proprioception
- Marked dysfunctions
- Subtle dysfunctions
- Abnormal tissue integrity
- Range of joint movement
- Muscle guarding or spasm
- Trigger points
- Altered spinal mechanics
- Muscle tone and development
- Rehabilitation

Always begin any treatment by quietly approaching from the side, and spend time communicating with and talking to the horse as you stroke and pat its neck or shoulder. Never go straight to the head.

It is fascinating that over 23 centuries ago, Xenophon, in his book, *The Art of Horsemanship* (1979 translation, pp. 34–35), wrote:

'The man that takes care of the horse should know that both in this matter (grooming) and in everything else which has to be done, the very last places at which he should approach to do it are in front and behind; for if the horse means mischief, these are the two points at which he has the advantage of a man. But by approaching him at the side you can handle him most freely and with the least danger to yourself.'

In my own experience there are key regions that need to be unwound *initially* to enable the whole spine to function correctly. To begin with, the occipito-atlanto-axial complex needs to be considered, followed by the cervicothoracic and lumbosacral junctions.

I therefore usually begin my osteopathic treatment at the poll, through to the withers and then to the pelvic region. From riding horses, I am personally of the opinion that unless the horse is free through the poll, neck and shoulders, they can never come through from behind correctly into balance.

These techniques are performed on both the right and left sides and obviously the practitioner will choose which hand is desired to facilitate their bias and treatment regime. Examination should begin on the symptom-free side, as the horse will be more receptive.

Continually observe the eyes, ears and mouth throughout the treatment, as these are always very expressive and excellent indicators, reflecting the horse's emotive responses. Ears back, eyes rolling and lips tense and curled are not signs of relaxation! There is also a 'pout' with the upper lip pursed forward. In our family we call this the 'Grandpa look', as it indicates a stubborn and rigid mood, which my eminent grandfather would display when he disapproved of our ideas or behaviour! This should not be confused with the unsure expression of the young horse, which may also extend the top lip but with less rigidity.

Positive responses will be seen with the horse chewing quietly and mouthing, yawning, audibly exhaling, lowering the eyelids and relaxing the ears.

Before commencing treatment, practitioners must familiarise themselves with Appendix A, which deals with the safety aspects involved in treating horses unsedated and sedated. It is particularly important that the practitioner ensures that the person holding the horse is *always* positioned on the same side as themselves, and the practitioner must communicate instructions clearly when necessary.

CERVICAL REGION

Overview

The practitioner will usually begin the treatment by addressing any dysfunction within the cervical region. This includes the occiput and the seven cervical vertebrae with the associated fascia and musculoskeletal tissue. Horses with cervical and poll mechanical dysfunctions may show resistance when ridden and exhibit any of the following signs: tension and shortening of the neck, high or low head carriage, intermittent tossing of the head, hollow outline and refusing to go on the bit, head tilting, reluctance to go forwards, tail swishing, teeth grinding, an inability to stretch over the topline resulting in a shortening of their natural stride length, inability to jump correctly, and an inability to perform certain dressage movements such as shoulder in and other lateral movements. There may be temperament changes and irritability, head shaking and head shyness, especially around the ears.

When ridden, they are usually stiffer and more restricted in turning the neck to the opposite side of the joint dysfunction. That is, if there are cervical positional changes with altered mobility on the left, they may be more restricted and reluctant to flex and bend to the right. The rider will comment that the horse is stiffer to ride on the right rein. This is not a golden rule but is a general occurrence.

National Hunt racehorses and event horses will often suffer from compression throughout the cervical spine from impact injuries when falling at a fence. A complex, compound dysfunction of impaction with rotation and lateral flexion of the cervical vertebrae results.

The aim of the osteopath is to improve overall function of the spine. To begin with, the practitioner releases dysfunction at the occipito-atlanto-axial complex, followed by the rest of the cervical spine. If the horse is head-shy and nervous, begin at the level of the third or fourth cervical vertebrae to gain the horse's trust as progression is made cranially towards the poll. Restoring normal joint function and desensitising and relaxing the associated muscle tissue and fascia in this region should allow the unwinding of the muscle chains to proceed throughout the horse.

Soft tissue techniques are used prior to all mobilisation, articulation or manipulation. As the tissues and joints respond, the horse will instinctively guide the osteopath as the unwinding of fascia and muscle chains occurs.

Be rhythmically guided through your treatment.

Techniques

1. *Soft tissue to the dorsal neck musculature.* The cranial hand stabilises the horse's head by resting on the nasal bone, while the caudal hand works deeply into the rectus capitis, nuchal ligament, splenius, rhomboid, trapezius and associated fascia along the dorsal neck musculature. Deep soft tissue techniques are applied with local inhibition of trigger points. Cross-fibre and longitudinal techniques are also used to stretch and desensitise the tissues (Figure 11.1).

2. *Mobilisation of the cervical spine.* Beginning at the occipito-atlantal region, the practitioner manoeuvres down the cervical spine, gently flexing and then laterally flexing the neck towards the shoulder. This is achieved with the cranial hand lightly placed on the dorsal nasal structures, flexing the head, gently pushing it towards the neck and using it as a lever to produce lateral flexion of the cervical spine. The caudal hand rests on the crest of the mane. The horse will follow the flexion voluntarily, in a rhythmic motion, if there are no restrictions or joint dysfunction (Figure 11.2).

3. *Relaxing and stretching the cervical spine.* Work along the nuchal ligament and associated dorsal cervical muscles, rhomboid and trapezius. Begin at the poll using deep circular and cross-fibre techniques with the thumb and fingers of the caudal hand (Figure 11.3a). This encourages the horse to lower and flex the cervicals, and soften, relax and stretch the topline (Figures 11.3b and 11.3c).

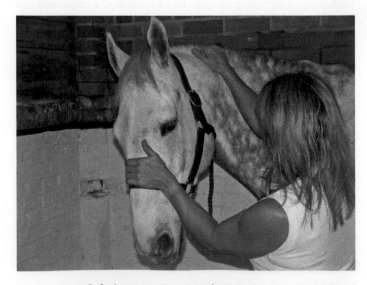

Figure 11.1 Soft tissue to dorsal neck musculature: cranial hand stabilises the head while the caudal hand applies soft tissue techniques.

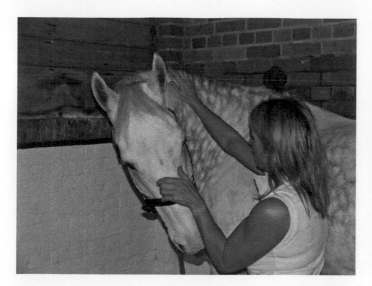

Figure 11.2 Mobilisation of cervical spine: use the head as a lever and gently laterally flex the neck.

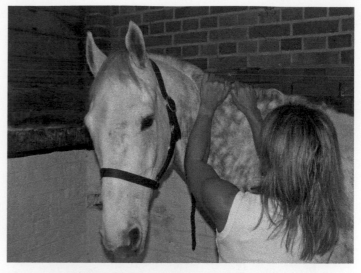

Figure 11.4 Springing the cervical dorsal line: gently and rhythmically spring the mane laterally away from the midline with both hands from the poll to the withers.

Continue with soft tissue techniques in a caudal direction along the dorsal neck musculature.

4. *Springing the cervical dorsal line (topline)*. Gently and rhythmically rock the dorsal musculature laterally, by gently springing the mane over with both hands from the poll to the withers (Figure 11.4).

5. *Soft tissue to the lateral neck musculature*. While stabilising the head with the cranial hand, use the palm, heel and fingers of the caudal hand to knead and massage the lateral cervical musculature, splenius, serratus anterior and associated muscles and connective tissue (Figure 11.5).

6. *Soft tissue and mobilisation to the ventral musculature*. Follow this with soft tissue massage and inhibitory techniques to the ventral musculature (Figure 11.6a). Especially work along the brachiocephalic muscle from origin to insertion to encourage flexion and lateral bending and release of any tension (Figure 11.6b). This muscle is one of the prime movers of protraction of the forelimb and

also flexes the head and neck laterally. Any restrictions of this muscle will shorten the stride length.

Use deep soft tissue massage and articulate with passive mobilisation along the cervical spine to remove adhesions, aiming to release and unwind the associated fascia and muscular tissue.

7. *Translocation of the cervical spine*. The practitioner stands facing the horse. With the palms of the hands either side of the cervical transverse processes, laterally oscillate each individual cervical vertebra between the hands (Figure 11.7). This allows assessment of the movement, as well as mobilising the joints. The horse may lower its neck as the practitioner works caudally down the neck.

The osteopath's experience and skill should lead them instinctively through the order and direction of treatment.

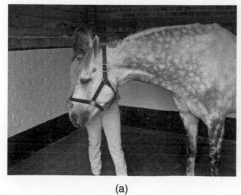

(a)

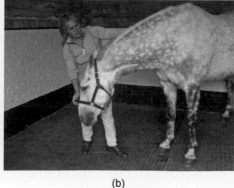

(b)

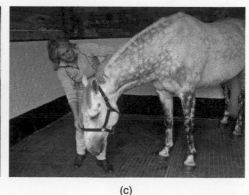

(c)

Figure 11.3 (a) Relaxing and stretching the cervical spine and associated tissues: begin at the poll using deep circular and cross-fibre techniques. Encourage the horse to lower its neck. (b) and (c) Relaxing the topline: the horse lowers its head and neck and stretches down.

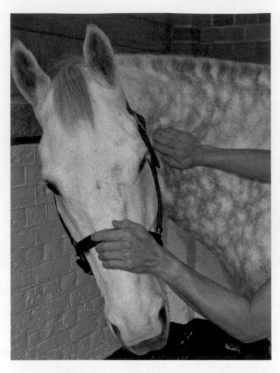

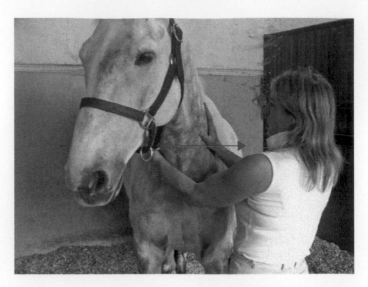

Figure 11.7 Translocation of cervical spine: with the palms of the hand on the cervical transverse processes laterally oscillate the individual vertebra assessing mobility.

Figure 11.5 Soft tissue to the lateral neck musculature: stabilise the head with the cranial hand and knead and massage the lateral cervical musculature with the caudal hand.

As has been emphasised before, the horse guides the practitioner. Never apply a technique if the patient is unwilling!

SHOULDER REGION

Overview
It is important to remember that the horse's thorax is in a muscular sling and must be able to swing between the

shoulders for optimum dynamic movement. There are no clavicular bones uniting the shoulder to the sternum.

Any restrictions around the shoulders and associated musculature will inhibit the extension of the forelimb. The gait will become unbalanced and the resulting stress can cause lameness.

Any reduction of movement in this region is seen as shortened protraction of the forelimb, with restriction through the withers, thus blocking the impulsion from the hindlimb. The horse has difficulty performing lateral movements and when jumping may dangle the forelimbs instead of snapping them up underneath the chest. When landing after a fence, the forelimbs take all the strain, along with the shoulder and neck. Bear in mind that at one point the entire weight

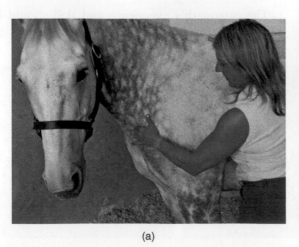

(a)

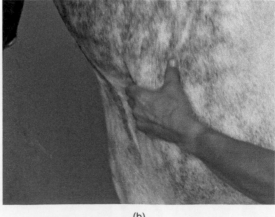

(b)

Figure 11.6 (a) Soft tissue to ventral cervical musculature: apply soft tissue and inhibitory techniques and encourage the horse to flex and laterally flex the neck. (b) Soft tissue to the brachiocephalic musculature: especially work along the brachiocephalic muscle using deep soft tissue techniques.

of the horse is taken on to one foot and the pastern is fully extended.

Causes of dysfunction through the peri-scapular tissue can be from restrictions at the cervicothoracic junction, concussive forces through the forelimb, compensations for foot pathologies, tendon or ligamentous injuries, poorly fitting saddles or restrictive riding.

There can be a distinctive blocked feel to the dorsal aspect of the scapula and withers. On palpation, the solid feel is as if one is palpating a wall. In some cases, for example a horse with navicular syndrome that is not yet clinically apparent, the tissues may show no improvement after treatment. Even after several structural treatments, function is never fully restored. This finding should immediately alert the practitioner, and referral back to the vet is essential to eliminate the possibility of pathology.

Deep soft tissue techniques are applied to the dorsal, lateral and ventral regions of the scapula, withers and shoulder. Supraspinatus and infraspinatus may be tender on palpation. The horse will often twitch along the skin quite dramatically. Inhibition should be applied to trigger points. Circular and longitudinal massage techniques should also be applied along the muscles including deltoid and associated muscles in the shoulder region.

Techniques

8. *Soft tissue to the scapula region.* Run the thumb along the cranial border of the scapula. Use the fingers to stretch the fascia medial to the scapula and progress ventrally. A deep probing will enable the lower cervical vertebrae to be reached (Figure 11.8).
9. *Deep soft tissue to lower cervical spine.* Change hand positions from the previous technique, flex and later-

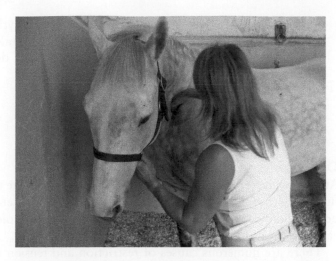

Figure 11.9 Deep soft tissue to the lower cervical vertebrae: flex and laterally flex the head with the cranial hand.

ally flex the horse's head with the cranial hand, and use the caudal hand to further probe medially towards the seventh cervical vertebra (Figure 11.9). The horse may exaggerate the flexion of the cervical spine, and spontaneous cavitations may occur as the neck is laterally flexed around towards the practitioner. Be cautious because, if the technique is too rapid or too deep, there is a tendency for the horse to turn and bite and in some instances rear up.

The shoulder can then be mobilised as long as there are no remaining adhesions within the pectoral and triceps muscles.

10. *Stretching and mobilising the shoulder.* With the carpus flexed and supported by the practitioner's inner arm, the humerus is used as a lever and the shoulder is stretched cranially and caudally (Figure 11.10). Functional and

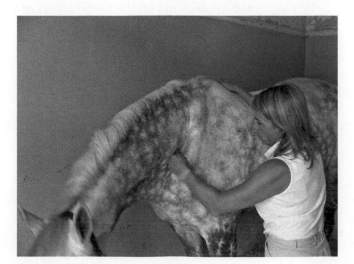

Figure 11.8 Deep soft tissue to the cranial border of the scapula and associated musculature: use the fingers to apply soft tissue medial to the scapula.

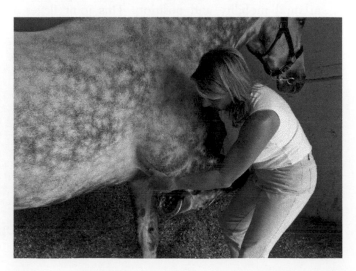

Figure 11.10 Stretching and mobilising the shounder: the carpus is flexed and supported and the humerus is used as a lever to stretch the scapula cranially and caudally.

harmonic techniques, along with sustained and rhythmic traction, can be applied. The practitioner must take care when flexing the carpus in case there are any degenerative changes.

CERVICAL REGION TECHNIQUES

Overview

At this point, return to the head and upper cervical spine to further release the occipito-atlanto-axial complex and temporomandibular joints and unwind the fascia of the hyoid, ears and facial muscles.

There are numerous causes of restriction and tension in this region: dental problems, such as sharp edges to the molars or mouth ulcers; ill-fitting bridles and bits; concussive falls, especially in National Hunt racing and eventing; being cast in the stable; stable vices such as weaving or windsucking; pulling back when tied up; hitting the poll on stable doorframes or on the roof of the trailer or horsebox; nasal congestion; head shaking – and many more!

Practitioners should be aware that horses do not have a transverse atlantal ligament. Young horses, especially foals, are very vulnerable if mobilised at the atlanto-axial joint, so great care and very careful palpation are essential when examining young stock. This is also why caution must be exercised when leading foals. If they pull back, the handler must move with the youngster as opposed to pulling them forwards, as there is a serious risk of injury to the cervical spine.

Techniques

11. *Occipito-atlantal mobility.* Re-examine the occipito-atlantal mobility and position. This joint flexes and extends the head, the 'yes' movement. Stand on one side of the horse with the caudal hand stabilising the neck as the cranial hand is placed on the nasal region and rocks the head in a nodding direction to assess flexion (Figure 11.11a).

To assess extension stabilise the neck with the caudal hand while the cranial hand cups the chin and lifts the head as far as the horse will allow (Figure 11.11b).

12. *Atlas technique.* Placing two or possibly three fingers within the space between the atlas and mandibular ramus assesses the atlas position. The width is compared between the two sides (Figure 11.12a). A wider gap between the two indicates that the wing of the atlas has rotated in a dorsal direction on that side.

The practitioner should be positioned on the side where the space between the atlas and the mandibular ramus is *narrower* and which may also be painful and tender on palpation. The caudal hand cups the wing of the atlas with the thumb in the atlanto-mandibular space. The cranial hand is placed on the dorsal nasal region and compresses and flexes the head (Figure 11.12b).

At the same time the slack is taken up and a subtle leverage is applied to the nose with the cranial hand laterally flexing the head, a high-velocity thrust is performed with the caudal hand in the direction of the opposite ear (Figures 11.12c and 11.12d).

As with all high velocity thrust (HVT) techniques the rhythm and timing are essential.

13. *Atlas dorsal technique.* If, on palpation, the atlas is higher on one side, a dorsal technique can be used. The practitioner will need to stand on a suitable object to position themselves correctly on the higher side. The horse is encouraged to lower the head. Contact is made by placing the caudal hand on the dorsal aspect of the

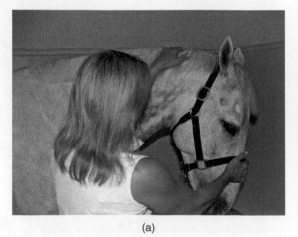
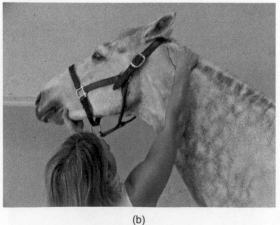

(a)   (b)

Figure 11.11 (a) Flexion of occipito-atlantal joint: the caudal hand provides a fulcrum on the neck while the cranial hand, placed on the nasal region, rocks the head in a nodding direction to assess flexion. (b) Extension of occipito-atlantal joint: cup the chin with the cranial hand and lift up the head to assess extension.

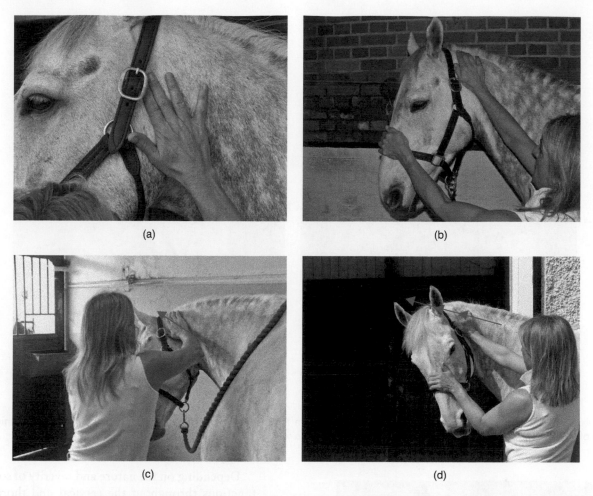

(a)   (b)

(c)   (d)

Figure 11.12 (a) Examination for atlas position: place fingers within the space between the atlas and mandibular ramus to assess symmetry between each side. (b) Atlas technique: the caudal hand cups the wing of the atlas. The cranial hand is placed on the nasal region to compress and flex the head. (c) Direction of thrust: this is obliquely towards the opposite ear. (d) Application of atlas technique: simultaneously compress and laterally flex the head with the cranial hand while the caudal hand applies a high velocity thrust in the direction of the opposite ear.

wing of the atlas. The pisiform is the point of contact, with the cranial hand supporting and reinforcing the caudal hand. Slack is taken up, and after a few springing movements of the arm a thrust is made in a ventral direction (Figures 11.13a and 11.13b).

14. *Axis technique.* Atlanto-axial mobility is rotational, performing the 'no' movement. When the axis is restricted, there is limited rotation and there may be pain and tenderness on palpation. A similar technique can be applied as used for atlas restrictions. Standing on the side that is restricted, the cranial hand is placed on the nasal region to use the head as a lever. Compress, flex and rotate the head to the ipsilateral side, while the caudal hand contacts the axis transverse process. A thrust is made obliquely across in the direction of the opposite ear as the head is simultaneously laterally flexed in one harmonious movement (Figure 11.14).

This technique can be applied along the cervical spine as necessary. For lateral dysfunction where the transverse process appears more prominent, the thrust would be made at a right angle to the vertebra across the midline.

15. *Lower cervical non-leverage thrust using momentum.* For the lower cervical spine the neck is not flexed. Contact is always dorsal to the cervical transverse process. The cranial hand is placed on top of the caudal hand for reinforcement. To introduce momentum and oscillation of the tissues, apply and release the contact point pressure. The thrust is then applied in the direction required, obliquely or medially across the midline (Figure 11.15).

Laurie Hartman (1985, p. 8) explains this technique as follows: 'The momentum effect in this technique is produced by applying and releasing the contact point pressure several times until a state of relaxation is sensed or until the momentum and oscillation of the tissues builds up adequate force at the contact point so that high application of force should not be then necessary.'

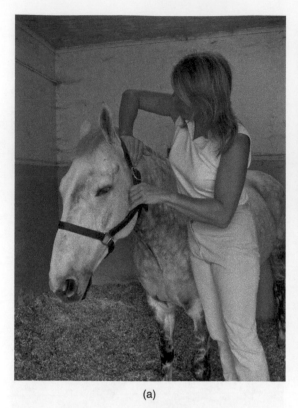

(a)

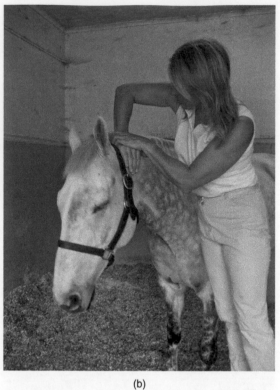

(b)

Figure 11.13 (a) Atlas dorsal technique: place the caudal hand on the dorsal wing of the atlas and reinforce with the cranial hand. (b) Application of dorsal atlas technique: gently spring and then thrust in a ventral direction.

Depending on the nature and severity of somatic dysfunctions throughout the cervical and thoracolumbar spine, the technique is generally performed after releasing the occipito-atlanto-axial junctions. However, some horses benefit from the lower cervical spine being

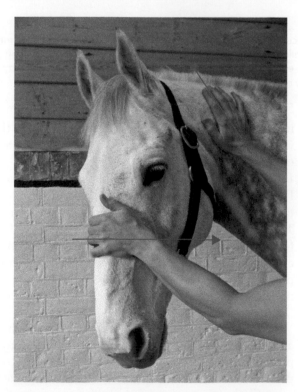

Figure 11.14 Axis technique: contact the axis transverse process and thrust obliquely to the opposite ear while simultaneously laterally flexing the head in one harmonious movement.

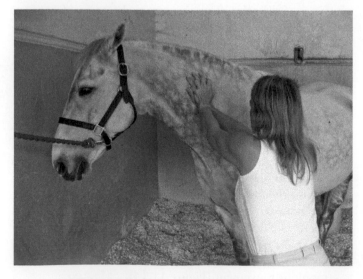

Figure 11.15 Lower cervical technique: contact is always dorsal to the transverse process. Introduce momentum and then apply the thrust in the direction required obliquely or medially across the midline.

initially articulated, which allows unwinding and tissue release to occur before they can tolerate the practitioner treating the upper cervical spine.

Following HVT techniques, the joints are rhythmically articulated to further encourage function and to assess the effect of the technique.

CERVICAL EXERCISES AND STRETCHES

Overview

The development of the dorsal neck musculature is a good indicator of mobility in the upper cervical spine. If it is very flat along the dorsal aspect of the first two cervical vertebrae, it suggests that the horse is blocking the movement. This is often because the rider is flexing the neck at the second and third cervical vertebrae in a false 'on the bit' illusion, instead of striving to get a true flexion through the poll with the horse working correctly through to the bridle. The horse is described as being behind the bit and does not engage through its back. Incorrect use of draw-reins and similar training aids will exacerbate this.

The practitioner can evaluate restrictions in the cervical spine and also actively mobilise the region using two methods. One is tempting the horse with food, and the second using the bridle to guide the horse to move its head and neck.

A carrot is used to encourage the horse to flex the cervical spine in different positions. Carrots are the most appropriate titbits to use as the horse can nibble the top and not reach the practitioner's hand. These exercises are valuable not only in the initial assessment of mobility but also as an indicator of improvement post-treatment.

Owners are always surprised to see how far the neck can laterally bend; they forget that a horse will voluntarily stretch to scratch the stifle or hip region if necessary! It is important to demonstrate the exercises to indicate the range of mobility and to show the correct procedure. The owner or rider can practise these tests at home once a week after the horse has been exercised and the muscles have been warmed up. With a young or 'nippy' horse, however, the exercise would have to be limited and very rarely used as one does not want to encourage the expectation of always receiving titbits!

There are many variations of these exercises. The following are probably the most indicative to cervical mobility and flexibility and are applied as part of the treatment regime following soft tissue techniques. Always compare both sides and gradually increase the stretch. The horse must never struggle to reach the carrot, and if it is having difficulty in any direction discontinue the exercise. The combined lateral flexion and rotation may look good but movement may be all from the lower cervical spine with the upper cervical spinal mobility limited.

Techniques

16. *Cervical carrot exercises and tests.* To test combined lateral flexion with rotation, a carrot is used to tempt the horse to turn its head and flex the neck around to the girth region, initially, and then, only if the horse is able, to the stifle and hip region (Figure 11.16a). This is repeated on both sides for comparison of mobility.

    The carrot is then held up higher to test for upper cervical spinal lateral flexion and to encourage rotation of the atlanto-axial joint. The head should remain as vertical as possible (Figure 11.16b). The horse may have to tilt its head instead of turning correctly if the region is restricted. There is frequently a significant difference between both sides.

    The carrot can then be held low to the floor and to the side to encourage lateral flexion and stretch of the cervical spine at a low angle (Figure 11.16c).

    The carrot is then positioned between the forelimbs so that the horse stretches over the topline to reach it, flexing the lower cervical vertebrae and thoracic inter-vertebral joints (Figure 11.16d).

    Finally the carrot is positioned directly in front of the nose and the practitioner encourages the horse to stretch out in a cranial direction to reach it (Figure 11.16e).

17. *Using a bridle to encourage mobilisation of the dorsal neck musculature.* From the ground the practitioner can show the rider how to mobilise the dorsal cervical musculature. With a snaffle bridle on the horse, the practitioner stands in front and gently encourages the neck to flex laterally and stretch. By observing the mane, the nuchal ligament and associated neck muscles can be seen to 'flick' over from the midline to the side of flexion and rotation (Figure 11.17a). The horse is then encouraged to laterally flex and rotate the neck to the other side. The mane is seen to 'flick' across the midline to the new direction (Figure 11.17b). With advanced horses, this mobility is essential for lateral movements such as the half-pass and sequence changes. It is important to visualise the nuchal ligament, remembering it is not just a rounded cord running at the crest from occiput to withers but has the harp-like lamellar part consisting of bilateral sheets extending down attaching to the cervical vertebrae and thus forming a powerful elastic structure that supports the neck and head.

Once the practitioner is satisfied that the cervical spine is mobile, attention can be concentrated on releasing tension around the skull, occipital and poll region.

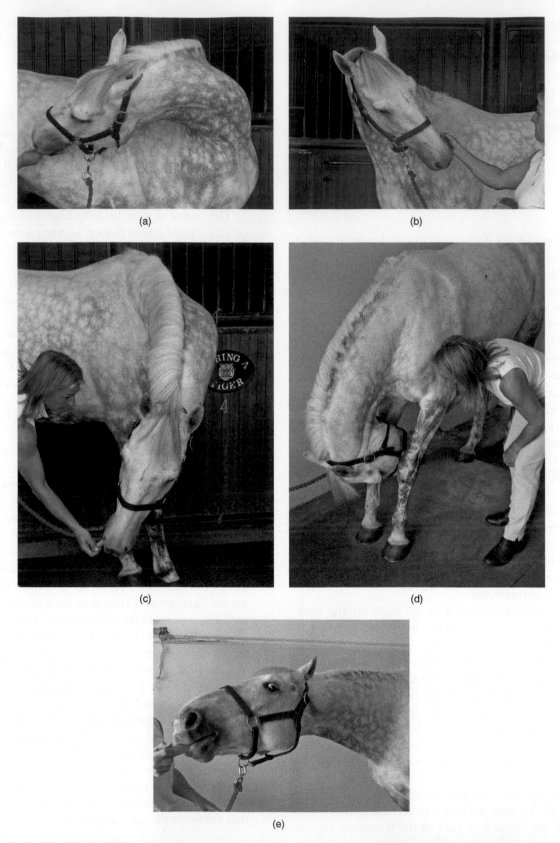

Figure 11.16 (a) Combined lateral flexion and rotation of cervical spine: using a carrot encourages the horse to turn its head to the stifle and hip region. (b) Upper cervical lateral flexion and rotation: hold the carrot higher to encourage rotation of the atlantoaxial joint. (c) Lateral flexion and stretch: hold the carrot low down to the side of the horse. (d) Stretching the topline: hold the carrot between the front limbs to encourage the horse to flex the lower cervical vertebrae and thoracic intervertebral joints. (e) Stretching in a cranial direction: hold the carrot out in front of the nose.

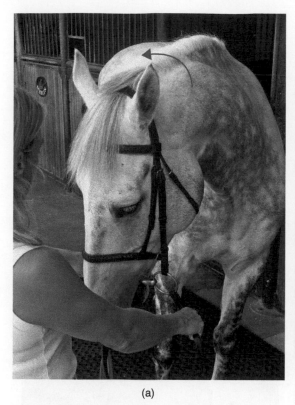
(a)

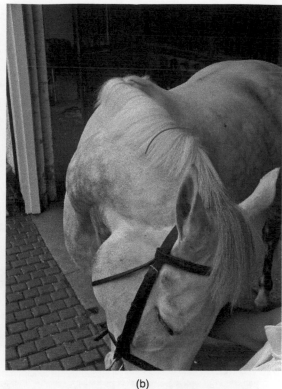
(b)

Figure 11.17 (a) Dorsal cervical musculature: using the bridle to encourage lateral flexion, there is a 'flick' of the mane to that side. (b) The neck is then laterally flexed to the other side: the mane 'flicks' across the midline to that side.

CRANIUM

Overview

There is what I call a 'headache' feel to some horses, around the frontal bone and poll. It is hard to describe but is a palpable tension with the skin seemingly fixed, tight and bound to the bone.

Techniques

18. *Cranium soft tissue techniques.* Begin soft tissue techniques at the poll, encouraging the horse to relax and lower the head (Figure 11.18a). Place the palm of the hand over the frontal bone and apply gentle rolling and circular strokes until the skin slides over the skull with ease (Figure 11.18b). Use friction and inhibitory techniques on any tense and tender regions.

Gentle tapping on the frontal bone is followed by soft tissue techniques and inhibition of trigger points in a rostral direction along the masseter muscles and facial crest (Figure 11.18c). Exactly as one would with the cheek bones of human patients, tap and gently pinch along the facial crest (Figure 11.18d). This seems to facilitate drainage and occasionally there is nasal discharge post-treatment.

As release occurs, gently palpate and stroke, in a rostral direction, the nasal bone and associated soft tissues (Figures 11.18e and 11.18f). This gently applied pressure may have the effect of encouraging the release of endorphins (see Chapter 9). Horses respond by relaxing. Watch the horse's eyes when performing these techniques: they usually relax the eyelids, and the eyes take on a softer expression.

19. *Harmonic mobilisation of cervical spine.* As the horse lowers the head, traction with harmonic mobilisation can then be applied. Cup the cranial hand under the horse's chin and rhythmically pull the chin cranially. At the same time, the caudal hand gently pushes on the frontal bone and occiput in a caudal direction, producing a rocking movement (Figure 11.19a).

Follow this by increasing the traction through the cervical spine. To achieve this the practitioner places the horse's chin on to his or her shoulder and leans backwards to increase the stretch. Sustained positional release techniques can also be used at this point by changing the direction of pull.

From this position the practitioner can then interlace the hands between the occiput and axis spinous process and take up the slack. Rhythmically springing in a ventral, cranial and rostral direction the harmonic mobilisation is continued (Figure 11.19b).

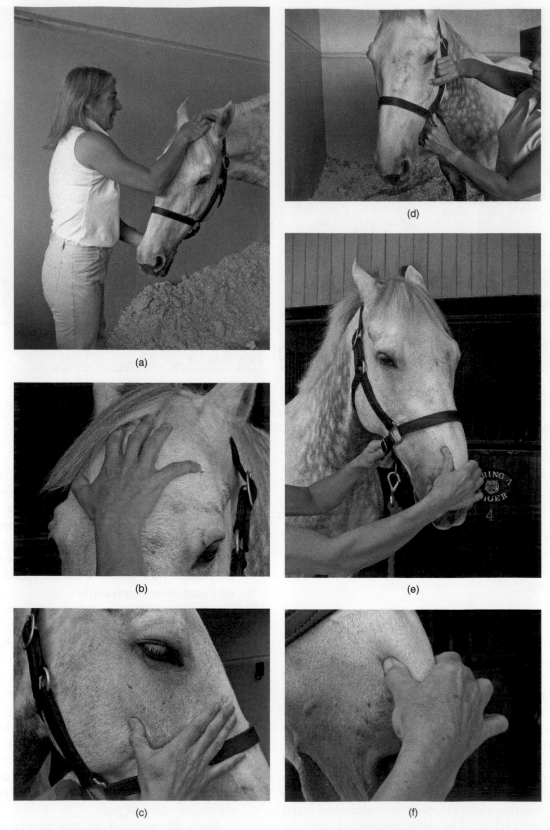

Figure 11.18 (a) Soft tissue technique to the cranium: begin at the poll, encouraging the horse to relax and lower the head. (b) Fascial tissue technique to the frontal bone: place the palm of the hand on the frontal bone and apply gentle rolling and circular strokes. (c) Soft tissue and local inhibition of trigger points: progress in a rostral direction along the facial crest and masseter muscles. (d) Release of facial tissue tension: gently tap and pinch along the facial crest. (e) Effleurage and inhibitory techniques to the nasal region: stroke the nasal region in a rostral direction. (f) Encourage the release of endorphins: gently palpate and stroke along the nasal peak.

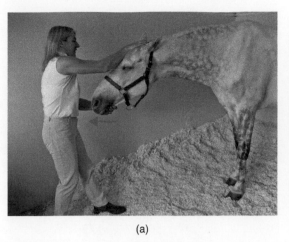

(a)

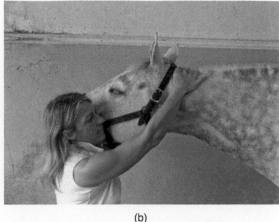

(b)

Figure 11.19 (a) Harmonic mobilisation of cervical spine: cup the chin with the cranial hand and rhythmically pull cranially as the caudal hand gently pushes the frontal bone caudally. (b) Rhythmical springing of cervical spine: interlace the hands between the occiput and axis. Rhythmically spring in a ventral and cranial direction.

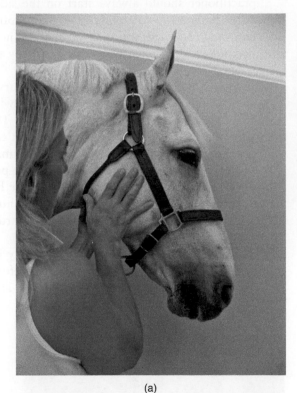

(a)

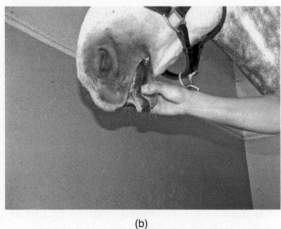

(b)

Figure 11.20 (a) Progression from mandible to muzzle: follow the contours of the mandible in a rostral direction. (b) Release of tissue tension around the muzzle: a gentle wringing movement is applied to the lower lip.

All rhythmic techniques are applied until the practitioner senses a softening in the quality and tone within the musculoskeletal tissue and fascia.

20. *Progression from mandible to chin.* With the thumbs follow from the mandibular angle the contours of the mandible in a rostral direction, using a longitudinal deep stroking movement (Figure 11.20a). On reaching the lower muzzle (chin), a gentle wringing movement is applied to the lower lip, addressing any tension palpated (Figure 11.20b).

21. *Soft tissue techniques to mouth and tongue.* Use a thumb or finger and with a circular movement massage the corner of the mouth (Figure 11.21a) before progressing towards the nasal and incisive region of the skull. The lips of a horse are very mobile and sensitive and can be easily mobilised by the practitioner. Circular rubbing of the underside of the upper lip, along the incisors and gums, and then lifting and stretching the upper lip (Figure 11.21b) have the effect of relaxing the horse if endorphins are released. The lower lip and gum region are similarly palpated. At this point the tongue can be mobilised if required but care must be made not to wrench or force the tongue laterally as it could be damaged on sharp teeth. Irreparable damage may also occur to the attachments if the tongue is pulled too vigorously.

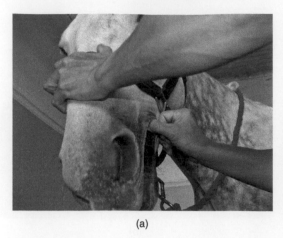

(a)

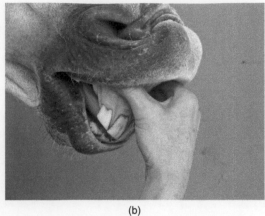

(b)

Figure 11.21 (a) Massage the corners of the mouth: use a thumb or finger and apply gentle circular and stretching movements to the corner of the mouth. (b) Massage to the underside of the upper lip and incisor region: circular rubbing relaxes the horse.

Gently squeeze and longitudinally stroke the nasal peak and nostril region and proceed to the masseter muscles and address any tender trigger points. A wringing and gentle pinching movement can then be applied along the facial crest in a rostral direction.

When working in this area, examine the rostral mandibular and maxillary region for signs of tissue damage from a noseband, headcollar and curb chain that might be affecting the horse's well being.

22. *Mobilisation of the ears*. The horse should stretch its head and neck down as treatment progresses. This is an opportune time to address any restrictions around the poll and ears (Figure 11.22a). The tension around the auricular muscles can be caused by many factors including cervical lesions, a tight browband or headpiece, ill fitted head collar, restricted riding and temperament issues. With patience, even the most headshy horse will allow the practitioner to gently mobilise its ears. The

practitioner should always start on the side that the horse finds more tolerable. One side is often not as tense and restricted, which shows that it is not always a psychological problem as owners frequently assume but is caused by tissue restriction.

Stretch and very gently mobilise the ears in all directions (Figure 11.22b). Pull the ears slowly in a lateral, cranial, caudal and ventral direction. Then gently abduct the ears. Massage the base of each ear and rotate them until the tissues respond. It is amazing how horses respond to these techniques, but the practitioner must take time and only proceed with the horse's cooperation. The forelock is then stroked and pulled in a rostral direction before progressing towards the temporomandibular joint.

23. *Temporomandibular joint*. TMJ symmetry is assessed and soft tissue tension is addressed before specific mobilisation and articulation techniques are applied.

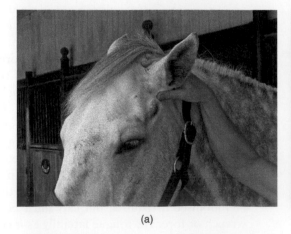

(a)

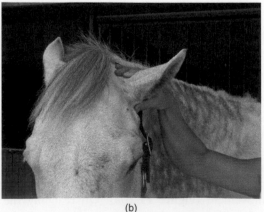

(b)

Figure 11.22 (a) Addressing restrictions around the poll and ears: begin on the side that the horse finds most tolerable to palpation. (b) Mobilisation of the ears: stretch and gently mobilise the ears in all directions.

It is important to make sure the teeth have been regularly rasped to allow the technique to be performed successfully.

Stand to the side of the horse and place the cranial hand on the nose over the naso-incisive notch. The caudal hand grasps the mandible at the chin, and the thumb is placed just inside the mouth in the interdental space, the diastema. Taking the mandible to one side and the nose to the other in a rhythmic motion produces a shearing and translocation movement (Figure 11.23).

If there is restriction in the joint, a specific manipulative technique is used. For example, if the right TMJ is restricted, the practitioner positions themselves on the non-restricted side, which, in this case, is the left side of the horse. Positioning the hands as described above, begin mobilisation using a shearing movement, then applying one quick, sharp thrust to the right with the caudal hand on the mandible, as the cranial hand on the nose simultaneously pulls to the left. This lever technique should restore normal mobility to the affected side.

24. *Hyoid and associated tissue*. Finally, the hyoid and its associated musculature and fascia are palpated in the centre of the intermandibular space. Myofascial release techniques are very effective, restoring the elastic tissue texture, combined with stretching and gentle mobilisation of the hyoid. The structures associated with the hyoid can be cupped in the caudal hand and a rhythmic 'push–pull' movement is applied while

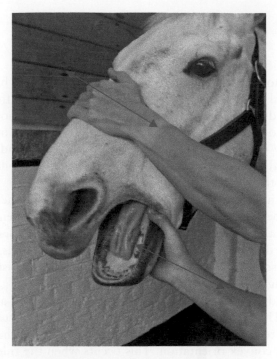

Figure 11.23 Translocation of the temporomandibular joint: taking the nose in one direction and the mandible to the other in a rhythmic motion produces a shearing movement. If there is a restriction, a short, sharp thrust is made in the direction of the restriction.

the nose is supported with the cranial hand. The ventral tissues are then longitudinally stretched using a stroking movement in a rostral direction (Figures 11.24a and 11.24b).

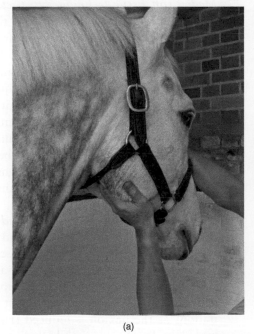
(a)

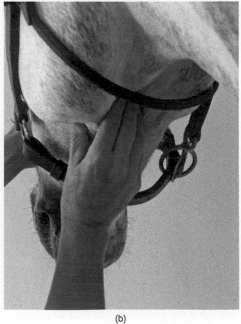
(b)

Figure 11.24 (a) and (b) Hyoid and associated tissues: apply myofascial release techniques finishing with lymphatic drainage.

PECTORAL GIRDLE

Overview

If the horse's stride pattern is compromised by any biomechanical dysfunction, the pectoral girdle is usually affected. This is due to concussive forces and limited protraction and retraction of the forelimb. Restrictions in this region, especially combined with cervicothoracic junction and lumbosacral junction limitations, affect the horse's ability to lighten the forehand.

The jumping horse will not be able to snap up the front feet, open through the spine and clear fences efficiently in front if this region is blocked. There will be difficulties with related distances and jumping through combinations, with the horse struggling to make the height, width and distance, resulting in faults and refusal to jump.

The dressage horse cannot lift up off the forehand and elevate. The withers are fixed and the dorsal neck musculature cranial to the withers region may be concave rather than the normal convex orientation. This occurs when the rider has 'pulled' the horse into shape instead of it developing self-carriage. The horse will be restricted when extending the paces, and within lateral work will be unable to fully adduct and abduct the shoulders, which may result in unlevel steps as the movements are performed.

A rider may try to compensate for this by shortening the neck, with the horse hollowing in front of the withers and extending through the lumbosacral junction. All that is achieved are detrimental biomechanical changes, resulting in even more dysfunction throughout.

On observation horses can look narrow through the chest, which is often described in the equestrian world as being 'as if both front legs came out of one hole'! With correct training and muscular development of the pectoral muscles, this will improve but only if the joints and surrounding tissues are amenable to change. Extensor carpi radialis may be underdeveloped, and brachiocephalicus may be tight, with the horse reluctant to stretch his head down, fully protract the forelimb and move his head laterally from the side of tension.

Deep inhibition, kneading, stretching and mobilisation techniques are used throughout the area.

Techniques

The practitioner uses a stroking movement with the palm of the hands in a ventral direction, following the sternocephalic and brachiocephalic muscles. From here the hands are naturally guided down towards the thorax, pectoral girdle and forelimbs.

25. *Soft tissue techniques for the pectoral and elbow region.* With the caudal hand resting on the withers for stability, the practitioner uses the cranial hand to massage the cranial superficial pectorals (descending pectorals)

(Figure 11.25a). Knead and stretch the tissues (Figure 11.25b) while progressing towards the caudal pectoral muscles. The manubrium of the sternum can be palpated in the midline. The practitioner then places the cranial hand on the cranial pectoral muscles or on the horse's neck for stability. The caudal hand continues treatment ventrally and in a caudal direction along the caudal superficial pectoral muscle (ascending pectorals). Finally, scoop up the tissues medial to the humerus, up towards the point of the elbow. Subsequently, the tissues should feel spongy and pliable.

26. *Soft tissue techniques to triceps muscle.* The cranial hand supports the pectorals at the chest. The caudal hand then gently clasps the triceps medially, with the thumb extended and positioned on the lateral aspect of the triceps. There should be a feeling of being able to 'wobble' the muscle. If there are restrictions within the tissue, the practitioner begins kneading with the fingers deeply medial to the triceps muscle, in a cranial direction (Figure 11.26). Trigger points are inhibited along the belly of the muscle, and soft tissue techniques are applied to the lateral aspect of the triceps before again 'wobbling' and stretching the muscle.

    In some respects, the triceps muscle tone and suppleness are good indicators of the muscular integrity throughout the body. The tone of the triceps must be compared both sides. Overdeveloped shoulder muscles indicate that the horse is pulling itself along instead of propelling from the hindquarters. Exceptions would be carriage and driving horses, which are obviously more developed through their shoulders.

27. *Medial soft tissue techniques to pectorals.* The caudal hand holds the forelimb up with the carpus flexed, and the cranial hand continues soft tissue techniques in the pectoral region at a deeper level. The cranial hand then holds the limb in the same position to allow even deeper soft tissue techniques to be applied medially to the elbow. It is important that the forelimb is not abducted or adducted but remains parallel with the body (Figure 11.27). The musculature here can be very tender and restricted and can be the cause of unlevel steps in the absence of any signs of pathology. It can be a very subtle dysfunction and requires skilled palpation.

28. *Deep soft tissue to the ventral and lateral musculature.* Deep inhibitory techniques and 'wringing' of the brachiocephalic and associated muscles along the lateral and ventral aspect of the neck are applied. There will be a natural response of flexion of the cervical spine laterally which often results in spontaneous cavitations as the flexion is induced (Figure 11.28). Care must be taken because while flexion occurs there is an instinct for the horse to nip and attempt to bite the practitioner.

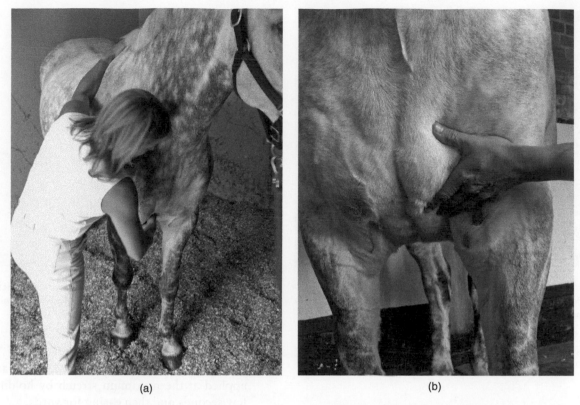

(a)

(b)

Figure 11.25 (a) Soft tissue to the pectoral and elbow region: the caudal hand rests on the withers for stability while the cranial hand applies soft tissue techniques to the cranial superficial pectoral muscles. (b) Soft tissue techniques: knead and stretch the tissues while progressing to the caudal pectoral muscles.

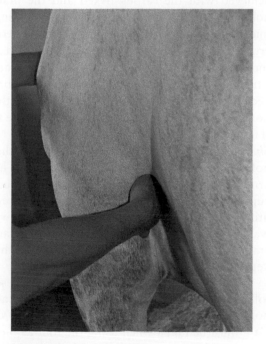

Figure 11.26 Soft tissue to triceps muscle: cranial hand supports the chest while the caudal hand applies deep soft tissue techniques medial to the triceps muscle.

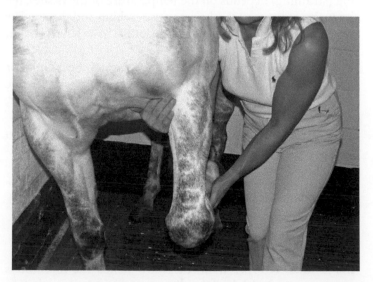

Figure 11.27 Medial soft tissue techniques to the pectorals: holding the leg up with the cranial hand allows deeper techniques to be applied with the caudal hand on the medial aspect. The leg must remain parallel to the horse's body.

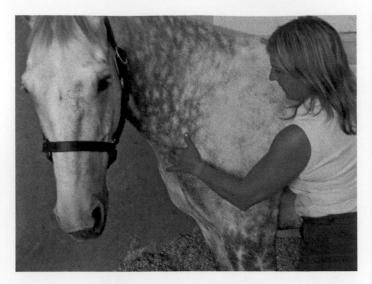

Figure 11.28 Soft tissue to the cervical lateral and ventral muscu-lature: spontaneous cavitations may occur as the horse voluntarily laterally flexes the neck towards the practitioner.

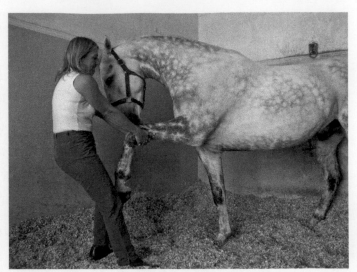

Figure 11.29 Cranial stretch to the shoulder – protraction: sustained traction can be applied. The limb must remain parallel to the horse's body.

SHOULDER GIRDLE STRETCHES

Overview

The shoulders are then stretched. Stretching is a technique to maintain suppleness and elasticity of the muscular tissue, thus enhancing joint mobility and range of movement. It must never be performed before the muscular tissue is warmed up, either by soft tissue techniques or with exercise such as ridden or lunge work.

Overstretching tears the fibres of the muscles, tendons or ligaments, which is a painful process. The risk of overstretch-ing (straining) depends on the temperature of the tissues, the intensity of the stretch, the rate of stretching and the number of repetitions. Cold tissues are susceptible to strains (Clayton 1991, p. 134).

If a horse cannot be exercised due to injury, heat lamps or massage can be used to increase the temperature of specific anatomical areas prior to passive stretching (Clayton 1991, p. 129).

It is important to begin with a small short stretch within the horse's tolerance, never forcing the issue and never jerk-ing the tissues at the finish.

Practitioners must always be very aware of their posture and have a stable base to avoid straining their own back when passively stretching the horse.

Techniques

29. *Cranial stretch*. With the elbow flexed the forelimb is supported with both hands proximal to the carpals. The practitioner gently leans back, rhythmically stretching the shoulder and associated tissue. The limb must not be abducted or adducted but remain parallel with the

horse's body (Figure 11.29). Sustained traction can be applied at the maximum stretch by holding still for a few seconds and then easing forwards.

The neck of the scapula is taken in a cranial direction while the dorsal border moves caudally as in protraction of the forelimb. The forelimb must always be placed slowly and gently on to the ground after the stretch.

30. *Caudal stretch*. In a reverse movement a stretch is achieved with the carpus flexed and the practitioner holding the hoof with the caudal hand, pulling rhyth-mically in a caudal direction whilst simultaneously ex-erting a caudal force with the cranial hand and ensuring the limb is parallel to the body. The cranial hand is po-sitioned either on or above the carpus. This brings the neck of the scapula in a caudal direction with the dorsal border moving cranially as in retraction of the forelimb (Figure 11.30).

31. *Short lever stretch*. A short lever stretch is achieved by holding the carpus fully flexed with the cranial hand and arm supporting the cannon bone, while the caudal hand cups the olecranon process of the ulna. The practitioner utilises his or her body weight by leaning slowly back-wards, while the caudal hand pulls the olecranon in a cranial direction (Figure 11.31). Once again, the limb is kept parallel to the horse.

Short lever stretches are used initially. These can be followed by long lever stretches with the practitioner holding the fetlock and foot and stretching the shoulder. Care must be taken when using the foot as the contact for a long lever. It may result with the horse snatching it back and unbalancing both itself and the practitioner. If the horse is resisting, the practitioner must not pull

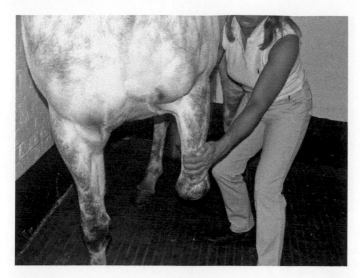

Figure 11.30 Caudal stretch to the shoulder – retraction: the limb must remain parallel to the body.

violently against it as the pectoral muscles and associated tissues could be damaged and torn.

CERVICOTHORACIC JUNCTION

Overview

This junction is one of the key areas that must be mobile if the horse is to be biomechanically sound. The treatment procedures so far illustrated do not necessarily follow a strict order. This technique can be applied very early on but is quite often more effective when the pectoral musculature and associated tissue are optimised initially. As treatment progresses, the mobility through the cervicothoracic

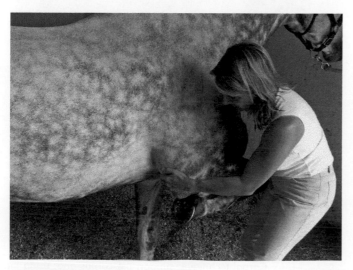

Figure 11.31 Short lever stretch: hold the carpus fully flexed supporting the leg with the cranial hand and cup the olecranon with the caudal hand to apply the stretch in a cranial direction.

junction should be assessed intermittently. Improvement of mobility through this region may be a good indicator of how effectively the horse is responding to treatment.

Technique

32. *Cervicothoracic junction technique.* Place the palm of the cranial hand on the manubrium of the sternum and associated pectorals while the palm of the caudal hand is placed on the withers (Figure 11.32a). A rhythmical pushing pressure is applied between the hands, alternately in a caudal then cranial direction (Figure 11.32b). There should be an impression of fluidity between the hands. The practitioner must palpate and differentiate the range of movement through the cervicothoracic junction. There is a distinct feeling of resistance, more like a 'blocking', when the junction is dysfunctional. The correct movement can be described as having a 'slinky' oscillating between both hands which, optimally, is a very light feeling. When restricted, it is as if one is pushing a wall. There are obviously numerous variations in between!

I learnt this excellent technique from Anthony Pusey when observing him treat a horse under sedation. I found that with practice it could also be applied very effectively and efficiently when treating the unsedated horse.

The thorax suspended within the muscular sling allows for abduction and adduction of the limbs in a way that has a significant influence on overall movement (Smythe and Goody 1993, p. 7).

FORELIMB

Overview

It is a logical progression to examine and mobilise the forelimbs at this stage of treatment. On initial palpation of the horse, any abnormalities of the forelimb, such as windgalls, splints or sidebones, should have been identified as these are all signs of concussion and stress on the limb.

Observe any asymmetry between the extensor carpi radialis muscles and palpate for tension and tightness. Osteopathic soft tissue work to these muscles can greatly enhance the horse's protraction, cadence and proprioceptive mechanism. Any mobilisation of the limbs will help reduce concussive forces through the body.

Low-velocity high-amplitude techniques are applied, that is, taking the joint through the complete range of movement slowly and rhythmically.

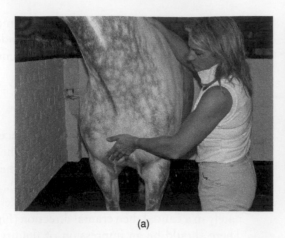
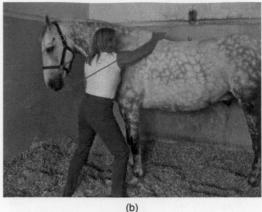

(a)   (b)

Figure 11.32 (a) Cervicothoracic junction technique positioning: place the palm of the cranial hand on the manubrium while the caudal hand is placed on the withers. (b) Cervicothoracic junction technique: a rhythmical pressure is applied between the hands. There should be an impression of fluidity between the hands.

Techniques

Begin with soft tissue techniques along the extensor carpi radialis. The knee or carpus moves in one direction, flexion and extension.

When flexed, 'a gap forms at the front between the radius and the upper row of carpal bones (radio-carpal joint); a second gap forms between the two rows of carpal bones (intercarpal joint). A third gap is hardly noticeable, that between the lower row of carpal bones and the metacarpus' (Smythe and Goody 1993, pp. 51–52).

Gapping these joints can be achieved in two ways (techniques 33 and 34).

Caution: Reminder to the practitioner that care must be taken when performing any of these techniques on young or older horses in case of developmental or degenerative changes.

33. *Carpal technique*. Support the carpus with the cranial hand and cup the fetlock with the caudal hand. Then, using the distal part of the limb as a lever, flex the carpals, applying a quick sharp flexion at the end of the range of movement (Figure 11.33).
34. *Carpal technique using the hand as a fulcrum*. The carpus is gently flexed over the cranial hand (Figure 11.34a). Then the same technique as used in technique 33 is applied, using a crisp, sharp, rhythmic movement at the end of the range of movement over the cranial hand (Figure 11.34b).

    Cavitation sounds from the carpal joints may be elicited.
35. *Friction techniques to the tendons*. The carpus is flexed and the superficial and deep tendons are palpated in a distal direction (Figure 11.35). Gentle friction techniques can be applied followed by a gentle oscillation of the tendons between the fingers.

36. *Mobilisation of fetlock and pastern joints*. The fetlock and pastern joints are mobilised by flexing (Figure 11.36a) and extending (Figure 11.36b) them using the hoof as a lever. There can be a dramatic difference between the ranges of movement of these joints in individual horses. This may be an indicator of the cushioning

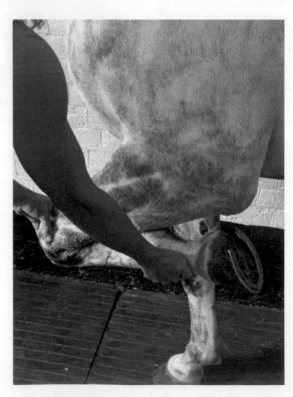

Figure 11.33 Carpal technique: support the carpus and, using the distal part of the leg as a lever, flex the carpals. If there are no contraindications apply a quick sharp flexion at the end of the range of movement.

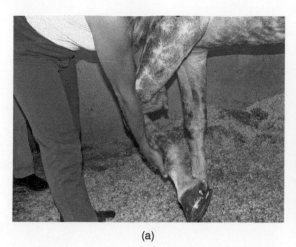

(a)

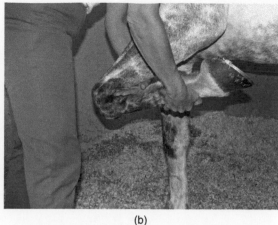

(b)

Figure 11.34 (a) Carpal technique positioning: using the hand as a fulcrum the carpals are flexed over the cranial hand. (b) Carpal technique: using the hand as a fulcrum, apply a crisp, sharp flexion of the carpals at the end of the range of movement over the cranial hand, assuming there are no contraindications.

and potential for jarring through the limb on impact with the ground.

Axially rotate the distal limb joints, and on finding restrictions use shearing movements in a medial direction (Figure 11.36c) followed by a lateral direction (Figure 11.36d) applying a sharper thrust in the direction of restriction.

The condition of the hoof and frog and the wear and type of shoes should be re-examined in more depth at this point. Always compare both feet. 'Asymmetry in foot size may be the result of trauma or congenital or developmental defects and reduced weight-bearing leading to contraction. In general, the limb with the

smallest foot is usually the limb involved with lameness' (Stashak 1995, p. 92).

THORACIC SPINE

Overview

The thoracic trapezius muscle and associated tissues are greatly affected by incorrectly fitting saddles. Muscular tone may be poor and uneven. There will be a tight, bound feel and the fascia appears 'stuck' rather than sliding over the deeper tissues when palpated. The thoracic spinous processes and the associated rib angles may be tender and painful. There could be an area of inflammation of the supraspinous ligament that is extremely sensitive when touched and the horse responds by dipping its back sharply. The practitioner will palpate a raised bump along the dorsal aspect of the spine but must not confuse this with prominent dorsal spinous processes in thin or poorly muscled horses. Areas of white hair are indicative of tissue damage and circulatory dysfunction induced by incorrect pressure from the saddle.

Techniques

37. *Lateral mobilisation of the thoracic spine.* The withers are easy to palpate and mobilise. First the withers are pushed away with the thenar eminence of both hands to achieve a lateral mobilisation across the midline (Figure 11.37a). The withers are then pulled with the fingers back across the midline (Figure 11.37b). Progression in a caudal direction can be made along the thoracic spine, pushing and pulling the tips of the spinous processes between the fingers and thenar eminence in a rhythmic motion.

Figure 11.35 Friction techniques to the tendons: gentle friction followed by oscillation of the tendons between the fingers is applied in a distal direction.

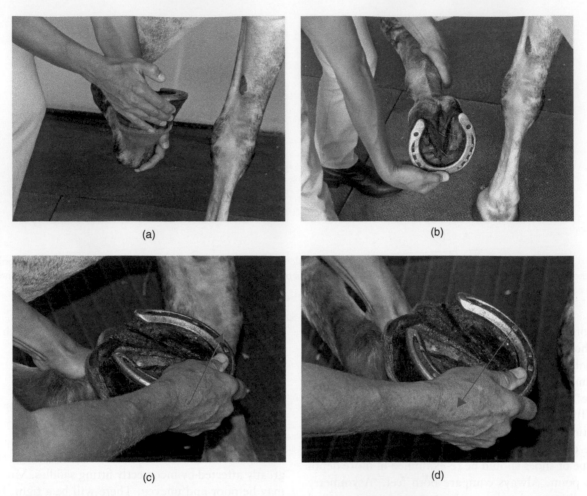

(a) (b)

(c) (d)

Figure 11.36 (a) Flexion of the fetlock and pastern joints: use the hoof as a lever and flex the fetlock and pastern joints. (b) Extension of the fetlock and pastern: use the hoof as a lever to extend the joints. (c) Shearing mobility of the distal joints: using the hoof as a lever move the joints in a medial direction. (d) Shearing mobility of the distal joints: move the joints in a lateral direction. On finding any restrictions apply a sharp thrust in the direction of the restriction.

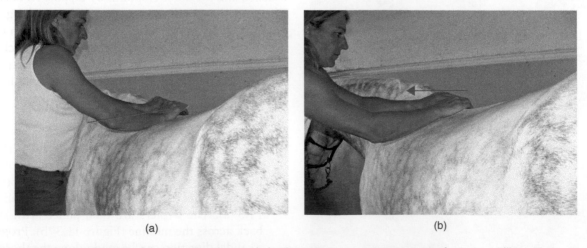

(a) (b)

Figure 11.37 (a) Lateral mobilisation of the thoracic spine: push the thoracic spinous processes away from the midline with the thenar eminence of both hands. (b) Lateral pull: grip the tips of the spinous processes with both hands and pull them across the midline. Rhythmically progress with the push–pull technique along the thoracic spine in a caudal direction.

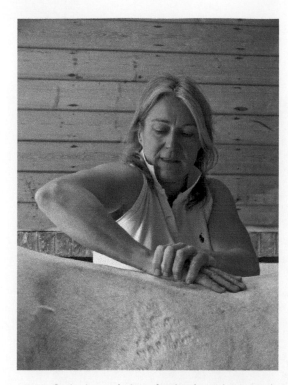

Figure 11.38 Springing technique for the thoracic spine: thenar aspect of caudal hand supported by the cranial hand contacts the dorsal aspect of the spinous process. A springing motion is produced.

38. *Springing technique for the thoracic spine.* Thoracic movement can be further assessed and mobilisation effected by springing along the thoracic spinous processes. The thenar aspect of the caudal hand is used as the contact point, with the cranial hand providing support and reinforcement. The practitioner's elbows are flexed to allow freedom of movement through the arms. A springing motion is then produced as the hands progress in a caudal direction along the thoracic spine (Figure 11.38).

39. *Push–pull harmonic technique along the thoracic spine.* This can be followed by another thoracic mobilisation technique. The practitioner stands alongside the horse with the cranial hand cupping the withers, and pulls and then pushes them in rhythm. The caudal hand pushes against the ribs in an oblique or medial direction across the midline, alternately releasing the contact in synchronisation with the cranial hand as it pushes and pulls the withers (Figure 11.39a). This push–pull technique progresses rhythmically along the thoracic spine in a caudal direction. The caudal hand can then use the tuber coxa as a contact point (Figure 11.39b).

This harmonic technique should be applied from both sides. The practitioner can stand on a suitable ob-

ject if height is required to perform these techniques (Figure 11.39c).

40. *Mobilisation using the tail as a lever.* The tail can be used as a lever, pulling the horse laterally as the cranial hand pushes against the ribs (Figure 11.40). This laterally flexes and stretches the thoracic spine and ribs on the contralateral side.

41. *Thoracic technique using a momentum-induced thrust with the tail as a lever.* At the point of any restriction, a momentum-induced thrust using the tail as a lever can be applied. Using the pisiform of the cranial hand, contact is made on the lateral aspect of the thoracic spinous process. The caudal hand uses the tail to elicit momentum through the spine by pulling and releasing with a rhythmic movement. The thrust is made with the cranial hand across the thoracic spinous process in synchronisation, with the tail being used as the lever.

This technique can be applied from the ground or standing on a suitable object to ensure the correct positioning is obtained (Figure 11.41).

Laurie Hartman (1985, p. 8) describes the momentum-induced thrust as follows: 'The main part of the leverage is applied and released several times in succession and the thrust is applied as the patient is in a relaxed phase or as movement builds up to a suitable level at the lesion point. This has the advantage that the patient and operator are gently on the move and the point of optimum tension can be much more readily felt by the operator's own proprioceptive mechanism.'

42. *Non-leverage thrust to the thoracic spine.* A direct non-leverage thrust can be applied if positional asymmetry and painful restrictions are palpated along the thoracic spine. The practitioner stands on the side of tenderness on a suitable object to obtain correct positioning for the height of the horse. The pisiform of the practitioner's dominant hand is the point of contact with the lateral aspect of the thoracic spinous process. The other hand stabilises and reinforces the contact, either by interlacing fingers or supporting the wrist of the contact hand (Figure 11.42a).

The slack is taken up and a thrust, using high velocity and low-amplitude force, is applied straight across the spinous process (Figure 11.42b). The springing recoil of the tissues appears to restore joint integrity and elasticity. Horses often respond by taking a deep breath, then exhaling with an audible sigh.

Post-treatment, the horse will look relaxed across the thoracic spine and the back appears raised and less hollow through the saddle region. The withers will seem less dominant and the overall stance is more within a 'square' on observation.

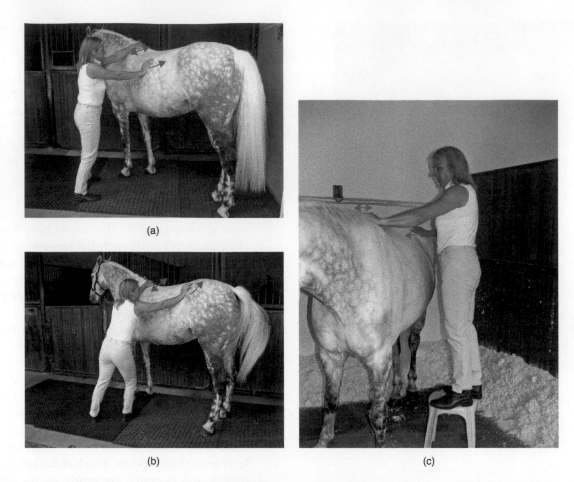

Figure 11.39 (a) Push–pull harmonic technique: the cranial hand cups the withers and pulls then pushes the withers in rhythm while the caudal hand pushes and releases against the ribs in synchronisation with the cranial hand. (b) Push–pull harmonic technique: the caudal hand then uses the tuber coxa as the contact point to push against. (c) Thoracic harmonic technique standing on a suitable object giving the practitioner height if required: the cranial hand contact can be on the withers or the caudal thoracic spinous processes to produce the harmonic technique while the caudal contact is on the tuber coxa.

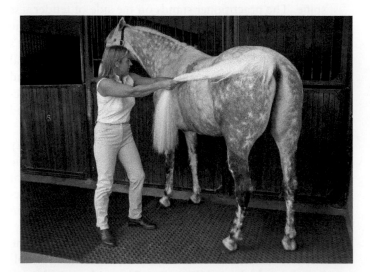

Figure 11.40 Mobilisation using the tail as a lever: pull the tail laterally as the cranial hand pushes on the ribs. This flexes and stretches the thoracic spine on the contralateral side.

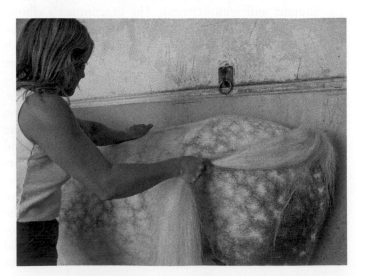

Figure 11.41 Momentum-induced thrust using the tail as a lever: contact with the pisiform is on the lateral aspect of the spinous process. Use the tail to elicit momentum and lateral flexion to allow the thrust to be applied across the spinous process as the slack is taken up.

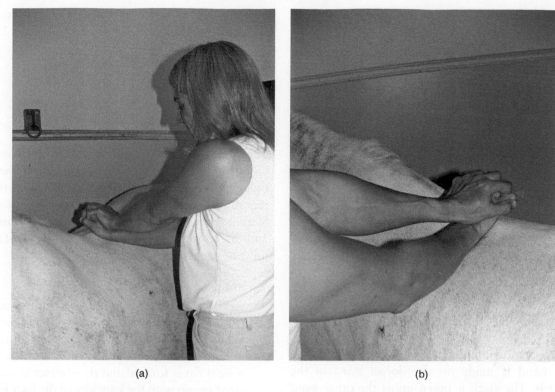

(a)   (b)

Figure 11.42 (a) Direct non-leverage thrust technique: the pisiform of the dominant hand contacts the spinous process while the other hand stabilises and reinforces the contact hand. (b) Direct non-leverage thrust technique: slack is taken up and, using high velocity and low amplitude force, a thrust is applied straight across the spinous process.

DORSAL RIB TECHNIQUE

Overview

The mobility of the ribs can be assessed in a similar fashion to the thoracic spine. Any of the thoracic mobilisations will inevitably have mobilised the associated ribs. Care must be taken, as horses can be especially sensitive along the ribs if there are any musculoskeletal dysfunctions within the region.

Techniques

43. *Low-amplitude thrust.* This is similar to thoracic technique 41, but the contact point is made with the pisiform of the cranial hand on the dorsal third of the restricted rib. The caudal hand uses the tail to elicit momentum but the leverage is kept to a minimum. The tail is used to flex the horse around the contact point and then only minimally oscillated. When the tissue tension at the point of contact is maximal, a high-velocity thrust is made in an oblique caudal direction (Figure 11.43).

44. *Non-leverage thrust technique.* A direct non-leverage thrust technique, as described in technique 42, is

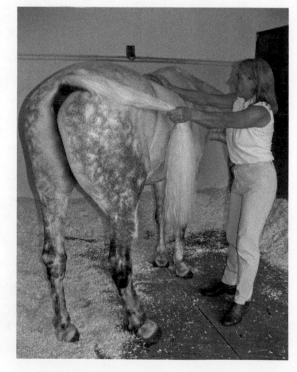

Figure 11.43 Dorsal rib technique low-amplitude thrust: the pisiform of the cranial hand contacts the dorsal third of the rib. The tail is used to elicit minimal momentum. A high-velocity thrust is applied in an oblique caudal direction across the rib.

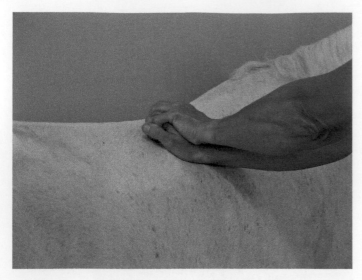

Figure 11.44 Direct non-leverage thrust: contact is on the dorsal third of the rib with the pisiform of the dominant hand. Introduce momentum then thrust, using velocity not force, in a ventral and caudal direction.

applied. The contact point with the pisiform of the dominant hand is made on the dorsal third of the restricted rib. The slack is taken up as the other hand reinforces the contact hand. The rib is gently bounced, which introduces momentum and then, as the tissues

respond, a thrust is made in a ventral and caudal direction using velocity not force (Figure 11.44).

LATERAL RIB TECHNIQUE

Overview
The lateral rib technique is especially useful when addressing girthing problems. Horses that resent the girth being tightened up are often very sensitive around the lateral rib region and surrounding tissues from rib 5 to ribs 8 and 9. Within the intercostal space there may be acute tenderness and the horse will be reactive on palpation. The osteopath must be cautious when examining this area.

Technique
45. *Lateral rib technique.* The practitioner stabilises their position by placing the cranial hand on the horse's withers. Locate the intercostal space dorsal and adjacent to the costochondral joints. With the caudal hand a tight fist is formed and the contact is made at the desired region with the knuckles of the four fingers (Figure 11.45a). The practitioner gently kneads into the space taking up the slack.

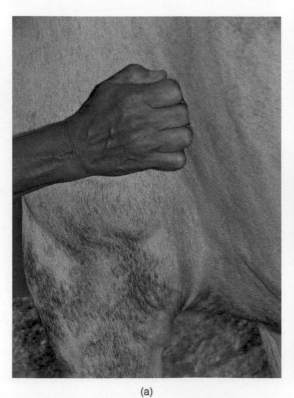

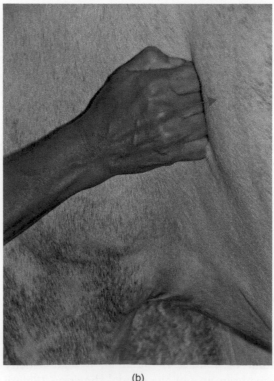

(a)   (b)

Figure 11.45 (a) Lateral rib technique positioning: use the knuckles to contact on the intercostal space dorsal and adjacent to the costochondral joints. (b) Lateral rib technique: gently knead into position taking up the slack and apply a high-velocity thrust in a medial, slightly dorsal direction between the ribs.

The horse will often resent this pressure and will move away. It is important to maintain a firm contact for the technique to be successful. Quite commonly the practitioner has to relocate the contact point but should not persist if the horse is becoming intolerant. If the horse reacts sharply to the contact, the practitioner can stabilise the horse's movement by holding the headcollar and keeping the head flexed towards them.

Timing is essential to optimise the horse's tolerance to the positioning. At the point at which the horse relaxes and the tissues are receptive, a high-velocity thrust with minimal force is applied in a medial and slightly dorsal direction between the ribs (Figure 11.45b).

This is quite an advanced technique that needs to be used precisely as horses respond instantly to it and can react suddenly. There is an immediate release of muscular tissue tension causing them to jump away as the thrust is performed. This is then usually followed by relaxation and lowering of the head while exhaling deeply and audibly.

Continue by once again gently oscillating the cervicothoracic junction as described in technique 7. The mobility will have improved and the horse relaxes into the movement, allowing the practitioner to continue on to the next procedure.

Note: Sensitivity of the tissues and resentment to the tightening of the girth is also an associated sign with horses that are suffering from gastric or duodenal ulcers. Any unexplained changes in behaviour such as the horse starting to wind suck or where performance is lack lustre with no obvious explanation should lead the practitioner to consider referral for veterinary opinion. The diagnosis is black and white in the sense that the horse either has ulcers or does not. Treatment for ulcers is effective and so for the horse's welfare this is an important differential diagnosis.

STERNUM XIPHOID

Overview

I often finish a treatment with a sternum xiphoid release technique. As must always be emphasised, however, there is no rigid routine to any treatment. The sternum xiphoid release, which is a harmonic technique, can be applied to lead the practitioner on to the next major region consisting of the lumbar spine and pelvic girdle.

Technique

46. *Sternum xiphoid release technique.* The practitioner rests the dorsal hand on the thoracic spinous processes, approximately between the ninth and twelfth thoracic

vertebrae. The palm of the ventral hand rests lightly on the abdomen at the xiphoid process in an arrowhead-shaped indentation, which can be viewed from the ventral aspect (Figure 11.46a).

The ventral hand then gradually and almost imperceptibly encourages spinal dorsal flexion by gently applying pressure with the fingers at the point of the arrow. The horse flexes, lifting up through the spine and, usually simultaneously, lowers the head and neck.

The palm of the ventral hand continues to apply gentle pressure in a dorsal direction while the dorsal hand simply rests on the thoracic spinous processes, creating an energy link between the two hands (Figure 11.46b).

A feeling of release is perceived between the practitioner's hands. I describe this as 'if releasing butterflies'!

The practitioner can if necessary play a more active role to encourage release by gently ironing and teasing the tissues at the point of the arrowhead. The hands may be reversed depending on the practitioner's preference and may be interchanged, if required, as the horse responds.

SPINAL REFLEXES

Overview

Horses need to be encouraged to flex through the thoracolumbar spine and lumbosacral junction as the dorsal chain is generally tight and tense compared with the ventral chain. This can be accomplished using spinal reflexes.

Flexion-inducing reflexes result in a separation of the thoracic spinous processes, which resembles a fan spreading open. The ligamentous tissue along the spinous processes and the supraspinous and interspinous ligaments will be stretched, along with the erector spinae musculature and fascia.

This can be explained to the owner and rider by opening the fingers of one hand in abduction as an example of the fan effect within the spinous processes. This will help them understand the stretch across the spine.

The abdominal muscles are also activated as these reflexes are performed. Good abdominal tone is as essential to the horse for stabilisation of the spine and posture as it is to us! Weak abdominal muscles are always a clear indicator that the horse is not working correctly through its back. The activation of these muscles as the spine is flexed should be pointed out to the owner. Additionally point out the region on the lateral aspect of the ribs where correct leg aids should be applied. This will help the rider understand how the horse responds by contracting and lifting the abdomen as the spine is flexed in response to these aids.

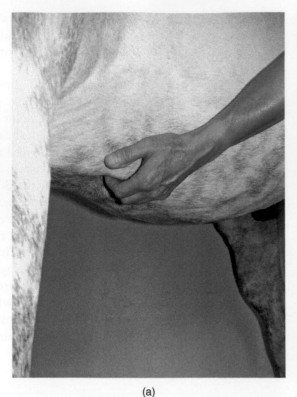
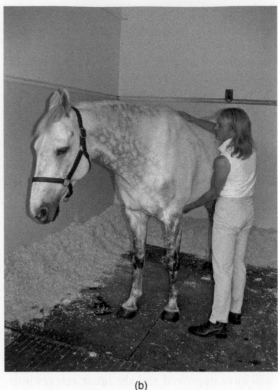

(a)   (b)

Figure 11.46 (a) Sternum xiphoid release: the dorsal hand rests on thoracic spinous processes while the ventral hand is placed on the xiphoid and gently applies pressure in a dorsal direction. (b) The horse gently flexes the spine: an energy link is felt between the hands and a feeling is perceived as if releasing butterflies.

The practitioner should stand to the side assessing its re-action and must apply the stimulus carefully as some horses resent the mobilisation through the spine and will buck and kick out. Palpation around the girth region may cause the horse to strike upwards with the front foot and or turn to nip the practitioner or handler.

I have noticed in practice that mares show more resistance to flexing the lumbosacral junction, so expectations should be modified and the technique performed gently. Always be politer with mares. They can very easily be provoked into kicking out at the practitioner!

The thoracolumbar and lumbosacral flexion reflexes are applied cautiously and gently to assess the ease of flexion throughout the spine as previously described in the pal-patory examination. Subtle dysfunctions in the cervicotho-racic, thoracic and lumbar regions may be observed.

As treatment progresses, the reflexes can be stimulated more vigorously, for example when addressing the lum-bosacral junction.

Finally, the thoracolumbar flexion reflex can be used near the end of the treatment session to re-examine and assess im-provement in the general mobility of the spine and activation of the core muscles.

Personally, I always begin by stroking the region I wish to stimulate and then, if the horse is receptive, increase the pressure deeper into the tissue. Some practitioners use a blunt instrument to illicit the reflexes. As a rule, I use my hand, unless the horse is unresponsive and dull to the reflex.

Techniques

47. *Thoracolumbar spinal flexion.* Standing by the shoulder of the horse, begin by stroking ventrally down the neck and pectoral muscles before resting the dorsal hand on the neck or withers. The palm of the ventral hand then gently strokes the abdomen from the sternum in a caudal direction to encourage flexion of the thoracic spine.

As the horse responds and is confident with the move-ment, the practitioner repeats the process, exerting more pressure each time until the horse fully flexes the spine within the limits of its ability. If the horse is not reacting adversely to the palm of the hand, use the fingertips to increase stimulation of the reflex. The abdominal mus-cles are observed tightening and, as the horse flexes, a totally different shape is seen as it lifts up through the withers and relaxes the cervical extensor muscles as the neck is lowered and stretched (Figures 11.47a and 11.47b).

48. *Lumbosacral spinal flexion.* The practitioner stands to the side of the horse's hindquarters rather than directly behind, where there is a risk of being kicked. Initially

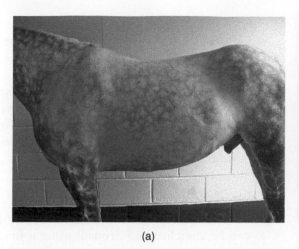
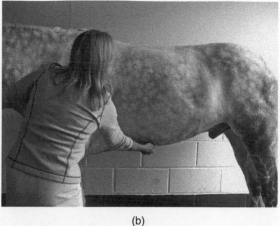

(a)   (b)

Figure 11.47 (a) Horse standing in relaxed position: note the white brick space under the abdomen. (b) Encourage thoracolumbar flexion: stroke gently in a caudal direction. The abdomen and topline lift up. Note the increased area of white bricks now visible under the abdomen.

stroke both hands either side of the sacrum in a caudal direction. Then, if the horse is receptive, run the fingers along the lateral borders of the sacrum and gluteal musculature, caudally, stimulating flexion through the lumbosacral junction (Figure 11.48). If necessary, the practitioner can stand on a suitable object to apply this technique.

49. *Lateral flexion of the thoracolumbar spine.* Lateral flexibility can be assessed by stroking the lateral thoracic region in a cranial to caudal direction with the fingers.

Begin with a light touch and progress to a deeper pressure within the limits of the horse's tolerance. There is contraction of the erector spinae musculature on the concave side to the stimulus, with stretching on the convex side (Figure 11.49). This should be applied from both sides and mobility compared.

50. *Thoracolumbar spine extension.* The technique must be applied gently as the horse will often resent this movement and react to its application. The practitioner places the fingers on the withers, either side of the spinous processes. Pressing down firmly in a ventral direction the hand is run down the spine in a caudal direction. The horse will dip its back and often hollow the neck in response to the stimulus (Figure 11.50).

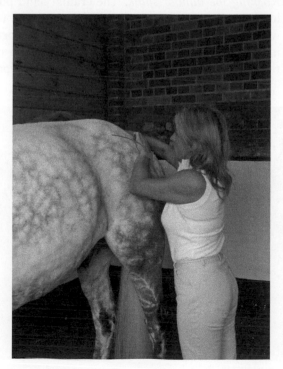

Figure 11.48 Lumbosacral flexion: run the fingers along the lateral borders of the sacrum caudally, stimulating flexion of the lumbosacral junction.

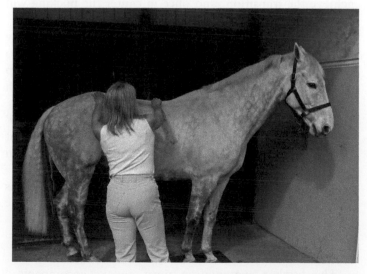

Figure 11.49 Lateral flexion of thoracolumbar spine: stroke along the lateral thoracic region in a cranial to caudal direction. There is contraction of the erector spinae on the concave side with stretching on the convexity.

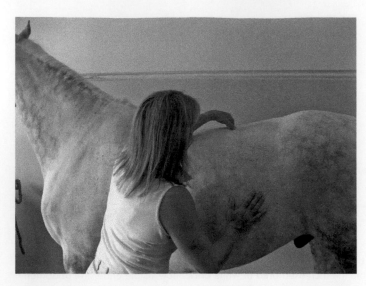

Figure 11.50 Thoracolumbar extension: press firmly in a ventral direction either side of the spinous processes as the hand progresses in a caudal direction. The horse will dip its back in response to the stimulus.

LUMBAR SPINE

Overview

Any restriction in the lumbar spine results in a feeling of tightness behind the saddle, and protraction of the hindlimbs may be compromised. The horse is unable to take the weight on to the hindquarters and swing correctly through its body. The outline remains straight with the weight on the forehand. It will often buck into the canter in response to the rider's aids. This seems to provide the impulsion needed to achieve the transition, and once in canter the bucking will usually cease.

When approaching a jump the horse will often throw its head up and rush, using speed instead of impulsion to clear the fence. In the air, instead of rounding over the jump described as the bascule, it will be flat and restricted through the spine.

The rider will often report that the horse feels 'blocked' behind the saddle, with resistance to carrying the weight behind, so throwing the centre of gravity more forward on to the forehand.

The integrity of the lumbar spine and associated tissues may be affected by any pelvic joint dysfunction. Fryette (1980, p. 94) stated that:

The lumbar examination must always accompany sacroiliac examination. The lumbar spine must be examined for muscular, ligamentous and fascia shortening, tension, mobility, tenderness, and position.

To perform some of these techniques, the practitioner may need to stand on a suitable stool or crate. Remember that it must not be something either you or the horse could be injured by.

Soft tissue techniques are applied to the lumbar, sacral and femoral musculature and fascia. Transverse techniques, stretching, inhibition of trigger points, deep kneading and friction, are just some examples that are applied depending on the findings at examination.

Techniques

51. *Functional technique*. The erector spinae musculature can be stretched and 'ironed' using a functional technique. The cranial hand is placed on the withers or caudal thoracic spinous processes. The caudal hand is placed on the region of the lumbosacral junction. Pressure is applied in a cranial and caudal direction, respectively, increasing the distance between the hands as the horse responds to the fascial drag produced between the contact points (Figure 11.51).
52. *Lumbar spine springing*. Springing of the lumbar spine is achieved using a similar technique to the one applied when springing the thoracic spine. The thenar eminence of one hand is reinforced with the other hand to produce the downward ventral motion. The contact point can be either the lumbar spinous processes or just lateral to the spinous processes (Figure 11.52).
53. *Rocking the lumbar spine*. The cranial hand pulls the lumbar spinous processes medially across the midline while the caudal hand pushes against the tuber coxa in a rhythmical movement. This produces an oscillation throughout the spine. The horse should respond by

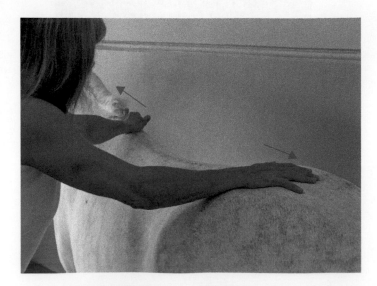

Figure 11.51 Functional technique to erector spinae musculature: place the cranial hand on the withers and the caudal hand on the lumbosacral junction. Stretch and 'iron' out the tissues.

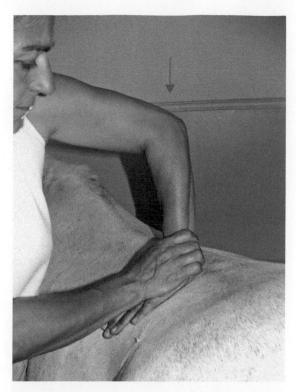

Figure 11.52 Lumbar spine springing: the thenar eminence of one hand is reinforced with the other to produce a springing motion along the lumbar spinous processes or lateral to the lumbar spinous process.

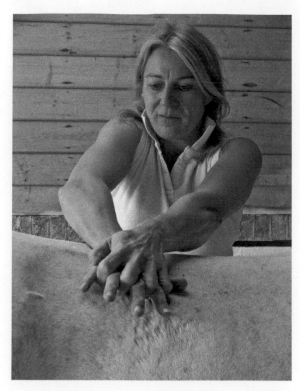

Figure 11.54 Direct thrust to lumbar spine: standing on the contralateral side to the restriction, use a pisiform contact over the region of the transverse process. Lean over and take up the slack before applying a sharp, high-velocity thrust in a ventral direction.

lowering its head as the muscle chains release and stretch (Figure 11.53).

54. *Direct thrust.* The practitioner stands on the contralateral side to the dysfunction, at a height that allows contact with the required area, to address any specific restrictions in the lumbar spine. The pisiform of one hand

makes contact lateral to the lumbar spinous process over the region of the transverse process and is reinforced with the other hand. The practitioner then leans over the horse using their body weight to take up the slack and, maintaining the pressure, applies a sharp, high-velocity, low-amplitude thrust downwards in a ventral direction (Figure 11.54).

HINDQUARTERS AND FEMORAL REGION

Overview

The lumbosacral junction is one of the key regions that need to be addressed. Before the practitioner specifically mobilises this junction, the pelvic and sacral musculature must be released as necessary.

Deep soft tissue techniques are applied along the gluteal musculature and fascia, working caudally towards the hamstrings and associated tissue. This can be followed by deep soft tissue and mobilising techniques, specifically around the greater trochanter of the femur.

Techniques

55. *Soft tissue to the femoral region.* The practitioner holds the tail with the caudal hand while using the thumb

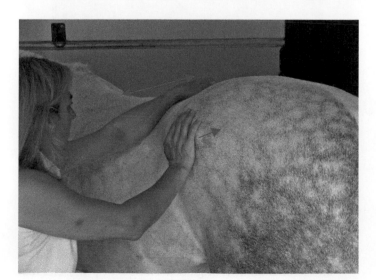

Figure 11.53 Rocking the lumbar spine: the cranial hand pulls the spinous processes medially while the caudal hand rhythmically pushes the tuber coxa.

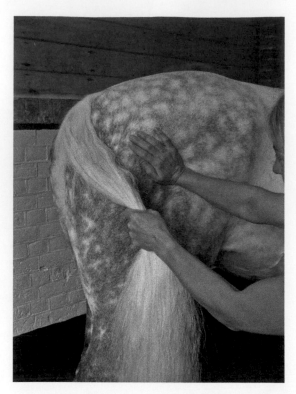

Figure 11.55 Soft tissue to the femoral region: the tail is held to stabilise the practitioner and hold the horse's attention.

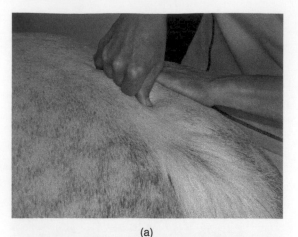

(a)

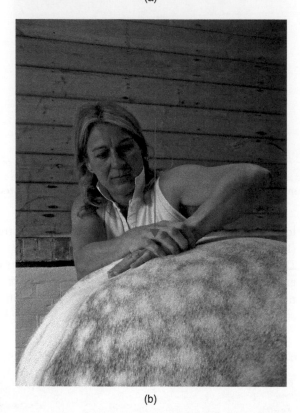

(b)

Figure 11.56 (a) Friction to the sacrum in a caudal direction. (b) Springing to the sacrum: contact the spinous processes and rhythmically bounce with the hands, springing along the sacrum in a caudal direction.

of the cranial hand to administer deep soft tissue work along the iliacus, tensor fascia lata and biceps femoris towards the greater trochanter where gluteus medius inserts. The thenar eminence can create a cup around the trochanter to apply a circular, deep, strong kneading technique around the hip joint. Holding the tail helps to stabilise the practitioner as the technique is applied.

To increase mobilisation of the hip, the tail is pulled laterally and cranially while the cranial hand counterbalances on the greater trochanter so that the quarters are pulled laterally towards the practitioner (Figure 11.55). One side is often more restricted, especially if there is asymmetry within the pelvic region.

SACRUM

Overview

There may be signs of underdevelopment in the sacral musculature, giving the horse a triangular appearance when observed from behind. The tissues may feel restricted and bound to the sacrum. This may or may not be in accord with other findings related to the sacroiliac joints or coccygeal vertebrae.

Techniques

56. *Soft tissue and mobilisation.* Friction along the sacrum in a caudal direction can be applied before mobilising the sacrum (Figure 11.56a). It is within this region that two of the powerful extensors of the hip biceps femoris and semitendinosus originate. These are the muscles that propel the horse forward, creating impulsion.

A springing technique can then be applied. The practitioner uses the hypothenar eminence of one hand as the contact point on the sacral spinous processes while reinforcing with the other hand. The hands are used to bounce rhythmically in a caudal direction, springing the sacrum (Figure 11.56b).

The sacrum may be fixed in a cranial or caudal position locked in extension or flexion with marked tenderness in the tissue fibres. A direct thrust can be applied to the region. Interlock the fingers and hands and gently bounce the sacrum as in Figure 11.56b. Apply a short, sharp thrust in a ventral direction on the caudal sacrum region in the case of fixed extension. In the case of fixed flexion, contact is made on the cranial sacrum region; apply the thrust in a ventral direction.

LUMBOSACRAL JUNCTION

Overview
If the spinal and caudal tissues are receptive, the lumbosacral junction can be mobilised by utilising the lumbosacral spinal reflex. This can be applied at any time the practitioner considers to be appropriate within the treatment programme for each individual horse.

Technique
57. *Lumbosacral flexion technique.* Stand to the side of the hindquarters and initially stroke the fingers either side of the sacrum in a caudal direction. If the horse tolerates this, proceed with a firmer, deeper stimulus, following the lateral borders of the sacrum and gluteals in a caudal direction (Figure 11.57).

If the lumbosacral junction is restricted, little flexion occurs initially and so the technique may have to be repeated when all the associated tissues are more receptive. When the junction responds to mobilisation, cavitation sounds along the spine are often heard which could be described as like the scales on a piano being played gently.

COCCYGEAL JOINTS

Overview
From the sacrum and lumbosacral region, the practitioner is naturally led to mobilising the tail. There can be a lot of emphasis on how the tail is carried. Remembering osteopathic principles, if the mobility throughout the tail and entire spine is good, the fact that the tail is carried to one side should not overly concern the practitioner. Arab horses naturally have a much higher tail carriage (one less lumbar vertebra than other breeds) and are often observed carrying the tail to one side, especially in walk. The dynamic and passive movement throughout the horse's structure will determine if the tail carriage is a significant factor or not.

The horse may be particularly sensitive about its tail being touched and will clamp it down. However, with patience and gentle palpation, it should eventually relax and allow the practitioner to mobilise the region.

A 'kink' may be palpated and care must be taken not to aggravate any old injuries when mobilising the tail.

Techniques
58. *Mobilisation of the tail.* Flex, extend and gently rotate the tail by holding the base of the dock (Figure 11.58).

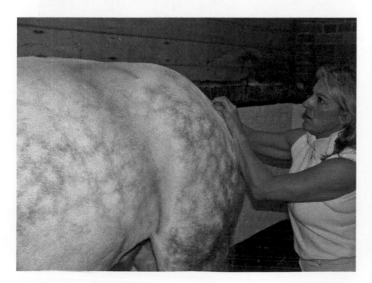

Figure 11.57 Lumbosacral junction technique: initially stroke the lateral borders of the sacrum then apply a deeper stimulus in a caudal direction to initiate full flexion of the junction.

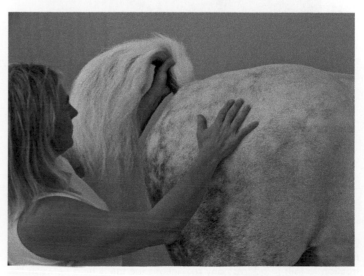

Figure 11.58 Mobilisation of the tail: holding the base of the dock, gently flex, extend and rotate the tail.

The sacrococcygeal joint can be tested for mobility by holding the tail in a flexed position while the cranial hand rests on the sacral region. Then flex and extend the tail dorsally, feeling for the movement at the sacrococcygeal junction.

59. *Articulation of coccygeal joints.* Each individual coccygeal vertebral joint can be articulated in flexion, extension, rotation and lateral directions. The practitioner progresses down the tail using a gentle shearing and rotational movement along the dock (Figure 11.59a). If

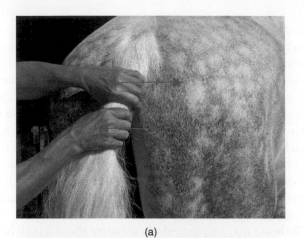

(a)

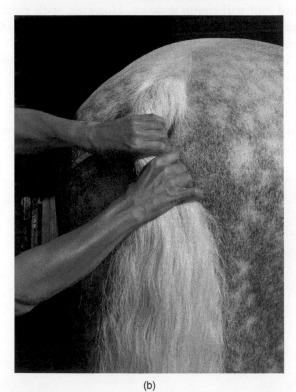

(b)

Figure 11.59 (a) Articulation of the coccygeal joints: progress down the tail using a gentle shearing and rotational movement. (b) Sustained traction to tail: to address any restrictions the tail is held between the hands, which gently pull in opposite directions in sustained traction, until the tissues respond.

there are any restrictions, gentle traction can be applied. The tail is held between the hands, which will be pulling in opposite directions in sustained traction until the tissues respond (Figure 11.59b).

60. *Traction to the tail.* Traction is then applied to the tail with both hands clasping the dock. The practitioner slowly leans back, taking up the tension as the horse counterbalances by leaning forwards in a cranial direction (Figure 11.60).

61. *Harmonic technique.* If at this point the spine is mobile and the horse is receptive, a harmonic technique can be introduced along with the tractional release being implemented. The tail is held in traction with the caudal hand while the cranial pushes rhythmically on the tuber ischii in a cranial direction (Figure 11.61a).

A rippling effect is observed down the spine, with the thorax freely moving between the shoulder blades and the horse lowering its head and stretching forwards (Figure 11.61b).

This technique will not be successful if there are any dysfunctions within the spine or pelvic region that have not already been addressed by the practitioner.

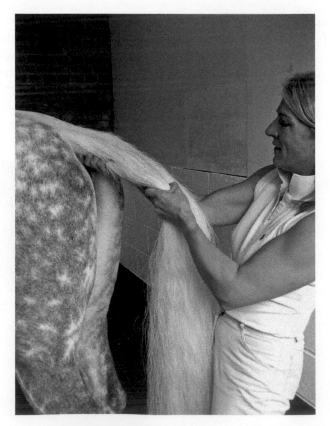

Figure 11.60 Traction to the tail: hold the dock with both hands and slowly lean back, taking up the tension as the horse counterbalances by leaning forward in a cranial direction.

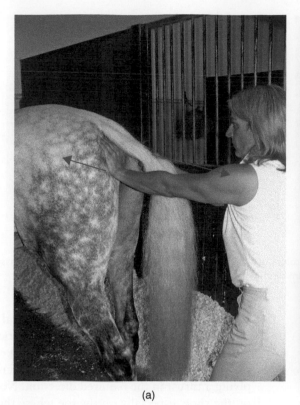 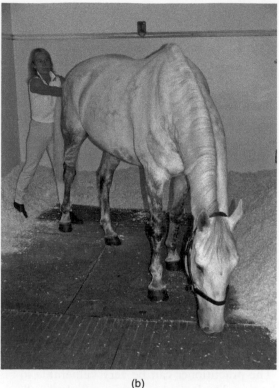

(a) (b)

Figure 11.61 (a) Harmonic technique: hold the tail in traction with the caudal hand while the cranial hand contacts on the tuber ischii and gently pushes rhythmically in a cranial direction. (b) A rippling effect is observed along the spine and the horse will lower its neck and stretch forwards.

HAMSTRING, ADDUCTORS AND CAUDAL MUSCULATURE

Overview

To use soft tissue and mobilisation techniques on the hamstring and adductor muscles, the practitioner can stand on the contralateral side; for example, the left side can be treated from the right.

Always be very aware of the horse's reaction, remembering how easily it can cow kick. Apply more traction to the tail for control and if necessary gently toggle the tail to keep the attention on you. It is very important that the horse is attentive to the practitioner. If they become distracted, you are more vulnerable to being knocked about or kicked. With practice, subtle tensions within the muscular tissue can be palpated that pre-empt sharper movements about to be performed by the horse!

Techniques

62. *Soft tissue to the caudal musculature.* Standing on the contralateral side, support and apply traction to the tail with the cranial hand and use the caudal hand to apply the soft tissue technique to the muscular tissue as required (Figure 11.62a).

The tension on the tail will help the horse to concentrate on you, and if they become fidgety gently toggle the tail to remind it of your presence (Figure 11.62b). There should be a palpable 'wobble' to the tissues, similar to the feel of the triceps muscles. Quite often there will be a 'stringy' feel to the tissues and fascia as one descends towards the Achilles tendon. This can be addressed using inhibition and wringing techniques.

If the horse is receptive, the practitioner can stand on the same side as the hamstring requiring attention and use longitudinal soft tissue techniques. The muscular tissue can then be stretched in a lateral direction followed by a 'wobble' of the muscle that is oscillating it between the thumb and fingers.

Before stretching the caudal muscles, the hindlimbs are examined.

THE HINDLIMB

Overview

As with the forelimb, the hindlimb is examined and any restrictions are addressed. It is more awkward to mobilise

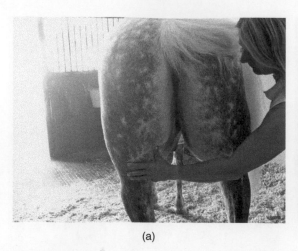

(a)

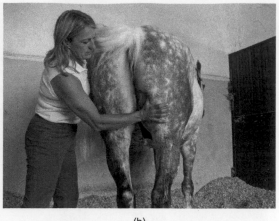

(b)

Figure 11.62 (a) Soft tissue to caudal musculature: stand on the contralateral side. Support and apply traction to the tail as soft tissue techniques are applied. (b) The tension on the tail will help keep the horse concentrated: a gentle toggle will remind it of your presence.

the hindlimb as a horse will tend to lean on the practitioner or pull and push the limb back and forth. Care must be taken if the horse has stringhalt, is a shiverer or wobbler, or has any stifle and hock pathologies.

Caution. The practitioner can be very vulnerable to being pulled about and kicked when examining the hindlimb. Never put the self or anyone else in danger of being injured: there is always another day to examine or treat if necessary!

Techniques

63. *Mobilisation of the pastern and fetlock.* Initially, lift the foot in exactly the same way as if the hoof was about to be cleaned out with a hoof pick. Unlike the forelimb, where mobilisation begins at the proximal joint, mobilisation of the hindlimb begins with the distal joints. This is more familiar to the horse and for the practitioner rather than suddenly palpating the stifle joint, an area that can be very sensitive to touch!

Extend, flex and axially rotate he distal joints (Figures 11.63a and 11.63b). If there are restrictions in the movements, the practitioner can gently take the joint to the point of restriction and toggle the joint before applying a thrust in the required direction. Note any wear on the shoe, especially on the toe where the horse may be dragging a toe or scuffing the hoof.

Assess the integrity of the tendons in a proximal direction as progression is made towards the hock joints.

64. *Flexion of the hock.* The hock can be flexed and extended, but remember that this also involves the stifle through the reciprocal apparatus (Figure 11.64).

The stifle and hock are synchronised in their movements by virtue of the ligaments and muscles that control them. When the stifle flexes, the hock flexes, and when the hock extends, the stifle extends. One does not function independently of

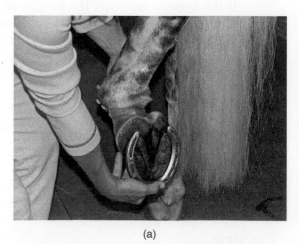

(a)

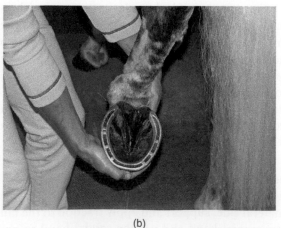

(b)

Figure 11.63 (a) Extension of the distal hindlimb joints: hold the toe of the hoof to use as a lever and extend the distal joints. (b) Flexion of the distal hindlimb joints: cup the hoof and use as a lever to flex the distal joints.

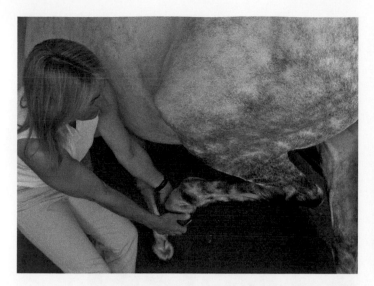

Figure 11.64 The stifle and hock are synchronised in their movements: hock flexion with stifle flexion.

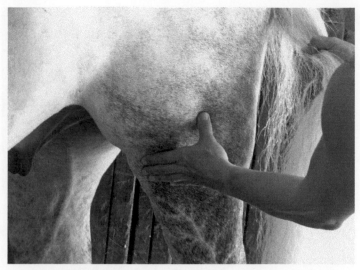

Figure 11.65 Palpation of the stifle joint: always stroke the hindquarters first before palpation and hold the tail to keep the horse's attention – this is a VERY sensitive region to touch.

the other because of the tendinous bands in front of and behind the limb (Smythe and Goody 1993, p. 82)

65. *Palpation of the stifle. Caution*: the stifle is an extremely sensitive region to palpate. Always begin by stroking the quarters and slowly but confidently progress down to the stifle and palpate. If the horse objects strongly, don't take risks. Leave the region alone!

The stifle may already have been assessed in the palpatory examination. However, at this stage of treatment the horse will be more familiar with the practitioner, and the stifle can be examined or re-examined as necessary. Slide the hand along the lateral vastus muscle in a ventral and cranial direction, and on reaching the stifle gently examine the region with the fingers (Figure 11.65).

Stretching the hindlimb can follow, but must only be applied after the soft tissues have been relaxed, as previously described.

Caution. These stretches should only be performed if the practitioner is very confident that the horse will not kick. They must never put themselves or the handlers at risk.

66. *Hamstring stretch*. In order to stretch the hamstring muscles, face the tail and hold the fetlock between both hands with the hock slightly flexed. The practitioner then steps back to about the mid-thoracic and shoulder region and applies gentle traction to the limb, ensuring that it is always parallel to the horse's body (Figure 11.66).

It is very important to have good posture and stability when performing these stretches as the horse will often pull the hindlimb back and can easily unbalance the

practitioner. It is always sensible to graduate the amount of traction according to the individual horse's tolerance. Over time the stretch can always be increased.

Sustained traction can be applied. At the moment of release, the practitioner slowly steps forwards in a caudal direction and, in harmony with the horse, lowers the limb to the ground. The limb should be placed on the ground slowly and not suddenly dropped, as the horse may lose its balance, react sharply and kick out.

67. *Abductor stretch*. The practitioner stands on the contralateral side of the limb to be stretched. Holding the foot, the opposite leg is then taken under the abdomen in a medial and slightly cranial direction (Figures 11.67a

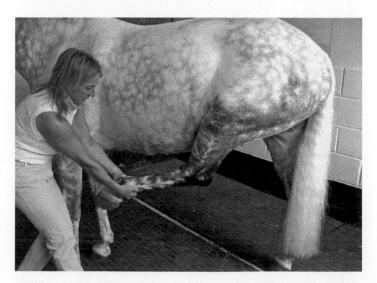

Figure 11.66 Hamstring stretch: the limb must remain parallel to the horse's body and the practitioner must maintain a good posture and balance when applying the traction.

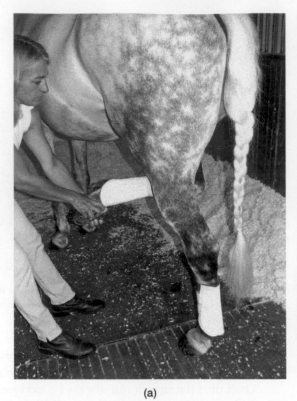
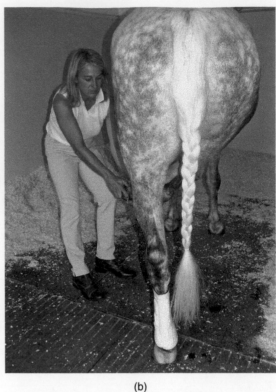

(a)   (b)

Figure 11.67 (a) Abductor stretch: stand on the contralateral side and stretch the leg gently under the abdomen. (b) Application of the stretch: the stretch is in a medial direction under the abdomen.

and 11.67b). This is performed on both sides and mobility is compared.

PELVIS

Overview

This substantial and very important region, the pelvic girdle, consists of two symmetrical halves made up of three bones, the ilium, ischium and pubis, which are fused together. The ilia join to the sacrum with strong ligamentous attachments, forming the sacroiliac joints. There is minute, if any, movement at these joints.

The sacrum, pelvis and sacroiliac joints can be traumatised in many different ways. This may be from falling, slipping, twisting, or continual stress from the required discipline as in, for example, the Quarter Horse performing sharp reining halts.

Some common causative factors include: cast in the stable; falling over or into jumps, especially when eventing or National Hunt racing; slipping on the flat or slipping into a fence; losing the hindlimbs underneath and landing on to the pelvis; hitting the pelvis against a doorframe when entering or leaving a stable; tripping up or down ramps; rearing and falling over backwards.

Initially a full clinical examination *must* be made by a veterinary surgeon in order to eliminate any pathology.

'When the horse has no history of trauma, diagnosis can be difficult. Excluding all possible sources of pain in the distal limb is frequently necessary before focusing on the pelvic region' (Dyson 2003, p. 491).

Sprain of the pelvic ligaments, restriction in the sacroiliac region or pelvic positional deviations may present as hindlimb lameness, which may be acute or intermittent. The horse may just be dragging a toe with reduced hindlimb movement, or there may be a noticeable hip hike on a straight line. This may be more apparent on a circle.

Osteoarthritis of the sacroiliac joints may be present despite symmetry of the tubera sacrale. It is usually a bilateral condition and is rarely associated with unilateral hindlimb lameness (Dyson and Murray 2003).

It is especially important for the practitioner to be aware that injuries to the pelvis may not be just the result of an external trauma. 'The forces involved in locomotion create predilection sites for stress fractures. These sites are associated with the concentration of forces involved in load bearing at speed and the biomechanics, innate structure and form of bone' (Pilsworth 2003, p. 484). Young thoroughbreds in training, for example, may develop dysfunctional symptoms without a history of a trauma or fall.

'Fractures of the ilial wing appear to be among the most commonly encountered types of athletic stress fracture in the skeletally immature thoroughbred racehorse' (Pilsworth et al. 1994, p. 486). The practitioner must be very cautious as the horse may not necessarily appear lame. 'Lameness often resolves rapidly within 24 to 48 hours and the horse then has a slight gait abnormality, walking with the back hunched up, but with no overt lameness' (Pilsworth 2003, p. 486).

Musculoskeletal dysfunction will affect biomechanical performance, and riders will complain that the horse has become reluctant and resistant when ridden. It is usually in canter that the problems are most apparent. There may be reluctance to canter on one rein. A buck may be used for the transition from trot to the faster gait as a means of creating impulsion. Cantering disunited or bunny hopping with the hindquarters croup high and continually breaking into trot may occur.

A horse will often begin refusing to jump or struggle to cope with related distances between fences, especially through combinations. The head carriage may be high and the back hollow with reluctance to propel from behind. There will be resistance and difficulty in performing lateral movements, such as half-pass and shoulder-in.

The tail may be carried to one side or clamped down. Discomfort may be expressed by swishing the tail when working, and the horse becomes bad tempered and nappy, refusing to go forwards.

Farriers may comment that the horse has become more difficult to shoe behind and shows a disinclination to stand on the painful, restricted side while the other hind foot is being shod.

The sacroiliac joints seem to be the most common region that owners and riders remember and latch on to. It is the asymmetry observed in the pelvic region that attracts all the attention. They have the impression that the 'pelvis was out and put back in' by the practitioner. This very misunderstood concept is an important issue that *must* be addressed, and it should be explained that this is an incorrect interpretation of the techniques applied.

Subluxation of the sacroiliac joint is comparatively rare (Rooney 1979; Haussler 1999).

When examining and palpating the pelvis, the horse must be standing squarely, on all four feet, on a level surface. A pelvis can have the appearance of being asymmetrical if the stance is not correct.

Similarly, if clipped there is a 'V' of hair that is usually left at the top of the dock and sacral area. This may not be central and so gives the illusion that the pelvis is asymmetric. Care must also be taken when examining a piebald or skewbald. White areas appear to be higher due to the contrast in colour. Don't allow your eye to be deceived into assuming that the pelvis is 'crooked'!

'Asymmetry in the height of the tubera sacrale is a common finding in horses in full work, free of lameness, although it may be seen along with poor performance or alterations in hindlimb gait. Apparent asymmetry may actually reflect differences in size of the dorsal sacroiliac ligament' (Dyson 2003, p. 491).

The pelvic area may show a high degree of variability within the anatomical features. Dr Narelle Stubbs (n.stubbs@uq.edu.au) has carried out numerous dissections of this region.

Any restriction or dysfunction in the spine resulting in the horse not engaging the hindlimbs and properly developing the correct musculature across the hindquarters will also give the appearance of asymmetry in the region.

Caution. Under no circumstances should the practitioner ever put himself or herself or the handler at risk. This especially applies to any pelvic examination. The horse's temperament and tolerance must be assessed at *all* times.

If the horse will not tolerate someone standing directly behind or there is any potential risk, an alternative method can be used. The practitioner can stand on a suitable object to the side of the horse and assess the symmetry of the tubera sacrale and tubera coxae from above. This may not be as accurate but it is safer.

It is especially important, when considering the pelvic region, to remind the practitioner of the osteopathic principles stated at the beginning of this chapter. If there is positional change and mobility is altered, then osteopathic treatment to restore the joint to normal movement is required. However, if there is positional asymmetry but joint movement is good, then the change in position can be ignored.

The pelvic symmetry will have been assessed in the palpatory examination but it is important that the practitioner re-examines the positional appearance of the pelvic bony landmarks.

'Clinical assessment of individual structures of the pelvic region by visual examination and palpation is not easy, especially in Warmblood and draft breeds, because of the large muscle mass of the hindquarters' (Dyson 2003, p. 491).

Re-examination of Pelvic Symmetry

68. *Horse must be standing square.* Begin by re-examining the symmetry of the pelvis from behind. This must be done on a level surface with the horse standing square on all four feet with the head and neck straight (Figure 11.68). This is not always easy to achieve! To encourage a square halt, a pull on the tail laterally will often assist in placing the feet. Alternatively lift a foot and place it in position. Patience is essential because as soon as the horse is standing square and the practitioner goes forward to begin the examination, the horse may well move.

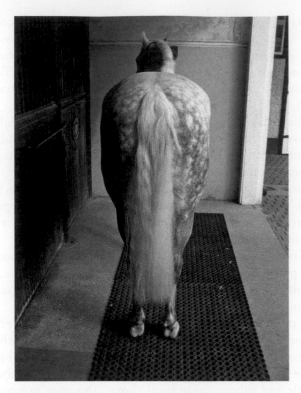

Figure 11.68 Examination of pelvic symmetry: the horse must be standing squarely with all four feet on a level surface and the head and neck should be straight.

69. *Assessment of tubera sacrale symmetry.* The practitioner must begin by approaching the horse from the side, gently stroking the lumbar spine and pelvis and gradually moving around to stand directly behind the horse. The fingers are then placed on the tubera sacrale to assess positioning in respect to each other in height (Figure 11.69). The pelvis is said to be asymmetric if one tuber sacrale visibly appears to be higher.

70. *Assessment of tubera coxae symmetry.* The tuber coxa orientation is then assessed using the index finger of each hand (Figure 11.70). The tuber coxa may appear higher or more cranial or caudal when compared with the other side.

   In an ideal situation two assistants can place an index finger on the craniodorsal aspect of each tuber coxa and extend the finger horizontally. Alternatively the tuber coxa can be marked with tape (Dyson 2003, p. 491).

71. *Assessment of tubera ischii symmetry.* Using the thumb of each hand, palpate the position of the tubera ischii (Figure 11.71). There may be an appearance of one being higher or cranial or caudal to the other.

   The pelvic positional findings for each of these structures are:

   • Dorsal/ventral: higher or lower on one side than the other.

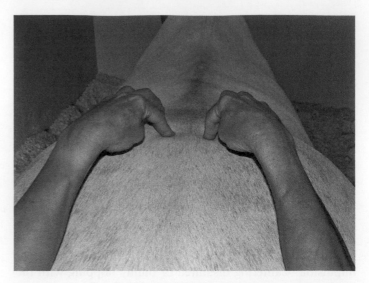

Figure 11.69 Assessment of tubera sacrale symmetry: place the fingers on the tubera sacrale to assess positioning in respect of each other in height.

   • Cranial/caudal: rotation of one side compared with the other.
   • Lateral deviation: from muscular contraction on that side.

   Following re-examination of the pelvis, stand to the side and just observe the whole horse, reassessing the stance and posture. If the pelvis is tilted cranially, the horse will look flat over the lumbosacral region and stand with the hindlimbs out behind. If the pelvis is tilted caudally, the horse will look arched over the quarters and will be standing under itself.

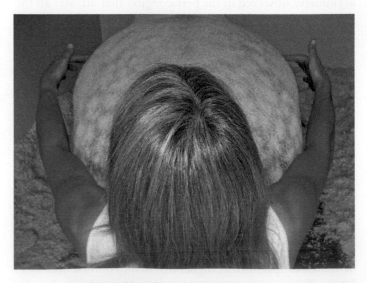

Figure 11.70 Assessment of tubera coxae symmetry: place the index fingers on the tubera coxae to compare positioning.

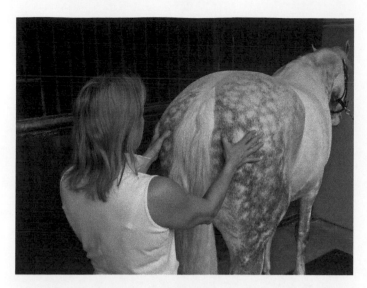

Figure 11.71 Assessment of tubera ischii symmetry: place the thumbs on the tubera ischii to compare positioning.

If there is pain, the abdominal muscles will be tight and the horse is described as being 'tucked up'. Clinical findings related to dysfunction of this region may include contraction, spasm and associated pain within the lumbar spine musculature. Contraction of the muscles with associated joint restriction around the femoral head and femoral region may also be present. Patterns of contraction and restriction either ipsilaterally or contralaterally may be observed.

Asymmetry found on examination may be anatomical, or the result of trauma to the region. For example, a horse careering and cantering around in the field abruptly slides to a stop at the perimeter fence causing the left hindlimb to slip underneath in a cranial direction. This may result in a strain of the left femoral musculature and restriction of movement within this region, with the pelvis appearing asymmetric, that is, lower and/or rotated on that side. There may be associated contralateral lumbar erector spinae contraction, restricted mobility at the lumbosacral junction, and cervical spine dysfunction as a result of the dynamic forces created from the abrupt movement.

With experience the practitioner will begin to recognise patterns and must decide the most appropriate treatment regime for every individual presentation. The most common finding is a subtle, positional asymmetry, resulting from altered musculoskeletal biomechanics throughout the spine and body. This could explain why the tubera sacrale, for example, may appear more level after osteopathic treatment.

The lumbar spine, sacrum and associated structures must be re-examined for other contributing factors. There may be a scoliosis, obvious muscular contraction or conformational anomalies.

PELVIC AND SACROILIAC JOINT TECHNIQUES

Overview

This is where it is *very important* to remember that structure governs function but it is the *mobility* and function of the region that is significant rather than the asymmetry and positioning.

The practitioner must have assessed the pelvis in conjunction with the lumbar, lumbosacral junction and associated musculoskeletal tissue. Asymmetrical pelvic positioning with normal local and spinal mobility, and with optimal muscular and fascial elasticity and tone, will *not* need manipulating.

Any associated soft tissue dysfunction must be addressed before specific mobilisation techniques are applied.

Reminder. For the pelvic mobilisation and thrust–spring techniques the horse should wear boots or bandages on the hindlimbs. This will protect the distal joints, as a limb may be struck with the contralateral foot as the procedure is performed. It is often sensible for the horse to have overreach boots on and if necessary put a form of leg protection on both front- and hindlimbs. Some horses really resent wearing boots and may lash out continually. In this scenario the practitioner must assess the risk of using any of the techniques without protection.

There must be a non-slippery surface with sufficient bedding to prevent injury as the techniques are performed.

Techniques

72. *Springing the sacroiliac joints.* To spring the sacroiliac joints, begin by standing to the side of the horse at an oblique angle to the pelvis, facing caudally. The fingertips of both hands are placed on or just medial to the ipsilateral tuber sacrale cupping this bony landmark. Using the fingertips to apply pressure, a springing movement is made in a ventral direction (Figure 11.72). This is repeated on the other side. On the side of restriction the pressure is applied more forcefully.

73. *Springing technique for sacroiliac joint.* If further mobilisation is required, the practitioner can stand on a suitable object. Using the thenar eminence of one hand and reinforced by the other, contact is made on the tuber sacrale. Using the body weight, spring and bounce the sacroiliac joint more vigorously in a ventral direction (Figure 11.73).

74. *Tuber coxa contact for pelvic mobilisation.* The tuber coxa may be used as the contact point for applying pressure with the fingers in a ventral and oblique direction to the pelvis to spring the pelvis (Figure 11.74).

The above two techniques can be used either for examination or mobilisation as required and then as

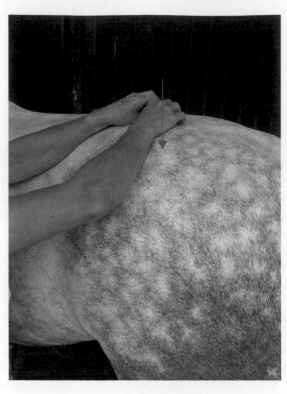

Figure 11.72 Springing the sacroiliac joints: the fingertips of both hands are placed on the ipsilateral tuber sacrale and pressure is applied with a springing movement in a ventral direction.

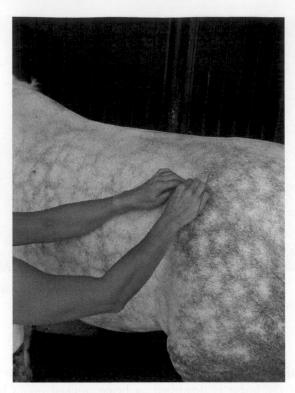

Figure 11.74 Tuber coxa contact for pelvis mobilisation: with the fingers on the tuber coxa, pressure is applied in an oblique ventral direction to spring the pelvis.

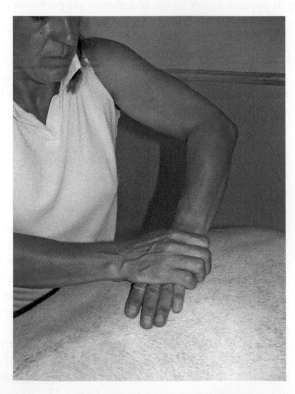

Figure 11.73 Springing technique for sacroiliac joints: stand on a suitable object and use the thenar eminence reinforced by the other hand to bounce and spring the joint in a ventral direction.

procedures to re-evaluate any improvement in mobility post-treatment.

75. *Dorsal thrust to the tuber coxa.* If the tubera coxae are asymmetric on palpation, the practitioner can use a dorsal thrust. Stand on a suitable object. Make contact using the hypothenar eminence of the caudal hand with the fingers pointing towards oneself on the tuber coxa that, on examination, appeared *higher* than the other side. The cranial hand then reinforces the caudal hand. The tuber coxa is bounced rhythmically in an oblique, lateral and ventral direction before applying a direct downward thrust (Figure 11.75).

76. *Cranial springing of the pelvis.* If, on examination, the pelvis gave the appearance of a rotation in caudal positioning, this technique can be applied. The fingers are used to apply a springing force on the *higher* tuber coxa at an oblique and ventral angle towards the practitioner. This springs the pelvis in a cranial direction (Figure 11.76a).

If the horse is very sharp and there is a risk of being kicked, the practitioner should stand on the contralateral side to the higher tuber coxa. From here, the hands and fingers reach across to make contact on the *higher* side and a springing force is applied in a ventral and cranial direction, stimulating the pelvis to spring in a cranial direction (Figure 11.76b).

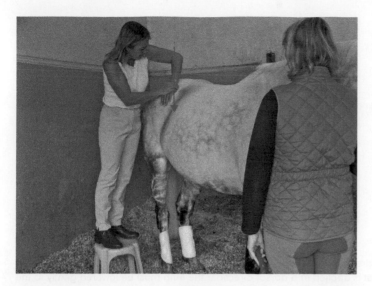

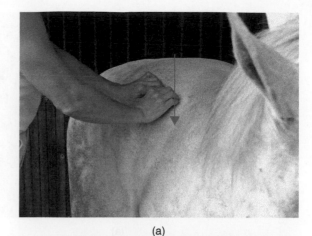

(a)

Figure 11.75 Dorsal thrust to tuber coxa: addressing the side on which the tuber coxa palpated *higher*, make contact with the thenar eminence. Rhythmically bounce the tuber coxa before applying a direct downwards thrust in a ventral direction.

77. *Thrust to pelvis using the hindlimb as a lever*. Preparation is very important with all the pelvic thrust techniques. They should only be applied near the end of the treatment programme when all the surrounding connective tissues have been assessed and released.

The side on which the pelvis appears *lower* and on examination is restricted and/or painful is the side from which the thrust is made. If the pelvis appears lower on the left, then it is on the left side that the handler stands and it is the left hindlimb that the practitioner uses as a lever to apply the thrust.

Facing caudally, take hold of the foot with both hands and gently flex the hindlimb. It is very important that the limb be held straight and not adducted or abducted (Figure 11.77a). Take up to the point of tissue tension and apply a sharp lift in a dorsal direction. A stabilizing contact can be used with the caudal hand on the pelvis to assist the thrust if required (Figure 11.77b). The limb is then gently lowered to the ground.

78. *Assisted pelvic thrust–spring technique*. The pelvic thrust–spring is a commonly used technique. The practitioner must be alert to the fact that the horse can become very aware of what is to follow and may be difficult to handle if this technique is unnecessarily applied at every treatment.

The idea is to spring and oscillate the sacroiliac joints and surrounding musculoskeletal tissue, resulting in a recoil release promoting improved mobility. It is *not* a repositioning or 'putting back' of the pelvis in the sense that the sacroiliac joints have been moved, as is so often incorrectly stated. The practitioner's aim is to thrust the horse on to the contralateral hindlimb so that

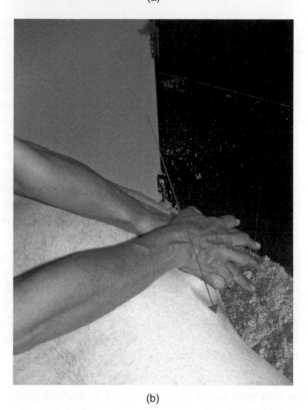

(b)

Figure 11.76 (a) Flexing the pelvis: contact is made on the tuber coxa that palpated *higher*; use the fingers to apply a springing force in a lateral and ventral direction. The pelvis flexes in a cranial direction. (b) If the horse is sharp and may kick, stand on the contralateral side to the higher tuber coxa and apply the springing force in a ventral and lateral direction.

it then springs back on to the ipsilateral side. The thrust is usually made on the side on which the pelvis appears lower.

As with all techniques one must work within the horse's limits of tolerance and never take risks. The thrust should *only* be applied if it is considered safe to do so.

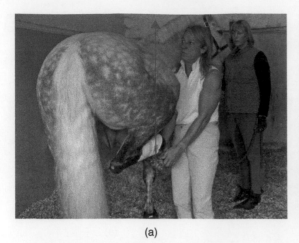
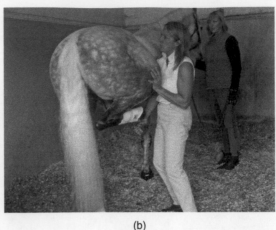

(a)   (b)

Figure 11.77 (a) Thrust to the pelvis using the hindlimb as a lever: addressing the lower palpated side, the hindlimb is held and flexed parallel to the pelvis. It must not be adducted or abducted. (b) A springing thrust is applied in a dorsal direction: the limb must be lowered gently to the ground once the technique has been applied.

The horse, standing evenly and squarely on the hindlimbs, is positioned diagonally across the stable with plenty of room for it to land on to the contralateral hindlimb following the applied thrust. The assistant holds the hindlimb up in an adducted and cranial direction under the abdomen, releasing it on command as the practitioner applies the thrust. The practitioner must stand to the side and be very aware of the high risk of being struck by the horse as it springs back on to the ipsilateral limb once the thrust has been made.

Contact is made on the femur and femoral region. Timing is essential as on command the assistant must immediately release the limb while simultaneously the practitioner applies the thrust in an oblique angle to the pelvis across the midline in a cranial direction (Figure 11.78). The assistant should wear gloves to hold the hoof and must be wearing suitable footwear.

It is very easy for the practitioner to be kicked performing this technique, and it is not always easy for the assistant to be quick enough in releasing the limb on command. It is for this reason I prefer and have adapted this one-person, unassisted technique.

79. *Unassisted pelvic thrust-spring technique.* The handler stands on the same side as the practitioner. On the side on which the pelvis appears lower, the practitioner lifts the hindlimb high up under the abdomen with the cranial hand. Contact is made with the caudal hand around the lateral condyle of the femur or within the femoral region depending on the balance of the horse. Timing is essential. The horse may be pulling the leg away from the practitioner who has to counterbalance this movement. At the moment at which there is a concentration

of forces at the sacroiliac joint, a thrust is applied using velocity and amplitude in an oblique direction to the pelvis across the midline in a caudal direction (Figure 11.79a).

The horse is momentarily off balance and should land with a spring on to the contralateral hindlimb (Figure 11.79b) and then immediately spring back on to the ipsilateral hindlimb (Figure 11.79c) before standing and relaxing. A successful release may result in a long audible exhalation from the horse.

Caution. The practitioner must step away quickly as soon as the thrust is applied. It is as the horse lands and springs back to the ipsilateral side that it may kick out. Good timing and safety are the keys to success.

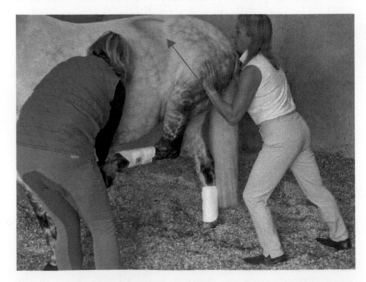

Figure 11.78 Assisted pelvic thrust–spring technique: it is important that the assistant holds the hindlimb parallel to the horse's body and releases it on command as the practitioner applies the thrust to the pelvis obliquely across the midline in a cranial direction.

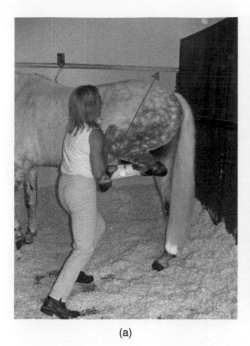
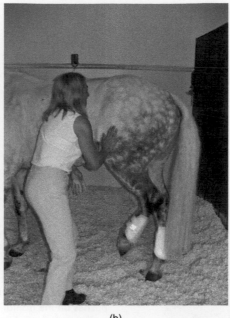
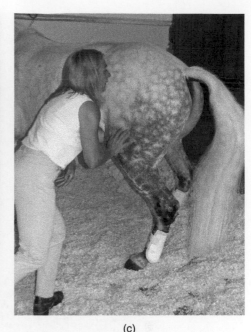

(a)   (b)   (c)

Figure 11.79 (a) Unassisted pelvic thrust–spring technique: the hindlimb is flexed and the caudal hand is in contact with the lateral condyle of the femur or around the femoral region. The thrust is applied obliquely across the midline in a caudal direction. (b) The thrust bounces the horse: it lands with a spring on to the contralateral hindlimb. (c) Finally the horse springs from the contralateral hindlimb back on to the ipsilateral hindlimb: an oscillation of the sacroiliac joints and surrounding tissues has been achieved.

Occasionally the horse just lands heavily on the contralateral side with no bounce or spring. The technique may have to be repeated to achieve the desired result.

Some horses are so sharp that they practically perform the technique themselves by snatching the limb away and landing on to the contralateral limb followed by springing back on to the ipsilateral side.

Always re-examine the sacroiliac joint mobility and the contralateral hip region. The tissues around the femur should be more pliable, with improved mobility throughout the hindquarters, lumbosacral and associated muscles and fascia.

Observed from the side, the horse will appear to be standing in a square and will look more 'up' through the withers and thoracolumbar spine. Owners often comment on the improved posture throughout the spine and how much more relaxed the horse seems.

COMPLETION OF TREATMENT

Overview

Depending on the initial osteopathic findings, there are several options available to complete the treatment. I usually end with one of the following.

Techniques

80. *Harmonic technique using the tail as a lever*. Having addressed the pelvis and hindquarters, use of the harmonic method described in technique 61 is appropriate.

The tail is held in traction with one hand while the other pushes rhythmically on the tuber ischii. A rippling effect is observed down the spine with the thorax freely moving between the shoulder blades. The horse will lower its head and neck, stretching and releasing in response to the rhythmic movement (Figure 11.80). The tail should be slowly released, allowing the horse to regain its full balance before the tail is gently placed back into the natural position.

81. *Sternum xiphoid technique*. The sternum xiphoid release, described in technique 46, could then be applied.

Place the dorsal hand on the thoracic spinous processes approximately between the ninth and twelfth thoracic vertebrae while the palm of the ventral hand is lightly placed on the abdomen in the region of the sternum and the xiphoid process, the slight indentation that can be felt and is shaped like an arrowhead.

When using this technique at the end of a treatment, gently apply pressure and allow the flow of energy to pass between the hands to induce relaxation (Figure 11.81).

82. *Cervical spine harmonic release*. The harmonic mobilisation described in technique 19 is an excellent way to finish a treatment if the horse is responsive.

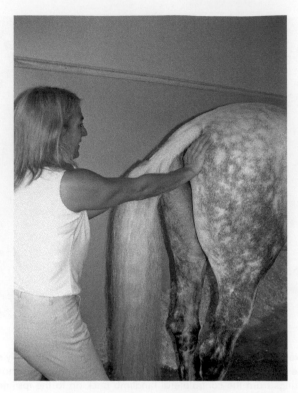

Figure 11.80 Harmonic technique using the tail as a lever: the tail is held in traction while the tuber ischii is rhythmically pushed in a cranial direction resulting in a rippling effect along the spine.

Cup the cranial hand under the horse's chin and rhythmically pull the chin cranially. At the same time the caudal hand gently pushes on the frontal bone and occiput in a caudal direction, producing a rocking movement (Figure 11.82).

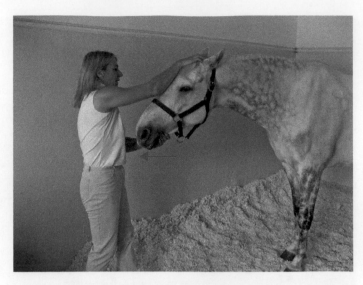

Figure 11.82 Cervical spine harmonic release: cup the chin with the cranial hand and rhythmically pull cranially as the caudal hand gently pushes on the frontal bone in a caudal direction.

83. *Traction throughout the whole spine to finish*. To increase the traction through the cervical spine the practitioner places the horse's chin on to their shoulder and gently leans backwards (Figure 11.83).

Finish by simply stroking the forelock in a rostral direction (Figure 11.84) and gently, slowly progress to the nasal region with a very light touch of the hand. Treatments should never end abruptly!

I often give the horse a carrot or some mints, if appropriate. A treat is always appreciated!

The techniques described in this chapter are intended to give a base for each practitioner to use, enhance and develop

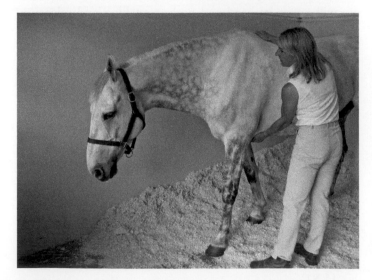

Figure 11.81 Sternum xiphoid technique: place the caudal hand on thoracic spinous processes and the cranial hand on the xiphoid. When applied at the end of a treatment, the practitioner simply allows the flow of energy to pass between the hands.

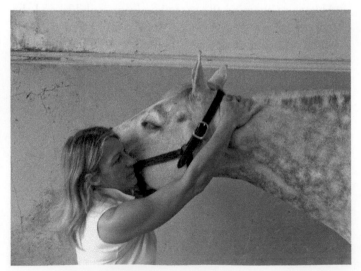

Figure 11.83 Traction throughout the spine: the practitioner places the horse's chin on the shoulder and gently leans backwards, applying traction to the spine, then releasing slowly.

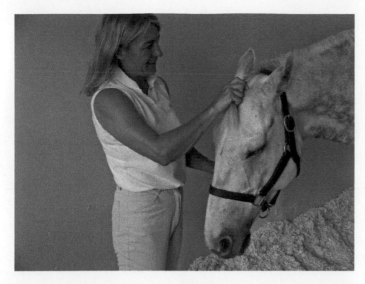

Figure 11.84 To finish treatment: slowly and gently stroke the forelock in a rostral direction.

their *own* individual treatment programme when treating horses.

Feedback from owners, riders and veterinary surgeons will help the practitioner continually develop and reflect on their osteopathic treatment regime: it is a constant learning curve.

One of the satisfying outcomes of treatment is how the horse's temperament can improve. Owners and riders will often telephone just to report to the practitioner how much 'happier' and more relaxed the horse is, both in the stable and when being ridden.

A few days of easy work, hacking or light schooling in large circles is very helpful post-treatment. There will be occasions when the horse is competing within a short period of treatment. Providing there are no contraindications, this should not be a problem. Performance is most likely to be enhanced after treatment, and successful results may follow.

It is impossible to dictate the interval or number of treatments required but it is always advisable to have a follow-up examination and possibly a treatment within one or two weeks from the initial consultation. Most problems make a significant improvement within three treatments. Intermit-tent checks may be advisable if the horse is participating in a strenuous sport or discipline. 'The decision as to the spacing of treatments is only arrived at by consideration of all the relevant factors relating to the chronicity, acuteness, urgency and practical factors of distance and advisability of travel' (Hartman 1985, p. 22). 'It is, nevertheless, a far more common mistake to overtreat than to undertreat' (Hartman 1985, p. 22).

REFERENCES

Buffon GLL (1753) *Histoire Naturelle*, **44** vols. Paris.

Clayton HM (1991) *Conditioning Sport Horses*. Sport Horse Publications, Saskatoon, pp. 129, 134.

Dyson S (2003) Pelvic injuries in the non-racehorse. In: Ross MW, Dyson SJ (eds) *Diagnosis and Management of Lameness in the Horse*. Saunders, St Louis, pp. 491–500.

Dyson S, Murray R (2003) Pain associated with the sacroiliac joint region: a clinical study of 74 horses. *Equine Veterinary Journal* 35, 240–245.

Fryette HH (1980) *Principles of Osteopathic Technic*. American Academy of Osteopathy, Carmel, p. 94.

Hartman LS (1985) *Handbook of Osteopathic Technique*, 2nd edn. Hutchinson, London, pp. 8, 22.

Haussler K (1999) Osseous spinal pathology. *Veterinary Clinics of North America: Equine Practice* 15, 103.

Pilsworth RC (2003) Diagnosis and management of pelvic fractures in the thoroughbred racehorse. In: Ross MW, Dyson SJ (eds) *Diagnosis and Management of Lameness in the Horse*. Saunders, St Louis, pp. 484–490.

Pilsworth RC, Shepherd M, Herinckx BM, *et al.* (1994) A review of 10 horses with fracture of the wing of the ileum. *Equine Veterinary Journal* 26, 94–99.

Rooney J (1979) Sacroiliac luxation. *Modern Veterinary Practice* 60, 45.

Smythe RH, Goody P (1993) *Horse Structure and Movement*. Revised by Gray P. JA Allen, London, pp. 7, 51–52, 82.

Stashak TS (1995) *Practical Guide to Lameness in Horses*. Lippincott Williams & Wilkins, Philadelphia, p. 92.

Stoddard A (1980) *Manual of Osteopathic Technique*, 3rd edn. Hutchinson, London, pp. 9–10, 14, 22.

Xenophon (1979) *The Art of Horsemanship*. Transl. Morgan MH. JA Allen, London, pp. 34–35.

Osteopathic Treatment of the Sedated Horse

12

Anthony Pusey and Julia Brooks

The conditions under which treatment is performed will depend on the site and nature of the problems presenting to the osteopath. Most cases, particularly if the onset of the problem is recent, can be treated very effectively while standing quietly in a stable or yard. However, in some instances, the use of sedation should be considered.

STANDING SEDATION

For problems that have been present for some time, lightly sedating the horse may be very helpful. Under these conditions, the horse is standing but it is relaxed and less reactive to external stimuli. It is then easier to perform indirect techniques that may require a position to be held for some time. It also enables treatment to be applied directly to the pelvis. The disadvantage is that all four legs should stay on the ground to steady the horse and so any treatment to the limbs should be done before sedating.

Effective sedation is achieved by using a combination of an α_2-adrenoceptor agonist and an opioid. α_2-Adrenoceptor agonists such as romifidine (Sedivet) downregulate the synthesis and release of noradrenaline, so reducing alertness and arousal. Detomidine may also be used. However, horses tend to be unsteady with this preparation, which encourages them to keep all four legs on the ground during procedures such as castration!

Although sedation with α_2-adrenoceptor agonists may seem profound, horses can still kick accurately when stimulated by touch, and an opioid is effective in reducing this sensitivity. Opioids act on μ-, κ- and δ-opioid receptors which are distributed widely in the central nervous system. Butor-phenol is a partial agonist, with varied agonist/antagonist actions at different receptors.

Neither drug affects the α motor neurones to the muscles, and patterns of dysfunction are unaffected in the sedated state. The correct dose is important and 1.5 ml romifidine and 1.5 ml butorphenol may be used to make the horse sufficiently relaxed for treatment but not oversedated such that balance is impaired. However, it should be individually tailored to the horse. A tough little pony may need more than a huge Irish draught horse. Chestnuts appear to need a higher dose mirroring their human counterparts who are said to be more difficult to anaesthetise. Ambient temperatures will also alter sedative effects.

It is helpful to record the dosage given for future consultations. However, this may need to be reviewed on followup. On initial consultation, pain and anxiety may increase the requirement for sedative compared with subsequent visits, which is in itself an indication of progress.

Achieving the perfect level of sedation owes much to the skill of the vet.

A note of caution here highlights diagnostic differences between the osteopathic and veterinary approach to musculoskeletal problems. A vet who does not regularly work with osteopaths will considerably omit the opioid part of the combination in the mistaken belief that a pain reaction is necessary to identify a level of pathology. Vets may be unaware that skilled palpation can detect alterations in tissue state and that prodding to elicit pain is unnecessary. The danger here is that, without the opiate, the hindquarters become very sensitive, which is undesirable when pelvic work is necessary!

Once administered, the sedatives reach their maximum effect within 5 minutes. However, it is often observed that, with effective treatment, sedation appears to become more profound well after this watershed. This is a good indication of the effectiveness of the treatment. The head will relax downwards and there may be some mucous discharge from the nasal passages.

Occasionally, as the sedative begins to take effect, the horse will walk forwards into the corner of the room. This appears to coincide with occipito-atlanto-axial joint dysfunction. Stiffness in this proprioceptor-rich area impedes the information available to the central nervous system for fixing the position of the body in space. With the slight, sedative-induced unsteadiness, this information is supplemented from the rest of the body in the forward movement, and by skin mechanoreceptor input from the head as it rests against the wall. As the strain in the upper cervical spine resolves, the horse no longer exhibits this behavioural pattern.

TREATMENT

The objective of treatment is the restoration of normal integrated function in the whole of the neuromusculoskeletal system. Particular attention is paid to those areas of dysfunction identified on observation and palpatory assessment, as well as results from the use of diagnostic tools such as thermographic imaging. All the osteopathic treatment modalities used in the human field can be applied to the horse with certain modifications (see Chapter 10).

The purpose of using sedation with treatment is to desensitise the horse at the level of the central nervous system (Figure 12.1). The approach described below is a guideline to treatment. The area treated and the order of treatment will vary with the site and nature of the problem and with the osteopath's individual preference for particular treatment modalities.

The head is a good starting point when initiating treatment.

CRANIUM

Injuries sustained in this area are often of the impaction variety. Impact of the occipital bone is common in horses that have fallen over backwards, and the frontal and nasal bones are vulnerable in falls at speed.

Following impaction injuries the frontal and occipital regions have a hard unyielding quality, and the normal sensation of flexion and extension movement in the cranial rhythm of these two bones is markedly reduced. The fascia of the cranium reflects this overall impression of solidity as it feels bound down to the underlying vault. These changes are often associated with increased tone in the suboccipital muscles. Occipito-atlantal joint compression is common. The aim of treatment is to restore symmetry and mobility to the tissues of the head and neck.

Technique

Inhibition

The close structural and neurological connections between the cranial bones can be used in treatment because changes in one area will have profound effects on related structures. The long nasal bones are useful in this respect, and inhibitory techniques here can be used to restore function to the head and neck. Initially, one hand adopts a monitoring role at the subocciput, with the thumb and first finger spanning the occiput between the ears. The other hand palpates down either side of the nasal bones to identify areas of changed tissue tone and texture. Having identified a trigger point, the thumb pushes in slightly on one side of the nasal bones while the index and third finger exert the same pressure on the opposite side (Figure 12.2). Slowly changing the amount of pressure exerted on a trigger point can achieve local

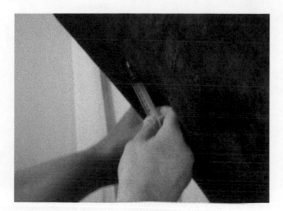

Figure 12.1 Sedation: with light sedative, the horse is relaxed yet responsive which is helpful for certain techniques.

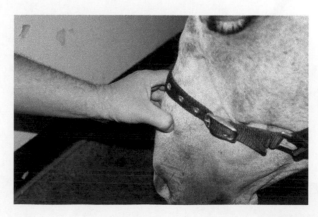

Figure 12.2 Trigger point inhibition: the thumb and fingers gently push into trigger points either side of the nasal bones while the effect on the subocciput is monitored.

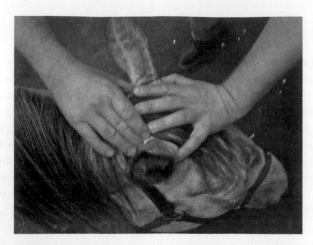

Figure 12.3 Occipito-frontal hold: one hand is placed over the sub-occiput, the other flat on the frontal bone with the middle finger positioned centrally and pointing up towards the poll.

tissue relaxation which is often reflected in a change in the suboccipital muscles. It is worth mentioning that horses are obligate nasal breathers so the pressure applied should not completely occlude the nasal passages!

If the nasofrontal hold is not tolerated by the horse, an occipito-frontal hold may have a better response. This involves placing one hand on the subocciput as before, with the other flat on the frontal bone with the middle finger positioned centrally and pointing up towards the poll (Figure 12.3). Trigger points in the fascia overlying the cranium can be inhibited. Direct soft tissue techniques to the temporalis and auricular muscles may be performed using both hands to 'scoop up' or lift the fascia from the cranium (Figure 12.4).

Functional technique

With the hands still in position on the subocciput and frontal bones, a functional tissue approach may be used. The hands

follow the lines of tension in the fascia, guiding the tissues in this direction and thereby taking them to a point of least tension. This position is held until there is a sense of relaxation and release in the tissues. The method can be taken further to incorporate cranial techniques. By following the cranial rhythm into flexion and extension ranges, restriction in this movement can be identified. Using the hands to reduce gradually the flexion/extension fluctuations in the frontal and occipital bones across the sphenoid, a still point is achieved and maintained until there is a general sense of release of tissue tension in the occipito-frontal region which may be reflected throughout the spine.

Parietal lift

Following the treatment of occipital and frontal regions, the lateral structures of the parietal and temporal bones are evaluated. As in humans, dysfunction gives an impression that the parietal bones are being dragged down towards the cranial base and seem welded to the temporal bones. This can be relieved by a parietal lift, using the thenar and hypothenar eminences. It is applied to the parietals each side and the practitioner pushes up vertically with firm, sustained effort (Figure 12.5).

Temporal balance

The temporal bones are formed by the solid petrous parts which are driven like wedges into the cranial base, and by the squama which form part of the vault providing a site of attachment for the muscles of the jaw and ear. The musculature of this region should be symmetric in development and orientation and should not feel bound down to the adjacent parts of the skull. The ears are useful handles for influencing the temporal bones. By holding one in each hand, an existing strain pattern in the soft tissues can be reproduced by gently

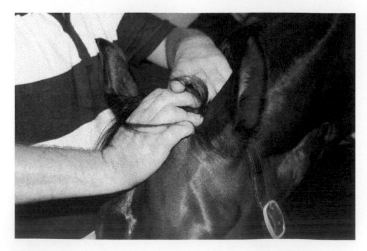

Figure 12.4 Fascial soft tissue: both hands can be used to 'scoop up' and lift the fascia from the cranium.

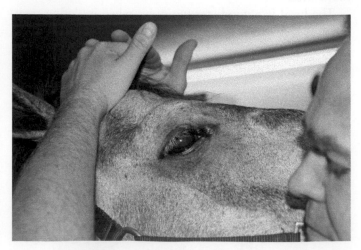

Figure 12.5 Parietal lift: a sustained lift uses the thenar and hypothenar eminences applied to the parietal bones each side and pushing vertically upwards.

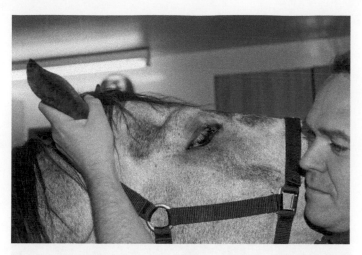

Figure 12.6 Temporal balance: holding one ear in each hand, the strain pattern can be reproduced by gently twisting and shearing the ears on the temporal bones. Traction can be used to disengage the temporal bones from the median structures of the cranial base.

twisting and shearing the ears, adopting a position of 'ease' in each range and holding this position until relaxation is felt in the tissues. An element of traction can also be introduced to 'disengage' the temporal bones from the median structures of the cranial base (Figure 12.6).

TEMPOROMANDIBULAR JOINT

The temporal bones are also involved with the mandible as the two bones join to form the temporomandibular joint. The mandible should hang in a relaxed fashion below the skull, rather as a basket is slung below a hot air balloon. The importance of this arrangement can easily be demonstrated on oneself by jumping up and down with the jaw clenched. Without absorption in the temporomandibular region, the shock waves appear to be transmitted straight into the skull. Muscle tension in this area also interferes with the normal retraction and protraction movements of the mandible as the head is flexed and extended on the neck during locomotion and grazing in addition to the lateral movements of the temporomandibular joints necessary for effective mastication. Treatment to this region should address any asymmetry, increase in muscle tone and changes in joint function.

Technique

Inhibition

Areas of local muscle tension around the mandible can be identified by exerting gentle pressure on the medial aspect of the mandibular body from the angle of the jaw to the mandibular symphysis in a way that has been likened to playing the piano. Treatment involves applying direct

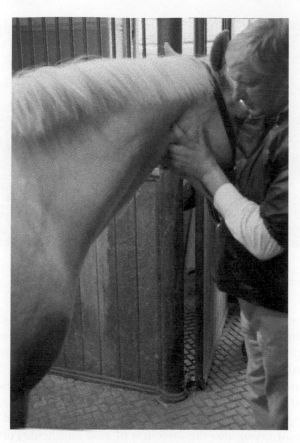

Figure 12.7 Inhibition: trigger points can be inhibited by applying direct pressure to soft tissues of the medial aspect of the mandibles.

pressure with the fingers to these trigger points (Figure 12.7). Successful outcome is indicated by relaxation of the mandible at the temporomandibular joints.

Soft tissue

The lateral musculature can be evaluated by sliding both hands along the lateral aspects of the mandibular rami to the point at which they join the temporal bones, assessing the symmetry and the quality and degree of bind of local soft tissues. Symmetry and quality of the cranial rhythm can also be palpated. Any tissue tension can be treated effectively by soft tissue work to these muscles, both cross-fibre and longitudinal stretch (Figure 12.8).

Traction

Direct traction of the temporomandibular joint can be produced by holding the angles of the jaw and slowly leaning backwards, and pulling down in a line from the ears in the direction of the ground, altering the angle of distraction as necessary (Figure 12.9).

Positional release

To treat the temporomandibular joints directly, positional release techniques are helpful. The dynamics of the jaw are

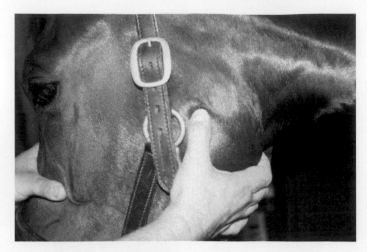

Figure 12.8 Soft tissue: cross fibre and longitudinal stretch can be applied to the muscles around the temporomandibular joint.

quite complex. The main components are opening and closing and lateral movements, but there are also accessory shearing ranges. By taking hold of the mandibular rami, a small degree of opening and closing can be tested. One direction will feel easier than the other and this represents the direction of 'ease'. Maintaining this degree of opening or closing, lateral movements to the left and right are tested and the joint taken into the direction of ease and held. Further elements such as cranio-caudal shear, rotation, distraction and compression are transposed on to this point in the same way. This establishes a position of minimum tissue tension which is maintained until there is a release of tension in the peri-articular structures (Figure 12.10).

Once satisfactory mobility has been achieved, it is often helpful to finish with craniofacial balancing. Sliding both hands on to the jaw so that the fingers embrace the joint and the palms rest lightly on the ascending mandibular ramus, the lines of any residual tissue tension are followed and this

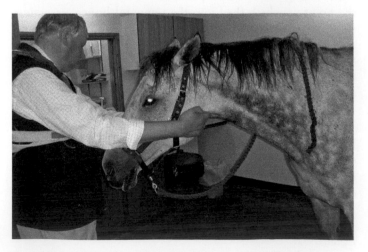

Figure 12.9 Traction: pulling down in a line from the ears and towards the ground produces traction at the temporomandibular joint.

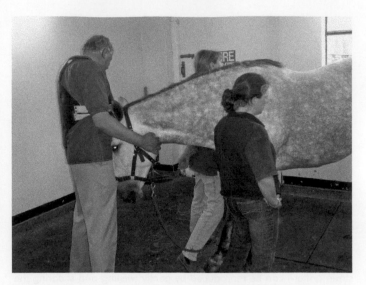

Figure 12.10 Positional release: combining vectors of temporomandibular movements with opening and closing and lateral movements, together with cranio-caudal shear, rotation and distraction or compression achieves a position of minimum tissue tension.

pattern is mirrored by the fingers until a point of minimal tension is reached. This position is maintained until there is a general sense of relaxation around the joint.

The temporomandibular joint and the occipito-atlanto-axial joint complex are intimately related anatomically, neurologically and functionally. The connection is often demonstrated to students by initially asking them to assess their own neck rotation, flexion and extension ranges. This is compared with the movement achieved when their teeth are firmly clamped on a spatula. The result is a noticeably diminished range when the muscles of the jaw are tightened over the spatula (Figure 12.11). The reduction in cervical movement which results from temporomandibular tension can be further compounded in horses by the use of some bits and devices designed to prevent the mouth opening. For this reason, balancing and relaxing the muscle tension of temporomandibular joint dysfunction is a good precursor to the treatment of the occipito-atlanto-axial complex.

UPPER CERVICAL SPINE

The upper cervical joints are the most mobile of the spine and are commonly affected by major trauma or multiple minor traumata. As a consequence, dysfunction in this region is not uncommon.

Occipito-atlantal Joints
Diagnosing the nature of an occipito-atlantal dysfunction both anatomically and in terms of chronicity is important in deciding the treatment approach to be used.

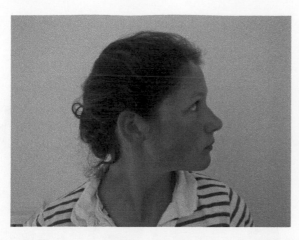
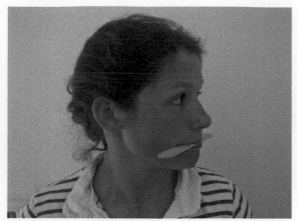

Figure 12.11 Upper cervical mobility and the temporomandibular joint: range of neck movement is considerably reduced when the muscles over the temporomandibular joint are tight.

Range and quality of movement at this level, particularly in flexion and extension, should be assessed and the symmetry and tone of the suboccipital region palpated. Positional elements of the occipito-atlantal articulation can be evaluated by placing the index and third fingers in the spaces between the prominent wings of the atlas and the mandible. A gap on one side which is greater than the other suggests asymmetry, and this can be reassessed later to evaluate the effect of treatment (Figure 12.12).

Inhibition and functional technique

The muscles of the subocciput should be palpated on both sides while attempting to flex and extend the occiput on the atlas. This can be done by resting the mandible on the practitioner's shoulder and by bending and flexing the knees and palpating for muscle reaction. With the acute problem

there will be a sudden cessation of movement in one or both ranges, often associated with local muscle spasm either unilaterally or bilaterally. From this position, inhibition of the suboccipital muscles using downward pressure of the fingers can be performed (Figure 12.13). This can be combined with a functional unwinding technique by bending and straightening the knees to establish a point of ease in the flexion/extension range and then using the hands in contact with the subocciput to introduce the secondary ranges of rotation, lateral flexion, translocation and compression/decompression (Figure 12.14). The resulting composite point of ease is maintained until there is a discernible, often quite sudden, relaxation of the muscles around the upper cervical joints. The horse may sigh deeply as the release occurs.

In the more chronic case, there is often an inability to extend the joint, reflecting the more common dysfunction

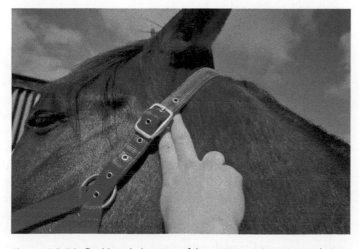

Figure 12.12 Positional elements of the occipito-atlantal articulation: a difference between the sides in the gap spanning the mandibular ramus and the wing of the atlas indicates occipito-atlantal joint asymmetry.

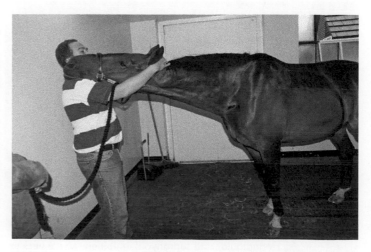

Figure 12.13 Suboccipital inhibition: acute upper cervical dysfunction can be treated using suboccipital inhibition.

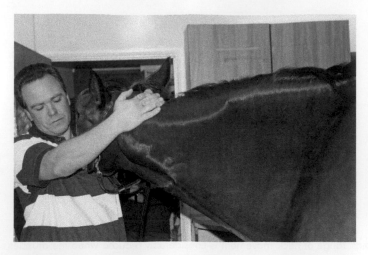

Figure 12.14 Suboccipital inhibition: this can be combined with a functional unwinding technique, building up the forces to achieve a position of minimum tension.

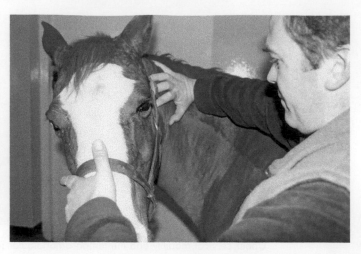

Figure 12.16 Atlanto-axial articulation: taking the nose round to the left and then to the right to check the range and quality of rotation can be developed into an articulation technique to improve rotation.

which involves a flexion of the occiput on the atlas. This makes it difficult to take the horse's head up on to the practitioner's shoulder. In these cases, treatment is started by inhibition techniques applied to the muscles running along the length of the mandible and around the hyoid apparatus (Figure 12.15). This aims to reduce the tension in the ventral structures of the upper neck sufficiently for the head to extend, so allowing it to be brought on to the practitioner's shoulder. The inhibition and functional techniques previously described can then be carried out. Extra vigilance is needed when checking ranges in this region because, with chronic occipito-atlantal dysfunction, trick movements are often well established and can give the impression of normal mobility. It is therefore essential that motion testing and treatment are undertaken in a slow and

sensitive manner without employing large ranges which would trigger the trick movement immediately.

Atlanto-axial Joint

The same type of complex trick movement occurs in atlanto-axial dysfunction. The joint can be assessed by sliding both hands over the articular pillars of C1/2 and palpating for local soft tissue binding. Leaving one hand spanning the area between C1 and C2, the nose can be taken around to the left and then, changing sides, to the right to check the range and quality of rotation which constitutes the most significant movement here. This can be developed into an articulation technique to improve rotation (Figure 12.16). Other techniques resemble those for the occipito-atlantal region such as local inhibition, compression, traction and sustained positional techniques.

Sustained positional release

Sustained positional release is a highly effective technique at this level. With the horse's mandible on the practitioner's shoulder, the hands can encompass the large wings of the atlas. Maintaining a quiescent hand position, the atlas is moved on the axis by virtue of changing the practitioner's body position in relation to the palpating hands, using the point of contact with the mandible as a fulcrum. This should start with rotation by moving in one direction and then in the other to establish which direction is easier. A degree of rotation in the direction of ease is maintained and then flexion or extension, lateral flexion left or right, compression or traction, and translocation are introduced depending on the ease of movement for each of these ranges. By building up these vectors to the point of minimum tissue tension and holding the position for around 90 seconds, there should be

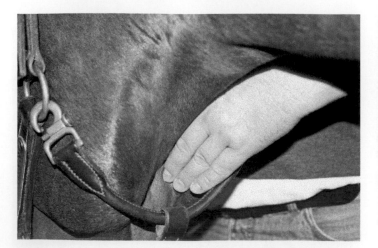

Figure 12.15 Mandibular and suprahyoid inhibition: where neck extension is difficult, treatment is started by inhibition of the muscles the length of the mandible and around the hyoid apparatus.

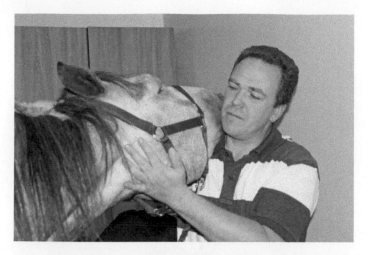

Figure 12.17 Atlanto-axial functional technique: maintaining rotation in the direction of ease, secondary movements are added to achieve a position of minimum tension which is held until relaxation of the tissues occurs.

a reduction of muscle tone which may be sudden or gradual (Figure 12.17).

If response of the soft tissues is poor, it is helpful for another practitioner to take up the slack at the root of the tail and exert gentle traction. This distraction often initiates a soft tissue response under the palpating hand at the top of the neck (Figure 12.18).

Soft tissue and inhibition techniques

Other techniques aimed more directly at the muscular component of the dysfunction include inhibition and kneading of the soft tissues of the suboccipital triangle. Attention should also be given to the ventral muscles which can be inhibited by lifting the horse's head on to the practitioner's

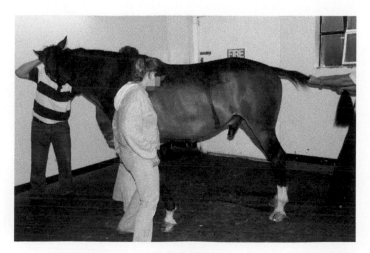

Figure 12.18 Triggering a response: if the response to functional technique is poor, another practitioner exerts gentle traction to initiate a soft tissue reaction at the top of the neck.

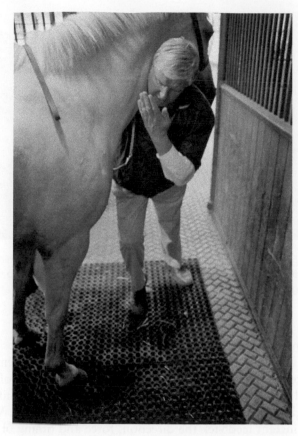

Figure 12.19 Ventral muscle inhibition: sliding the practitioner's shoulder into the ventral structures, upward pressure can be applied.

shoulder and then sliding this shoulder upwards along the mandibles and then immediately behind the mandible and into the soft tissues of the ventral structures of the upper one-third of the neck (Figure 12.19). Once in position, upwards pressure can be applied gradually. The horse often participates by pushing down on to the practitioner's shoulder.

MID- TO LOWER CERVICAL SPINE

Treatment directed at the rest of the neck is a natural progression from the occipito-atlanto-axial and temporo-mandibular areas. It is helpful to remember that the cervical spine follows the course of an inverted 'S' which, below C3, is an extension curve concave dorsally. This means that the transverse processes are situated more ventrally in the neck than might be imagined.

Soft tissue techniques

Soft tissue work, which includes longitudinal and cross-fibre stretching, can be used to treat cervical paravertebral soft tissues and ventral structures. With the mandible resting on the practitioner's shoulder the soft tissue reaction can

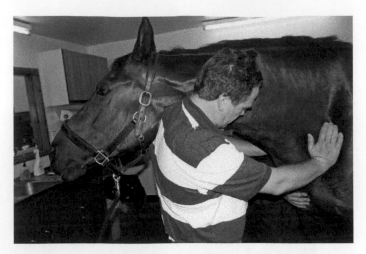

Figure 12.20 Soft tissue technique: direction, force and timing of longitudinal and cross fibre technique are varied in response to tissue changes.

be monitored by the apparent change in weight, position and movement of the horse's head. The head will often feel lighter as the soft tissues relax, and the movement of the head on the neck produced by the practitioner's shifting weight backwards and forwards will feel more fluid. With this instant feedback the direction, force and timing of soft tissue treatment can be varied constantly for optimum effect (Figure 12.20).

Articulation

Having worked from the superficial down to the deep soft tissues, joint articulation can be performed. The position of the horse's mandible on the practitioner's shoulder is maintained and the hands used as a fulcrum on the desired level of articulation. The impetus for movement is produced by the practitioner's shifting weight from one foot to another for lateral flexion, or bending and straightening the knees for flexion and extension, while a combination of the two produces rotation (Figure 12.21). It is important to be slow and rhythmic and to use small ranges of movement initially, during which soft tissue reactions are monitored continually. Variations in force and direction of articulation can be made in response to these tissue changes.

In order to encourage ventro-dorsal movement, the practitioner's shoulder is run along the ventral surface of the neck, gently pushing directly upwards at each articular level to identify any areas of resistance. At a point of resistance this upward pressure should be increased and the horse will often assist by pushing down on to the shoulder (Figure 12.22).

Articulation involving translocation with a degree of lateral flexion can be directed to the site of restricted movement. With one practitioner's shoulder supporting the

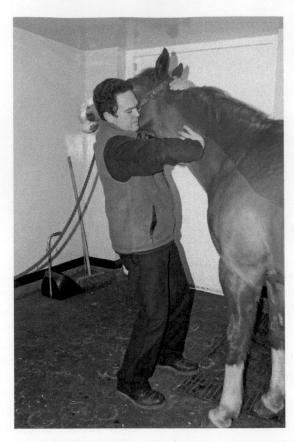

Figure 12.21 Articulation: using the hand as a fulcrum, different planes of movement are introduced by shifts in practitioner's weight bearing.

head and exerting a degree of traction, another practitioner positioned at one side of the neck embraces the transverse processes with both hands and pushes rhythmically from side to side (Figure 12.23).

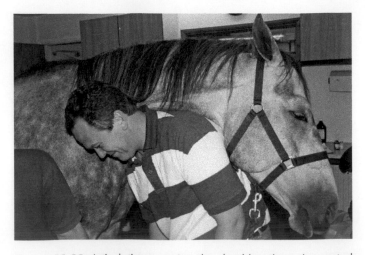

Figure 12.22 Articulation: running the shoulder along the ventral surface of the neck until an area of resistance is felt, gentle upward pressure is used to achieve ventrodorsal movement.

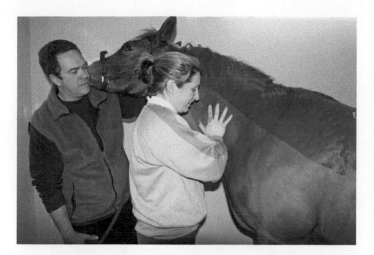

Figure 12.23 Translocation articulation: with one practitioner supporting the head and exerting traction, the other applies pressure to the transverse processes in a side to side movement.

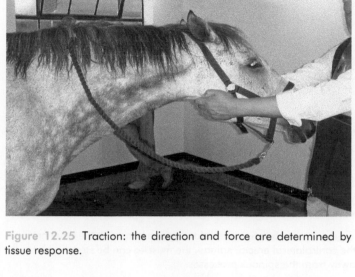

Figure 12.25 Traction: the direction and force are determined by tissue response.

Cervical traction/compression

Cervical spine injuries commonly result in a compound dysfunction of compression with rotation. These types of injury respond well to traction. This can be applied with the head either on the practitioner's shoulder or cradled under an arm with one hand under the mandible and the other on the subocciput and then slowly leaning backwards (Figure 12.24). Traction with upper cervical extension can be produced by holding the angles of the jaw and again leaning backwards (Figure 12.25). With the application of traction the tissues respond quickly. It is important to go with the flow by letting the direction and force of the traction be determined by tissue response. The horse may pull backwards slightly and the neck visibly stretches with relaxation of the soft tissues in the neck. When no more change can be felt, a second practitioner taking up the

slack in the tail and exerting gentle traction may stimulate further reaction. When a point is reached that appears to be static in terms of tissue change, traction is released gently.

Occasionally there is no reaction to traction. In these cases response can be stimulated by direct compression of the cervical spine from the vertex of the head (Figure 12.26). Again, as with traction, if a positive response is felt and the muscles of the neck relax, maintain the degree and direction of pressure until no more change occurs.

THORACIC SPINE

Soft tissue techniques to the neck can be extended into the thoracic paravertebral tissues and are very similar to the human approach to this region. It may be helpful to stand

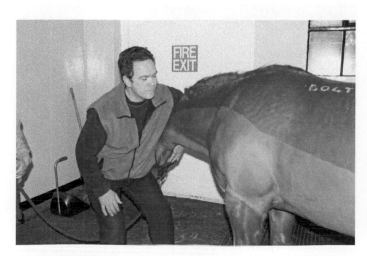

Figure 12.24 Traction. With the head cradled under one arm leaning back exerts traction through the cervical spine.

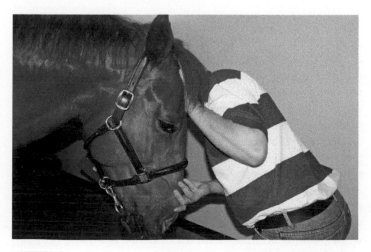

Figure 12.26 Compression: the cervical muscles may be relaxed by direct compression from the vertex.

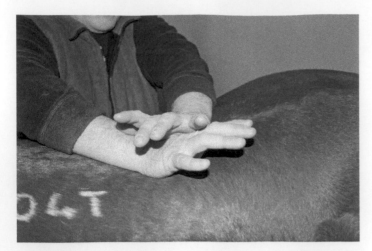

Figure 12.27 Soft tissue: reinforcing one hand with the other hand on the contralateral erector spinae, the muscles can be stretched laterally away from the spinous processes.

on a bale or crate in order to obtain purchase on the areas to be treated. Care should be exercised on this rather vulnerable perch for although a sedated horse is relatively quiet it is still capable of movement.

Soft tissue techniques

Starting at the cervicothoracic level, cross-fibre stretching can be carried out along the whole length of the thoracic spine. Positioning the thenar eminence of one hand just on the far side of the spinous process and reinforcing this hold with the other hand, the erector spinae muscles can be stretched laterally away from the spinous processes. Starting superficially and gradually going deeper, the degree and ease with which the soft tissue yields under the hands should be monitored and the treatment directed particularly to those areas that are resistant to pressure (Figure 12.27).

Thoracic springing and articulation

As an adjunct to this soft tissue work, individual joint articulation can contribute to improving mobility in the thoracic spine. As with soft tissue techniques a bale or crate may be used to stand by the side of the horse so that direct downward pressure can be exerted on to the spine. Areas of stiffness can be identified by placing the fingers of the cranial hand into the interspinous space and monitoring tissue resistance as the other hand pushes gently down on to the caudal spinous process (Figure 12.28). Having identified an area of restriction, the hands are placed on the transverse processes either side of the spinous process. The body weight is transmitted downwards through the forearms while pushing cranially with the near side hand and caudally with the other in a cross-handed thoracic spring technique (Figure 12.29). From this position the angle of the ribs can

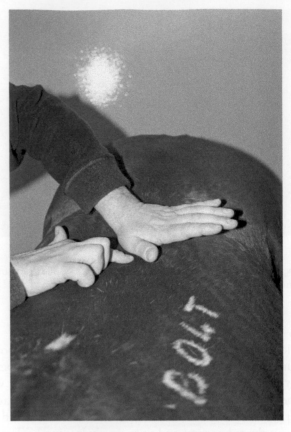

Figure 12.28 Thoracic articulation: by palpating the interspinous space and pushing gently down on to the caudal spinous process, movement can be assessed.

be accessed with one hand holding back on the spinous process while the other maintains a steady pressure on the rib angle in a lateral direction away from the midline (Figure 12.30).

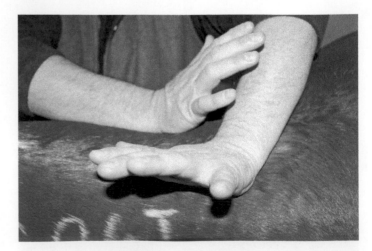

Figure 12.29 Dorsal springing: body weight is transmitted downwards, pushing cranially with the nearside hand and caudally with the other in a cross-handed thoracic spring technique.

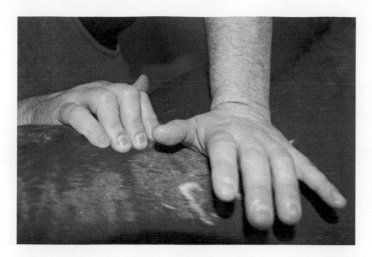

Figure 12.30 Rib articulation: with one hand holding back on the spinous process, the other maintains a steady pressure on the rib angle in a lateral direction, away from the midline.

Soft tissue

Periscapular soft tissue is of great value once the midline structures have been treated (Figure 12.31). There are a number of important muscles in this region which need to be supple for the cervicothoracic spine and forelimbs to function optimally.

1. Trapezius: cross-fibre and longitudinal soft tissue here (Figure 12.32) relaxes the topline of the cervicothoracic region which needs to be supple to allow the head and neck to stretch away from the thorax during locomotion.
2. Ascending pectoral muscles: by standing at the side and reaching around to the front with one hand and countering on the horse's elbow with the other, an effective

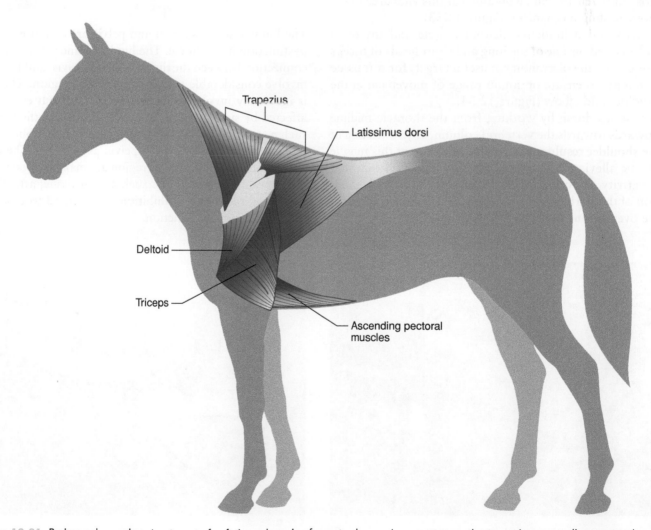

Figure 12.31 Periscapular region: treatment of soft tissue here is of great value and encompasses the trapezius, ascending pectoral muscles, triceps, deltoid and latissimus dorsi.

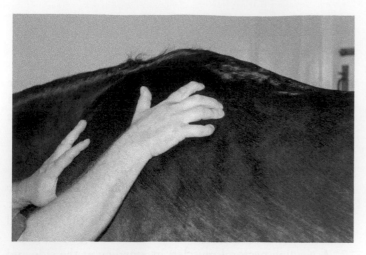

Figure 12.32 Trapezius: cross-fibre and longitudinal soft tissue here relaxes the topline of the cervicothoracic region.

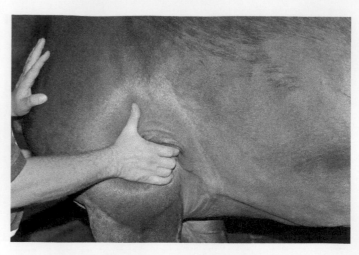

Figure 12.34 Triceps and deltoid: these muscles respond well to soft tissue technique.

cross-fibre release can be obtained at this vital area of the thoracic sling mechanism (Figure 12.33).

3. Triceps and deltoid: the deltoid muscle and the often well defined outline of the long and short heads of triceps rising from the olecranon are useful targets for soft tissue technique to ensure optimum range of movement at the shoulder and elbow (Figure 12.34).

4. Latissimus dorsi: by working from the thoracic midline upwards towards the vertebral column, any restriction at the shoulder resulting from increased tone of this muscle can be alleviated. Localised areas of increased tone and sensitivity can often be identified here, and local inhibition of these trigger points may have a dramatic effect on the overall tone of the muscle (Figure 12.35).

LUMBAR SPINE, SACRUM AND PELVIS

The lumbar spine, sacrum and pelvis are common areas of dysfunction in the horse. The lumbar spine is the only bony connection between the thorax and the pelvis, and falls often involve considerable torque through this region. The pelvis is inevitably involved in this type of injury. It can also be affected by sudden forces transmitted through the hind legs such as may occur when putting a leg into a rabbit hole or ditch and may well result in pelvic asymmetry. The causes and nature of injuries in this region are many and varied, and a wide range of techniques such as soft tissue, articulation, positional release and inhibition can be used to desensitise and restore normal function.

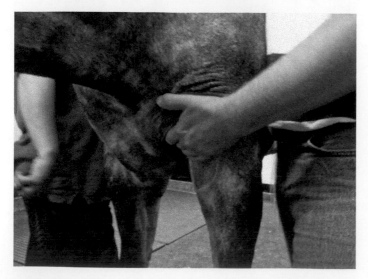

Figure 12.33 Pectoral soft tissue: reaching round to the front with one hand and countering on the horse's elbow with the other, an effective cross-fibre release of the ascending pectoral muscles is achieved.

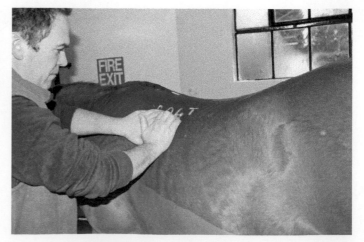

Figure 12.35 Latissimus dorsi: working from the thoracic midline upwards towards the vertebral column, soft tissue and inhibitory techniques have an effect on muscle tone.

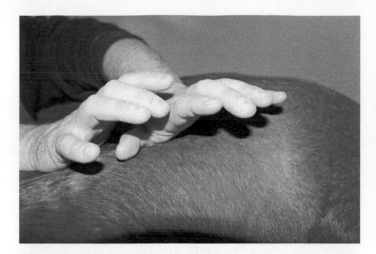

Figure 12.36 Soft tissue and articulation: one hand pushes on the ipsilateral side of the spinous process while the other pushes laterally on the contralateral soft tissue to combine articulation with soft tissue technique.

Soft tissue technique

To apply this effectively the practitioner should be in a position to apply pressure dorso-ventrally as well as craniocaudally. A stout box or bale may be helpful depending on the relative size of practitioner and horse.

Paravertebral soft tissue lateral stretch

This is similar to thoracic erector spinae techniques but, as the lumbar spine is unencumbered by the restrictions imposed by the ribs, it is easier to combine the technique with lumbar spine articulation. From the side of the horse, the thenar eminence of one hand is placed on the contralateral erector spinae just lateral to the tip of the spinous process, and covered with the other hand. By leaning forwards the practitioner's body weight is transmitted vertically down and laterally to effect lateral stretch. By moving the uppermost hand to the side of the spinous process nearest to the practitioner and pushing downwards and laterally in time with the soft tissue work of the other hand, an element of articulation can be introduced (Figure 12.36). This should be undertaken rhythmically and, by varying the speed of movement, the natural harmonic rate of the tissue can be determined. This is the rate at which the body responds optimally, avoiding too fast a rate which irritates the tissues and too slow which has little effect on tone. Changes in tissue states should be monitored continuously and may require changes in pressure and direction of the technique. This treatment can be extended over the sacrum, laterally into the glutei and downwards into the hamstrings (Figures 12.37 and 12.38).

Articulation

Lumbar spine articulation can be performed using a technique similar to the cross-handed springing of the thoracic

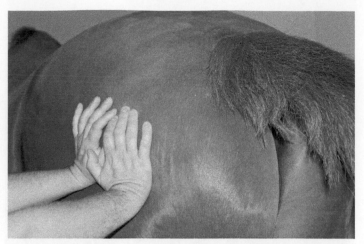

Figure 12.37 Soft tissue technique: cross-fibre stretch can be extended from the lumbar spine into the glutei.

spine and involves identifying areas of stiffness and then encouraging movement by pushing down on the transverse processes on either side of the spinous process.

Fascial release techniques

Fascial release techniques, by which relaxation and symmetry are restored to the soft tissue of the lumbosacral complex, can be achieved using the tail. The tail is intimately associated with the muscles and fascia of the lumbosacral spine as the sacrocaudalis dorsalis muscles of the tail form a continuum with the stabilising multifidus muscles of the lumbar spine. It can be used to identify and release strain patterns in the lumbar and sacropelvic region.

Standing to the side of the sacrum, the tail is held about 8 cm from its root, with the other hand resting over both tubera sacrale above the lumbosacral joint and over as much of the rest of the sacrum and pelvis as can be spanned comfortably. By lifting the tail, the sacrum will extend on the

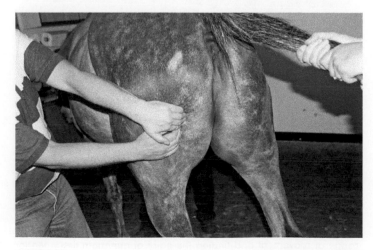

Figure 12.38 Soft tissue technique: cross-fibre stretch can be applied to the hamstrings.

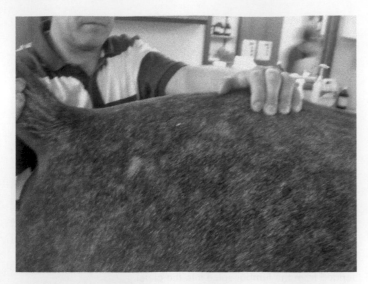

Figure 12.39 Articulation of the lumbosacral joint: by lifting the tail, the sacrum will extend on the caudal lumbar vertebrae.

caudal lumbar vertebrae (Figure 12.39). Dropping the tail will flex the sacrum with respect to these vertebrae. The range and ease of motion and the quality of the end point of movement at the lumbosacral junction should be noted. The soft tissues may move in one direction much more easily than the other, and so the tail should be taken into the easy range, either flexion or extension, until an end point is reached. From this point, testing is repeated using sidebending and rotation left and then right followed by translocation dorso-ventrally and laterally. For each range the direction of least tension is held. Having built up these vectors to a point of minimum tissue tension, the root of the tail is squeezed, initially gently and then with a gradual increase in pressure (Figure 12.40). This may be sufficient to produce relaxation in the tissues of the sacro-pelvis. The release of tension is

felt by the palpating hand positioned over the lumbosacral complex, and is often accompanied by traction as the horse shifts its weight-bearing forwards.

Traction

If the horse does not respond to squeezing the tail, it may be necessary to apply some direct spinal traction via the tail with the aim of stimulating a tissue response. This is a combined effort on the part of both participants, as traction is initiated by the practitioner and facilitated by the horse which shifts its weight forwards. The tail position is maintained at the previously established point of ease and the slack in the soft tissues is gradually taken up by slowly and gently leaning back (Figure 12.41). Traction is gradually increased until the horse begins to pull forwards. This tendency should be countered. At this stage, help is often required as the forward momentum is considerable and appears to bear no relation to the size of the horse (Figure 12.42). During this process, the horse may begin to shift its pelvis quite dramatically as it changes weight-bearing from one hind leg to the other (Figure 12.43). The traction is maintained through these changes until the horse ceases to pull forwards. If the horse does not shift its weight forwards a response may be stimulated by a second practitioner performing a positional release at the occipito-atlanto-axial joint (Figure 12.44). With the mandible on the practitioner's shoulder, movement ranges are tested and a point of ease identified and maintained. The subsequent sense of relaxation often acts as a sudden switch which causes the horse to pull firmly against the traction exerted by the practitioner at the tail.

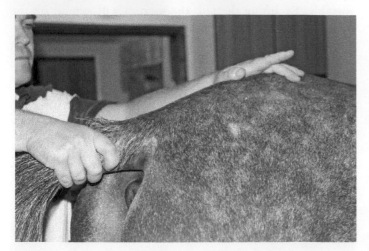

Figure 12.40 Functional technique: taking the tail through each range of movement and finding the point of minimum tissue tension the root of the tail is squeezed, gradually increasing the pressure until the tissue relaxes.

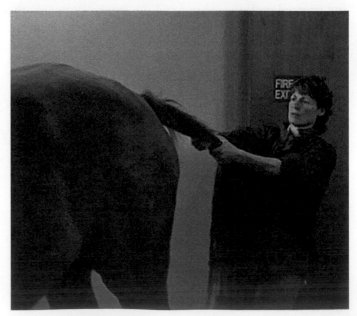

Figure 12.41 Traction: with the tail position at minimum tension, traction is applied by slowly and gently leaning back.

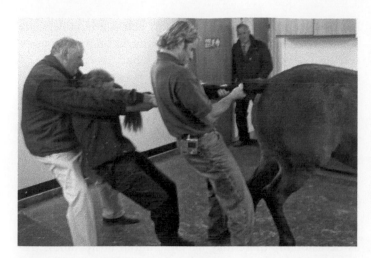

Figure 12.42 Traction: a number of people may be required to counter the forward shift in weight-bearing. Ponies often pull harder than their larger counterparts.

At all times the direction and force of the traction must be in response to the signals from the horse. Once the horse stops responding, the grip on the tail should be gradually released.

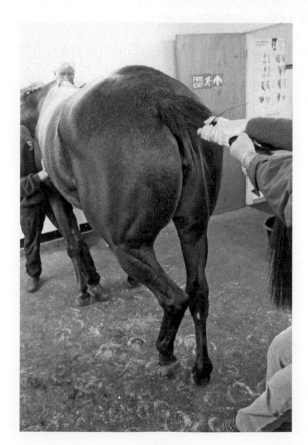

Figure 12.43 Traction: there may be dramatic shifts in weightbearing to stretch the pelvic soft tissues. Photo courtesy of Jonathan Cohen MSc (Ost).

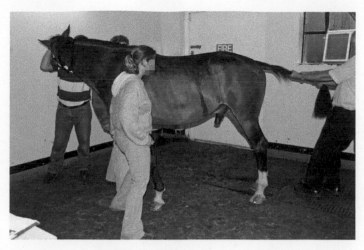

Figure 12.44 Traction: forward weight shift may be stimulated by simultaneously relaxing the suboccipital area with a positional release technique at the occipito-atlanto-axial joint.

Throughout this process there should be a sense of continual stretch. If at any stage there is swishing or clamping of the tail against the perineum, treatment should be suspended for a few moments. The tail is then gripped again and the sequence restarted. If the feeling of resistance persists, the procedure should be abandoned and a different approach used.

Pelvic lift

The pelvic diaphragm is another structure that can affect the function of the lumbosacral spine, pelvis and hindlimb and, as in humans, the pelvic lift technique is very effective. Holding on to the tail and moving it to one side the practitioner's shoulder is manoeuvred into the musculature of the perineum between the ischial tuberosities and steady cephalad pressure is exerted (Figure 12.45). This not only

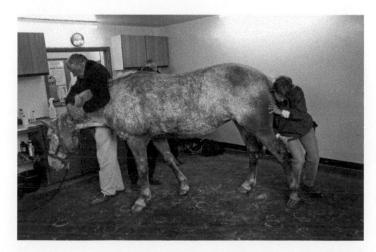

Figure 12.45 Pelvic lift: the practitioner's shoulder is manoeuvred into the musculature of the perineum between the ischial tuberosities and steady pressure in a cranial direction is exerted while monitoring tissue tension via the tail. Photo courtesy of Jonathan Cohen MSc (Ost).

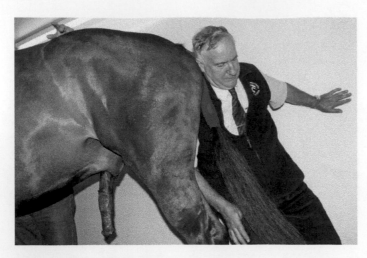

Figure 12.46 Pelvic lift: when the site and direction of pressure produces a tissue response, the horse often pushes backwards, necessitating counter pressure.

relaxes muscles of the pelvic diaphragm but also introduces compression and flexion at the lumbosacral joint which can improve mobility.

From this position, trigger points along the ischium can be identified by pushing the shoulder against the medial aspect of the tuber ischii and sacrotuberous ligament. Pressure can be altered in direction from a purely lateral pressure and changed in an arc to push in a more cephalad direction. When the site and direction of pressure produces a tissue response, the horse often pushes backwards, appearing to sit on the practitioner's shoulder and necessitating further counterpressure from the practitioner (Figure 12.46). This

is heavy work and a lumbar support belt is advisable. Care should be taken when using this technique on mares in season as, on very rare occasions, they have been known to respond with their hind legs!

POST-TREATMENT CARE

Once treatment has been completed, it is helpful to allow the horse to rest for 15 to 20 minutes. During this time, there may be fasciculation of the muscles in the areas treated, indicating continuing tissue changes. After this time the horse may be moved, but sharp turns should be avoided as occasionally there may be some initial unsteadiness. Although drinking is permitted, it is sensible to avoid giving food for 2 hours. Owners should be advised to remove hay nets from the stall or lorry. Box rest for the first 24 hours is helpful, assuming the horse will tolerate this, in order to allow tissue changes to continue without being challenged by energetic high jinks in the field.

Depending on the nature and longevity of the problem, the horse is followed up after an interval of 1 or 2 weeks, during which they should be confined to a small paddock to reduce the possibility of injury in the early stages of the treatment. Later, rehabilitation programmes between treatments play a vital part in recovery.

The number of treatments required will depend on the nature of the problem but around three or four treatments is routine. Follow-up consultations and possibly treatments are advisable during the rehabilitation period.

Examination and Treatment under General Anaesthetic

13

Anthony Pusey and Julia Brooks

INTRODUCTION

The 1970s were devoted to exploring an osteopathic approach to treating horses and experiencing enormous satisfaction at the changes that could be made. However, the treatment modality used had its limitations, particularly in dealing with problems of a more complex and long-standing nature.

Later in the decade, the Leicestershire osteopath Arthur Smith brought the idea of osteopathic treatment under general anaesthetic to my notice. Together with a local vet, he had treated a number of racehorses successfully under these conditions.

It was in Germany that the opportunity arose to examine and treat an anaesthetised horse whose problem had been resistant to other forms of treatment. The lady owner, dressed in figure-hugging jodhpurs, used her veterinary nursing experience to assist the vet in administering the anaesthetic. Her husband filmed the proceedings on his new video camera. It was immediately clear that, under these conditions, we could more easily determine the potential for movement on a joint-by-joint basis and that treatment was easier and more effective. It was also possible to focus on areas that were difficult to access in the standing horse.

Reviewing the video later, techniques used on the horse lying on its back or on its side showed a striking similarity to human practice and we discussed other procedures that could be borrowed from the human field. The owner's only comment on the film was to exclaim with horror that, had she known that her bottom was so big, she would have put herself on a diet some weeks previously!

With time and experience, the benefits of treatment under general anaesthetic for certain cases became more and more obvious, and problems that had formerly appeared to be intractable were resolved.

RATIONALE FOR TREATMENT UNDER GENERAL ANAESTHETIC

There are a number of reasons why this might be the treatment of choice, quite apart from the fact that horses look more like our human patients when lying on their backs!

Effects of Injury

Horses are large animals that often perform at high speed under the weight of a rider. Huge forces are generated and can do extensive damage when something goes wrong, especially during a fall. Under general anaesthetic some fairly large and specifically directed forces can be applied in order to reverse the effects of these injuries without having to counter the muscular activity involved in keeping the horse upright. It is also much easier to do a slow, methodical examination of each joint complex. This method makes it possible to check that the articulation moves in the expected range rather than with a well established trick manoeuvre, which involves accessory movements and participation of joints at other levels in order to achieve what passes for normal motion. It is astonishing how often an area seems to function reasonably well when watching a horse move, but in fact moves abnormally on a segmental check under general anaesthetic.

Site of Injury

Another advantage of this procedure is that certain areas such as the cervicothoracic region, lying deep within the structures of the shoulder girdle, are much easier to access. The variety of techniques possible is also much greater and can range from specific mobilisation for a localised problem to extensive fascial unwinding techniques for widespread complex dysfunction.

Presentation

There are a number of clinical indications which suggest that treatment under general anaesthetic is the approach of choice. For example, a history incorporating phrases such as 'My horse has always been stiff', or that it has 'always moved in an odd way' or has 'never been able to maintain a topline' suggests long-term dysfunction.

The typical clinical picture is of a horse that functions below its potential and suffers recurrent, acute problems on increasing work or a minor trauma. Examination of active movements and palpation frequently reveal long-standing compensatory patterns with involvement at a number of vertebral levels. These cases may respond to osteopathic treatment of the standing horse in the short term, but problems will often return with very little provocation.

Active Movements

One important and consistent sign in cases benefiting from treatment under general anaesthetic can be observed in the transition of movement from walk to trot. These horses typically prepare themselves for changing pace by straightening their head and neck to splint the cervicothoracic area and then launch themselves into the trot. This means that rather than a smooth transition into the faster gait, there is a jerky two-phase movement of a hop (elevating the forelimbs to splint the cervicothoracic region) and skip (propelling the body forwards to generate momentum so that the legs can follow on rather than participate in the movement).

Infra-red Thermography

Infra-red thermography is a useful diagnostic tool for visualising muscular activity and autonomic nervous system responses. Some cases present with marked and extensive surface temperature changes which are the manifestation of a short-term problem that has not yet created compensatory patterns of movement. These will usually respond to treatment of the standing horse. Other more subtle findings on thermographic scans point to the existence of a more complex problem that will require treatment under anaesthetic. Typically, these cases show slight cooling at the top of the neck, indicating upper cervical dysfunction which, over time, has compensated for adverse neuromusculoskeletal changes.

Other thermographic patterns suggesting long-term problems are disruptions to the normal warm dorsal stripe extending from the withers to the coccyx. This is explained by reduced activity and a corresponding reduction in heat production of the erector spinae as a consequence of stiffness and pain. Changes in the segmental supply by the sympathetic nervous system in response to injury also contribute to this cooling effect (Figure 13.1).

PREPARATION

In long-standing problems, the horse adapts to dysfunction by developing alternative patterns of posture and movement which involve changes in muscular activity and joint function. Treatment under general anaesthetic is much more effective if some of these secondary changes are addressed in the weeks before the procedure. Generally, three or four treatments in the standing horse are advisable to strip back the layers of compensation to reveal the bedrock of the primary problem.

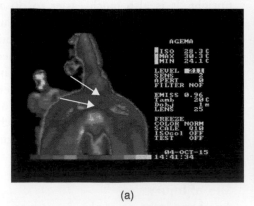
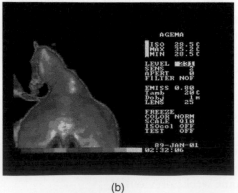

(a) (b)

Figures 13.1a and 13.1b Infra-red thermography: looking at the back from above and behind the tail, the dorsal stripe is present in the horse on the right (orange). This is disrupted in the scan on the left (arrows), indicating long-term dysfunction of the dorsal erector spinae.

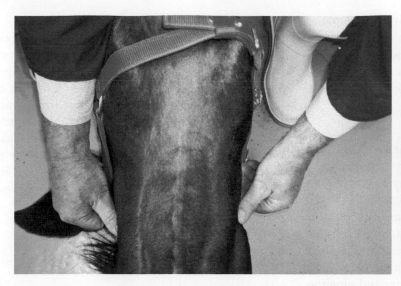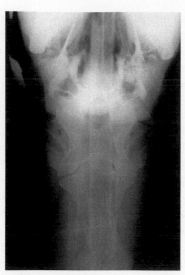

Figure 13.2 X-ray cervical spine: this is a sensible precaution as the neck is a common site for fractures and congenital malformations. Positional changes maintained by abnormal muscle tone can also be visualised.

PRECAUTIONS

As in human practice, anaesthetics carry a small risk. However, the anaesthetic is light, the horses are systemically well and there is no invasive surgery involved. Sensible precautions include a full fitness workup including blood tests, mainly to exclude infection. A cervical x-ray is always undertaken as treatment often involves the neck, which is a common site of injury and occasional congenital malformations. This has the advantage of visualising any apparent positional asymmetry of the joint complexes, particularly in the upper cervical spine (Figures 13.2a and 13.2b).

To complete these tests and to ensure that the horse has not eaten in the hours before the anaesthetic, it is recommended that it should arrive at the clinic on the day before the procedure. Although horses have no mechanism to vomit, which is a danger with anaesthetics in humans, a full stomach may rupture as the horse drops to the ground.

GENERAL ANAESTHETIC

Types of Anaesthesia

There are a number of ways to achieve general anaesthesia (Appendix H). This is largely determined by the environment, the availability of the equipment and the procedure to be carried out. As far as osteopathic examination and treatment are concerned, the anaesthetic used does not abolish local muscle reflexes and so tissue diagnosis is still possible.

The two principal forms of general anaesthesia are intravenous and inhalation.

Intravenous anaesthesia

Intravenous anaesthetic is not ideal for osteopathic treatment. One drawback is that it is much shorter acting and so it is necessary to be sure, before the start, of the area to be targeted and the result required. There is limited opportunity for joint-by-joint assessment or time-consuming techniques such as fascial unwinding. However, it is cheaper, is not labour intensive, and does not require complicated equipment or a particular environment (Figure 13.3).

The procedure itself begins with pre-medication, usually in the form of a combination of analgesic and sedative given intramuscularly to quieten the horse. This is followed 20 minutes later by induction, which involves a dissociative agent given intravenously to achieve amnesia, analgesia and

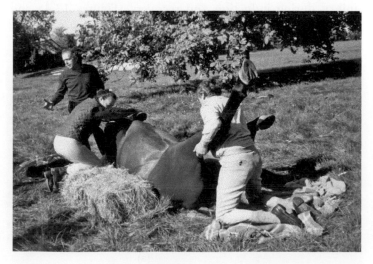

Figure 13.3 Intravenous anaesthetic: this can be used in a variety of settings and does not require much equipment. However, it is short acting, allowing only limited time for diagnosis and treatment.

loss of consciousness. This will give around 20 minutes of anaesthesia after which the horse becomes conscious quite quickly, often signalled by a stiffening or sudden movement of one or more limbs. Anaesthesia can be maintained for longer by incremental doses of the induction agent.

Inhalation anaesthesia

This is the preferred option as it can be maintained for longer to allow an unhurried, methodical examination and treatment. The procedure starts in the same way as intravenous anaesthesia with pre-medication and induction. However, once induced, anaesthesia is maintained by anaesthetic gases via an endotracheal tube. The advantages are that constant anaesthesia can be maintained and treatment can continue uninterrupted. The disadvantage is that it involves quite cumbersome equipment such as gas cylinders and monitoring devices and is therefore only practical in the environment of an operating theatre. The endotracheal tube may be of some minor inconvenience when examining the neck.

Where to Do It

Intravenous anaesthesia can be carried out almost anywhere that allows space for manoeuvring, but carries a high risk of injury to horse and practitioner. Field anaesthesia is not advisable as there may be a brief period of excitation during the recovery phase. Restraint must be exercised at this stage and the horse should not be allowed to run uncontrolled in an open space. The procedure may be carried out in a large loose box where the horse can come round quietly in a peaceful environment.

Inhalation anaesthesia requires more space to accommodate equipment and is best performed in operating theatres. These are often padded areas to reduce the possibility of injury during induction and recovery (Figures 13.4a and 13.4b).

What You Need

Many of the examination and treatment procedures take place with the horse on its back. Lifting equipment such as a winch is useful for manoeuvring the horse. Its position can then be maintained using hay bales or inflatable cushions.

Treatment techniques may involve lifting various body parts, and it is useful to be able to employ your own body weight by using a rope rather like a windsurfing harness. The headcollar should be left on the horse to allow a purchase point for the rope. As well as an anaesthetist, it is helpful to have another pair of hands to assist in techniques.

OSTEOPATHIC EXAMINATION AND TREATMENT UNDER GENERAL ANAESTHETIC

Positioning

Once anaesthetised, the horse is placed on to its back and supported in this position by a couple of airbags or hay bales either side of the withers. For certain techniques it may be necessary to roll the horse on to its side, which is readily done by deflating a cushion or removing a bale. Bringing the horse back into the supine position is not so easy, and so forward planning to avoid too much weight lifting is advisable.

Observation

Once in position, the process of examination can begin. The horse should lie squarely with the well muscled back as a platform. In fact, a horse with problems will rarely be able to do this. Many of the horses with long-term dysfunction have poorly developed erector spinae muscles as a result of pain and stiffness. Instead of having a broad, muscular surface to lie on, there is a sharp ridge of spinal processes which makes it difficult for the horse to lie straight and tends to make it fall to one side or the other. The horse may even adopt a

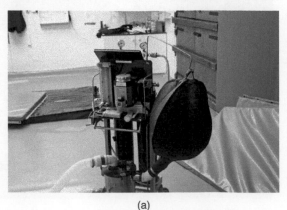

(a)

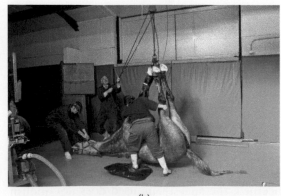

(b)

Figures 13.4a and 13.4b Inhalation anaesthesia: for osteopathic treatment, this is the method of choice and is performed in an operating theatre with space and appropriate equipment. Photos courtesy of Jonathan Cohen MSc (Ost).

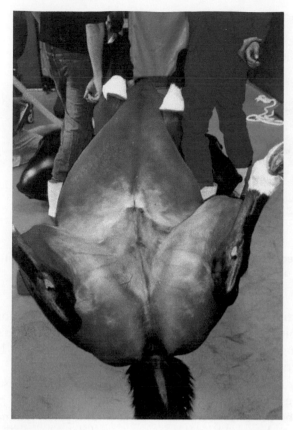

Figure 13.5 Supine: the horse may be unable to lie squarely on its back because of musculoskeletal asymmetry.

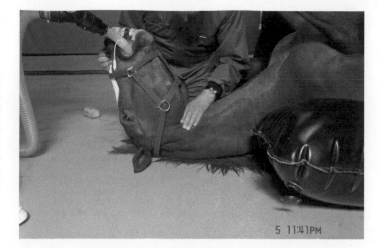

Figure 13.6 Occipito-atlantal joint: the main movement at this level is flexion–extension. The range should be full with a well defined end point.

twisted posture as it lies on its back (Figure 13.5). The fascial and muscular patterns that develop following injury and subsequent compensation produce a functional scoliosis that is maintained even under full anaesthetic. It is a testament to the willing nature of horses that they will often try to work for the rider while coping with a large degree of dysfunction.

The legs should be suspended symmetrically above the body in a relaxed fashion. Again, asymmetry of muscle development and joint flexibility means that this rarely happens. One or other of the forelimbs and/or hindlimbs may be held in relative protraction or retraction to give a disorganised, asymmetric look to the supine horse.

Palpation

For the palpatory phase of assessment, the supine horse very much resembles human patients. A thorough, region-by-region examination can be made by testing the appropriate movement ranges. The testing should be done slowly and carefully because, even in the anaesthetised state, a joint with long-term dysfunction will have developed so-called 'trick movements'. This is where the joint has adapted to incorporate accessory ranges of motion and to involve other vertebral levels in order to compensate for neuromusculoskeletal changes, and may appear to achieve a better range of movement than in fact exists.

Occipito-atlantal Region

Kneeling beside the top part of the neck, the muzzle is lifted to flex the head on the first cervical vertebra while observing and palpating the range and quality of the movement (Figure 13.6). There should be a smooth, easy sensation of tissue change with a well defined end point as the joint complex reaches its limit of movement. A common departure from normal function is the introduction of lateral plane activity in addition to flexion. The head may deviate laterally, either immediately on lifting the head or at some point during the range testing, if mobility is limited on one side of the joint complex more than the other. Occipito-atlantal impaction is a common injury that results in marked restriction in flexion. Movement is taken up lower down the cervical spine instead, making flexion feel abnormally easy.

Occipito-atlantal extension is also assessed. Normal movement should be free and easy with an obvious end point. Any rotation or sidebend mixed in with the extension is abnormal (Figures 13.7a and 13.7b). This may be monitored by palpating the suboccipital region.

Atlanto-axial joint

This region is particularly important for rotation and is often compromised in a fall at speed on to the head where the top of the neck is subjected to a twisting, compressive force. Movement should be assessed to the right and left, using the muzzle as a lever. At the end of the range, the mandible should lie almost parallel with the floor on either side when all the joints are moving normally, as the rotation range at the atlanto-axial joint alone is estimated at around 110° (Figure 13.8). Unilateral or bilateral restriction should be noted.

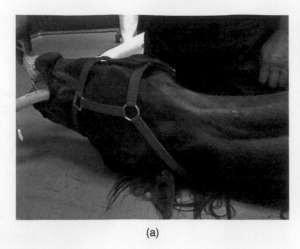

(a)

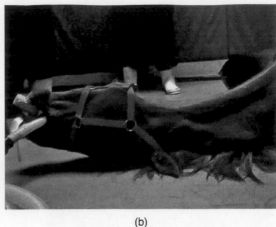

(b)

Figures 13.7a and 13.7b Occipito-atlantal joint: rotation or sidebend mixed in with the extension is abnormal (shown on the left in a pre-treatment assessment). Normal movement should be free and easy with an obvious end point (shown on the right, post-treatment).

Temporomandibular joint

The temporomandibular joint is intimately associated with the upper cervical spine. The connection is not only mechanical but also neurological as its nerve supply originates from the spinal trigeminal nucleus of the brain stem which extends into and interconnects with the dorsal horn of the upper cervical cord. Opening and closing movements are augmented by side-to-side shift and cranio-caudal glide to give an elliptical range necessary for chewing. Joint dysfunction and asymmetry in tone and bulk of the overlying muscles are common findings.

Kneeling at the head of the horse, the head is lifted on to the practitioner's lap. From this position the range of movement of both right and left articulations can be evaluated and compared with one another.

Holding the mandible with one hand and the nasal bone in the other, these two components can be moved in opposite directions to produce a lateral shift at the temporomandibular joint. This should be an easy movement achieving a surprisingly large range. Mobility should be assessed in both directions (Figure 13.9).

By taking hold of the angle of the jaw on both sides and lifting straight up towards the ceiling, cranio-caudal glide can be assessed. Distraction should take place symmetrically and smoothly at the temporomandibular joints (Figure 13.10). Horses with long-term neck problems or dental problems may be very restricted in one or both of these articulations.

Hyoid region

With the head still on the lap the hyoid apparatus can be evaluated. This can be done initially by palpating the structures of the floor of the mouth including the muscles between the mandibular rami which attach to the hyoid. The tissues

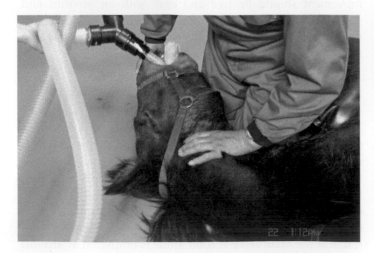

Figure 13.8 Atlanto-axial rotation: at the end of the range, the mandible should lie almost parallel with the floor.

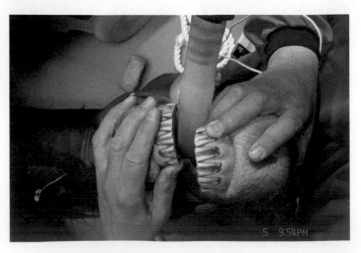

Figure 13.9 Temporomandibular joint: lateral shift should be of equal range and ease of movement in both directions.

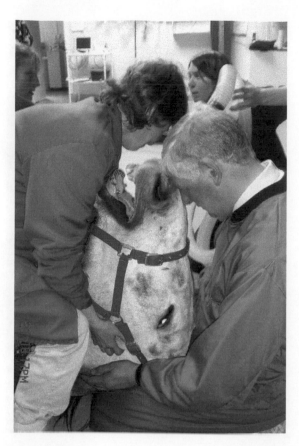

Figure 13.10 Temporomandibular joint: cranio-caudal glide is assessed by lifting the angle of the jaw straight up towards the ceiling. Distraction should be smooth and symmetric.

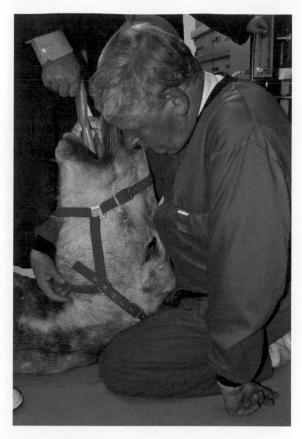

Figure 13.11 Hyoid apparatus: this can be assessed by using the tongue into which it inserts. Photo courtesy of Jonathan Cohen MSc (Ost).

should be yielding under pressure of the fingers, rather than having the firm, resistant quality that indicates dysfunction. This can be tested further by using the tongue, as the lingual process of the basihyoid inserts into its root. The tongue is grasped and gently pulled straight upwards and to each side while noting the ease of these movements (Figure 13.11).

Third cervical to sixth cervical

While assessing flexion, extension, sidebend and rotation ranges in the upper cervical spine, it is important to observe how the movement is transmitted through the neck into the middle and lower cervical spine. A common site of restriction is found in the mid-cervical spine, probably because this area tends to buckle under the weight of the body during a fall. These strains often coexist with acute lumbosacral and sacroiliac dysfunction.

The mid- to lower cervical spine can also be tested for mobility by applying traction to the whole neck. This is easiest to achieve by encircling the practitioner's waist with a rope with the ends slipped through the headcollar. By slowly leaning back, the degree of 'give' in the tissues of the spine can be assessed (Figure 13.12).

Leaning back, the head and neck lift slightly from the ground and a sense of sequential separation of the vertebrae should be obtained. The quality of this separation, ranging from reluctant to easy, should be noted, as well as any lateral deviation indicating that one side of the spine is more restricted than the other. Typically, in cases of poor cervical function, the head feels very heavy and stretches with little elasticity. There is often a marked change in this sensation after treatment, when the neck feels much lighter and stretches easily throughout its length.

If two practitioners are available, one person can palpate the neck for the quality of distraction and local soft tissue reaction while the other applies traction. Other movements can also be assessed. Sidebend is tested by sideshifting the neck at each level and feeling for passive motion quality and sense of 'give' in the local paravertebral tissues while the head and neck are slightly raised and a degree of traction is maintained (Figure 13.13).

Thoracic girdle

Careful examination of the cervicothoracic region is particularly important. Its anatomical position, lying deep beneath the powerful muscles of the thoracic limb, makes it a difficult

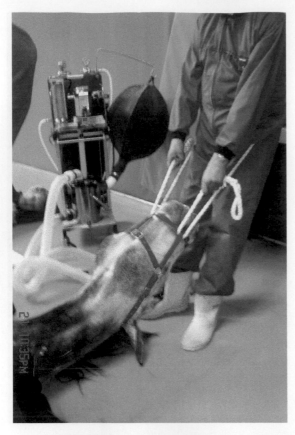

Figure 13.12 Mid-cervical spine: distraction in this region can be tested by slowly leaning back against a rope harness to exert traction.

area to treat in the standing horse. Problems here are characterised by poor scapulothoracic function. The scapulae bind to the thorax, restricting the ability of the rib cage to roll in the muscular sling which is suspended between the forelimbs. This impairs easy protraction and retraction phases of forelimb action and results in a short, choppy gait.

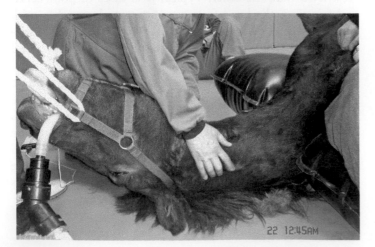

Figure 13.13 Mid-cervical spine: one practitioner can monitor soft tissue reaction in the neck and introduce movements at different segmental levels while a degree of traction is maintained.

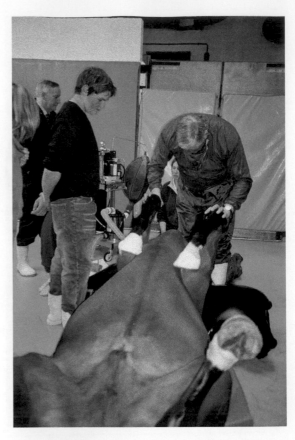

Figure 13.14 Thoracic girdle: protraction and retraction ranges can be tested by rocking the forelimbs backwards and forwards.

Examination starts with forelimb movement. Standing astride the neck of the horse, the forelimbs are suspended above the thorax, flexed at the knees. With hands placed on the horse's knees, the limbs are pulled towards and pushed away from the practitioner's body. The degree of protraction and retraction of each forelimb can be evaluated by watching and feeling how the movement is transmitted through the leg and scapula and into the thoracic wall, thoracic inlet and cervical fascia (Figure 13.14).

Limited retraction is a common finding, either unilaterally or bilaterally (Figure 13.15). However, the limbs may retract abnormally easily. This is typical of a compensatory or 'trick' manoeuvre where accessory ranges of movement may be introduced and some structures may be overworking, particularly in the distal limb joints, to give an apparently full and easy motion.

It is important not only to look at the limb movement itself, but also to observe the degree of soft tissue 'give' in the scapula, cervical spine and thoracic inlet structures while performing passive retraction.

Protraction is often severely limited by fascial tethering at the ventral aspect of the cervicothoracic spine and thoracic inlet and by the soft tissue binding of the scapula onto the thoracic cage (Figure 13.16). However, protraction

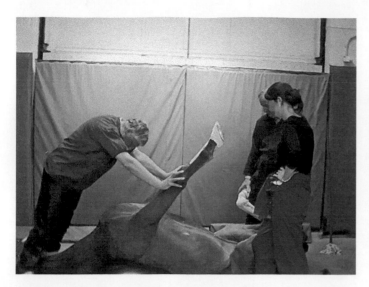

Figure 13.15 Thoracic girdle: limited limb retraction is a common finding.

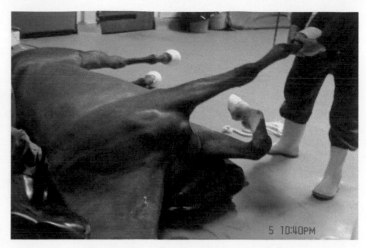

Figure 13.17 Thoracic limb: the interaction of the limb with the thorax can be examined in a sidelying position.

which seems easy may be the result of compensatory increased movement in the soft tissue and articulations of the forelimb while the structures of the thoracic girdle have poor mobility.

Abduction and adduction can be tested by pushing the knees towards and away from each other and noting the ease and quality of movement in both forelimbs.

Full assessment of every joint of the foot and limb is also possible and is much easier than in the standing horse.

Another way of examining the interaction of the limb with the thorax is to partly deflate one of the supporting air bags so that the horse lies to one side at 45° to the horizontal.

Taking the uppermost forelimb by the hoof, the leg is straightened and the soft tissues from the foot, up the limb

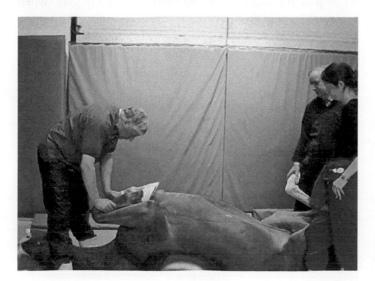

Figure 13.16 Thoracic girdle: protraction is often limited by fascial tethering at the ventral aspect of the cervicothoracic spine.

and into the scapular muscles and thoracic paravertebral tissue are palpated. Often, areas of gritty, inelastic tissue will be found, indicating chronic dysfunction of the periscapular muscles. The range and quality of movement of all the joints of the forelimb can be assessed.

Using a light hold on the foot, the limb is rocked in an oscillating movement to obtain a general sense of the ease of motion of the scapula on the thoracic cage. The relationship between limb and thorax can be investigated further by applying traction through the limb at varying degrees of protraction and retraction (Figure 13.17).

Thoracic spine

With the horse still on its side, it is also possible to evaluate the thoracic spine movement from the withers to the thoracolumbar junction.

Kneeling to face the horse's back, the lateral aspect of the spinous processes from T6 to T18 is pushed down gently. The amount of 'give' that occurs from the downward pressure provides an indication of quality of the soft tissue state and intervertebral joint mobility (Figure 13.18). This can be investigated further by palpating the paravertebral regions of the thoracic spine while another practitioner exerts a direct pull on the straightened forelimb. This evaluates the degree of fascial drag into the limb from T6 to T14 and identifies levels of restricted mobility.

Lumbar spine

With the horse supine and supported by cushions, the pelvic and lumbar movement can be examined. The hindlimb may be fully extended, a position which is maintained by a complex ligamentous apparatus, or flexed where this mechanism can be disengaged by flexing the fetlock and applying pressure with the practitioner's knee on to the posterior surface of the horse's tibia.

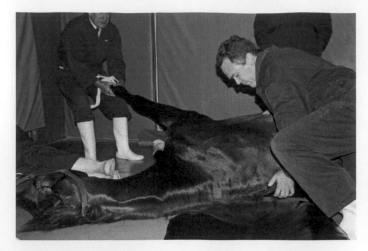

Figure 13.18 Thoracic spine: gentle pressure on the spinous processes is used to assess joint mobility.

Standing behind the tail with the hindlimbs flexed, and holding a foot in each hand, the legs can be rocked forwards into protraction (Figure 13.19). This is much the same action as is used to test lumbar flexion in the sidelying human patient. Flexion should be taken up through the hocks, stifles and hips and then transmitted through the ilia into the lumbar spine. A common finding is a reduction in flexion range where the restriction appears to be located at the usually mobile lumbosacral joint. If, on flexing the hindlimbs, they seem to overflex easily from the hips, this suggests the presence of a trick movement which may be masking an underlying lumbosacral and pelvic dysfunction.

Abduction and adduction ranges of the hip can be assessed by separating the hindlimbs and bringing them together (Figure 13.20). This movement should also be transmitted through the pelvis and into the lower lumbar spine.

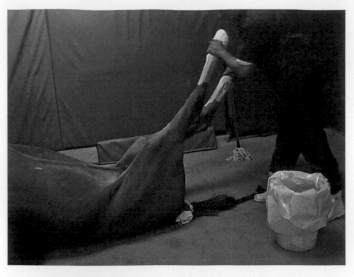

Figure 13.20 Pelvic girdle: adducting each hindlimb across the midline and comparing the ease and range of movement gives an indication of sacral and pelvic function.

Rotation through the lumbar spine can be determined by taking both hindlimbs together to one side and then the other, checking for range and quality of movement (Figure 13.21).

Sacrum and pelvis

The movement of the sacrum and pelvis are closely associated with the function of the lumbar spine. This is the powerhouse of the horse, generating forward propulsion. Holding the tail, slack is taken up by leaning backwards slowly and then exerting traction (Figure 13.22). In the normal horse, stretch will be felt progressing through the sacrum and lumbar spine into the thoracolumbar region. In a horse with pelvic dysfunction, movement will appear to stop at the sacral level and there will be no 'give' when traction is applied.

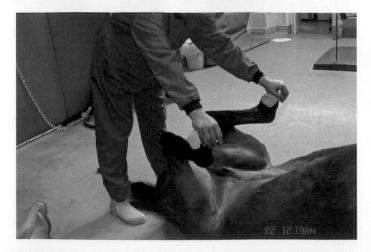

Figure 13.19 Lumbar flexion: rocking the hindlimbs backwards and forwards, movement should be transmitted through the limbs and pelvis and into the lumbar spine. A common finding is restriction in flexion range at the lumbosacral level.

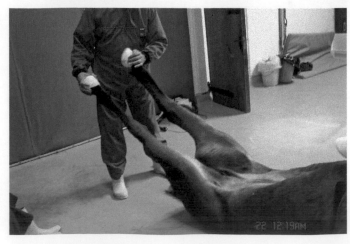

Figure 13.21 Lumbar spine: rotation of the lumbar spine can be assessed by taking both hindlimbs to one side and then the other.

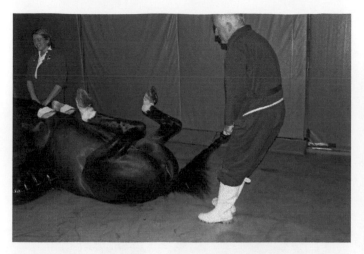

Figure 13.22 Pelvic girdle: leaning backwards, traction is exerted through the sacrum and lumbar spine and into the thoracolumbar region. With pelvic dysfunction, movement appears to stop at the sacral level and there will be no 'give' when traction is applied.

A common pattern of dysfunction is a sacral torsion, where one ilium will appear to be held relatively forwards or back compared with its counterpart on the other side, and movement will be restricted. The human equivalent is often described as an anterior or posterior ilium. An assessment is made by taking hold of the hoof of one flexed hind leg and rolling the ilium forwards and backwards and comparing the ease of movement and the range with the limb on the other side.

It is also possible to assess sacral and pelvic movement using straightened legs. Each hindlimb is taken in turn and moved across the midline (adduction) and away from the midline (abduction). One side is compared with the other for ease and range of movement (Figure 13.23). This articulates the limb with the pelvis and introduces movement of the

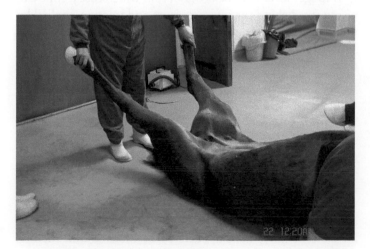

Figure 13.23 Pelvic girdle: adducting and abducting the limb introduces ventro-dorsal movement of the ilium and will help identify torsion strain patterns through the pelvis.

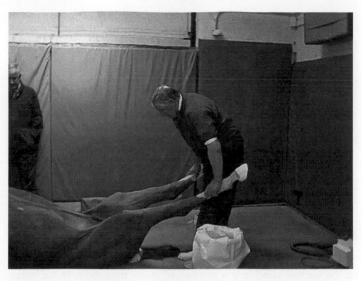

Figure 13.24 Hindlimb: pressing down on the cannon bones, the range of retraction can be assessed while observing the changes in the ventral fascia of the pelvis and abdomen.

ilium in a ventro-dorsal range, and will highlight any torsion strain patterns through the pelvis.

Using the hind legs, pressure is exerted on both cannon bones, pushing slowly down in the direction of the floor to check retraction ranges of the limbs. The ease of movement and the tension that this manoeuvre creates in the tissue of the abdomen and ventral pelvis are evaluated (Figure 13.24).

Treatment

Many of the principles of treatment are similar to those applied to the standing horse (Chapter 12). Indirect approaches, such as functional techniques, are particularly effective under these conditions. A joint or body part can be taken through each range of movement in directions that offer the least resistance to achieve a position of ease where there is minimum tissue tension. Where this principle is applied to the whole body with a practitioner at each leg finding the point of ease, the final resting position may recreate the vectors involved in the original injury (Figure 13.25). Direct techniques, where a joint is moved to the point of restriction and taken through this barrier using stretching or manipulation, are also effective in the recumbent horse. Alongside these, soft tissue techniques, inhibition and articulation are used.

There is a need to be flexible about the approach. Deciding where to start will be very much an experimental task. If treatment to one area does not achieve the desired tissue effect, there is no point in flogging a dead horse! The interconnectivity of the spine, both mechanically and neurologically, means that osteopathic intervention in other regions often has a significant effect on the recalcitrant level. It will then

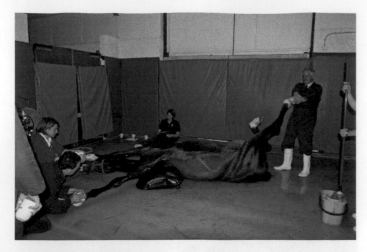

Figure 13.25 Treatment: functional techniques are useful. Building up the vectors to achieve a position of 'ease' may recreate the forces involved in the original injury.

be possible to return to this segment and make the required changes.

The treatment procedures outlined below provide a framework which will need to be varied from case to case. A typical sequence of treatment is described which moves around the body and may revisit some areas more than once. This is a more realistic illustration of a clinical case rather than listing techniques region by region.

Hyoid apparatus

The hyoid apparatus forms a sling between the mandibular rami. It also has an insertion into the base of the tongue, which means that the tongue can be used to influence the cartilage, ligaments and muscles of the region. It is an important structure in that it is closely related to the upper cervical spine.

The horse's head is lifted on to the practitioner's hand or lap and the upper cervical region is palpated to monitor tissue change. A second practitioner then grips the tongue and tests for the end point of the movement in all ranges. A little traction can be exerted in the direction of the restriction. Alternatively, a functional approach can be taken by moving the tongue through all its ranges, finding a position of least tension and waiting for tissue relaxation in the hyoid region which can be evaluated by palpating the intermandibular space (Figure 13.26).

Temporomandibular joint

The temporomandibular joint is another structure of importance when treating the upper cervical spine. Restrictions here may be resolved in a number of ways. The head can be held steady on the osteopath's lap with a firm two-handed hold on the subocciput. Another practitioner then grasps the mandible, close to where it articulates with the temporal

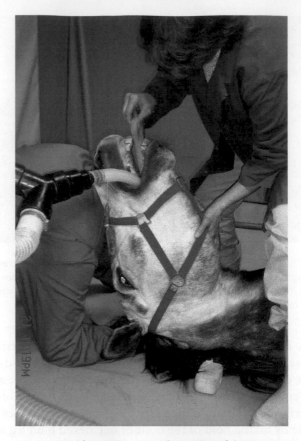

Figure 13.26 Hyoid apparatus: gentle traction of the tongue may be used in the direction of restriction. Alternatively, a functional technique can be used to find the position of minimum tissue tension, maintaining this position until tissue change occurs.

bone. From here, a rhythmic upward traction is introduced until relaxation of the soft tissues and symmetry of function in the joints on both sides have been achieved (Figure 13.27).

A longer lever may be necessary, in which case a rope can be put just behind the lower incisors and traction applied by pulling gently up on the rope in the direction of the ceiling. This distraction can be sustained or a rhythmic traction-and-release sequence can be performed (Figure 13.28).

Occipito-atlanto-axial region

The headcollar should be checked to ensure that it is a reasonably tight fit and unlikely to slip off. Using a rope passed around the practitioner's waist and through the headcollar, gentle, rhythmic traction is applied to distract the head and neck. The cervical spine should stretch easily and sequentially from the upper to the lower vertebrae. If restrictions of cervical joints exist, the head often feels very heavy and inelastic. If movement appears to be blocked and there is an obvious focus for this resistance, a short, fast tug can be applied at a specific level (Figure 13.29). Cervical traction is repeated to check whether function has improved.

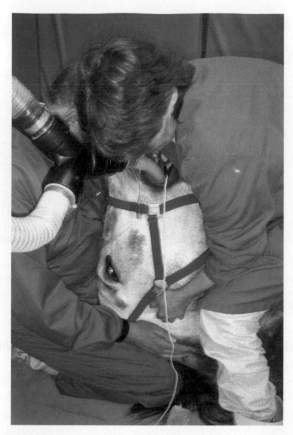

Figure 13.27 Temporomandibular joint: with the head stabilised, rhythmic traction can be applied to the mandible to improve temporomandibular function.

Thoracic limb girdle

It is important to ensure freedom of movement of the forelimb and scapula with the thoracic cage as this facilitates a long, easy stride length. A functional approach is useful here. Two practitioners each take a straightened forelimb.

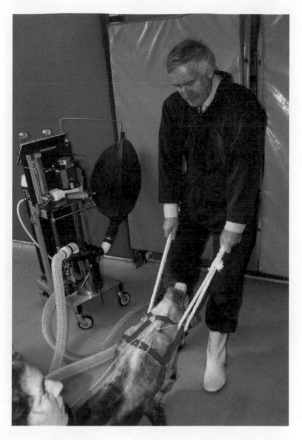

Figure 13.29 Cervical spine: using a rope, body weight can be used to exert gentle rhythmic traction. For a joint complex which is resistant to traction, a short, sharp tug technique can be used.

Both limbs can be taken through each range of movement in a complex manoeuvre involving the individual joints of the forelimbs, scapulohumeral, scapulothoracic and thoracic inlet regions until a point of minimum tension is achieved, described as the point of ease (Figure 13.30).

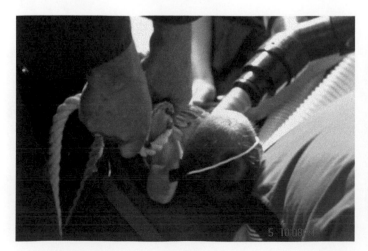

Figure 13.28 Temporomandibular joint: greater leverage can be achieved by using a rope behind the incisors or canines and gently pulling straight upwards.

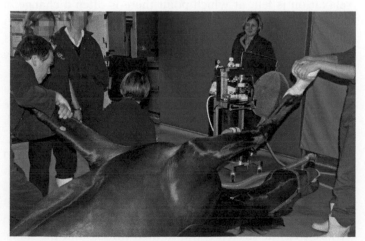

Figure 13.30 Thoracic girdle: each practitioner takes hold of a forelimb and moves it through all ranges of movement to find the point of ease. This is maintained until tissue change is felt.

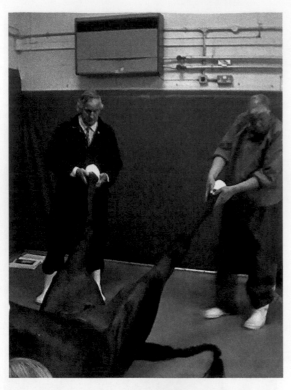

Figure 13.31 Pelvic girdle: each hindlimb is taken to the point of ease. This is maintained until tissue change is felt.

Hindlimbs, sacrum and pelvis

As for the forelimbs, a functional approach may be used with the hindlimbs to improve the mobility of each of the peripheral joints, the hips and the sacroiliac region (Figure 13.31).

This approach can be extended to include all four limbs simultaneously in what could be described as a 'whole body unwind'. The position of ease is maintained until a sense of relaxation is felt, at which point there is often a change in breathing pattern. It is interesting to note that the position of the body at the point of minimum tension often reflects the direction of the forces occurring in the original injury (Figure 13.25).

The lumbar spine and midline structures of the pelvis can be encouraged to function better by using the tail. A rope around the practitioner's body is used like a belt, through which the tail is wrapped. By leaning backwards and then re-laxing, a rhythmic traction can be applied though the sacrum and lumbar spine (Figure 13.32). This causes the pelvis to rock into relative flexion and extension, which produces stretch and relaxation in the lumbar spine. While this is be-ing performed, the upper cervical spine can be monitored to ensure that the stretch is transmitted throughout the spine. A degree of cervical traction can be exerted simultaneously by a second practitioner, which increases the dorsal stretch produced by the flexion phase of the pelvic movement. The

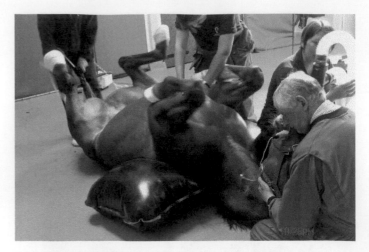

Figure 13.32 Midline structures: traction of the midline structures can be applied using the tail. From the sub-occipital region, transmission of movement throughout the spine can be monitored and additional traction may be applied at this end.

level of any block in the transmission through the spine can be readily identified.

Sacroiliac dysfunction and rotation strains of the lumbar spine may be treated using the limbs. Straightening the hind legs and taking them over to one side and then the other puts a stretch through the sacroiliac and lumbar region (Figure 13.33). This can then be exaggerated by applying a short, sharp tug to the uppermost leg. This tug technique can also be applied to the distal joints of the limb.

Specific lumbar joint stiffness can be targeted in a way that resembles human technique. If the left side requires mobilisation, the straightened left leg is brought in an arc to the right. The whole pelvis rotates around in response to this. Elements of flexion or extension can then be introduced by moving the leg in a cranial or caudal direction until the

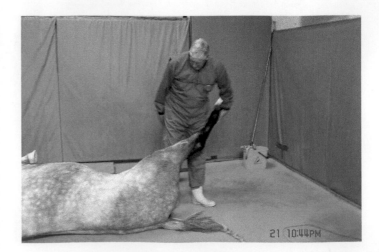

Figure 13.33 Pelvic girdle: the sacroiliac and lower lumbar spine can be mobilised by taking the hindlimb across the midline. A tug technique may be applied to the individual joints of the limbs.

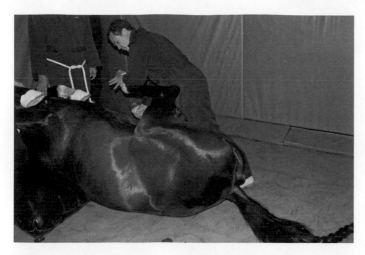

Figure 13.34 Lumbar spine: a specific lumbar vertebral joint complex can be mobilised using the hindlimb to articulate or deliver a short thrust.

forces focus on the joint in question (Figure 13.34). Placing hands on the proximal part of the limb, rhythmic downward pressure towards the floor can be applied to mobilise the lumbar vertebral joint. A short downward thrust movement may also be used.

Caudo-cranial spinal traction

This technique is aimed at improving the transmission of movement through the whole spine. At one end, the horse's head is positioned on the lap and a firm hold is taken on the occiput. At the other end, a practitioner starts up a rhythmic traction using the tail, by leaning back and then releasing. The practitioner at the head end holds back on the occiput as the traction reaches the upper cervical spine, which facilitates a decompression force from below on to this area (Figure 13.35). Compression with rotation strain patterns

are common and, with increasing traction, the body will begin to roll gradually one way or the other. The practitioner at the head end must decide when to let the head and neck follow this rotation by monitoring soft tissue response in the upper cervical spine.

Shoulder girdle and thoracic spine

Having assessed the effect of general traction throughout the spine, it is important to review the thoracic girdle. This may be done with the horse in almost a sidelying position. Partly deflating one of the supporting cushions, the horse is positioned at 45° to the vertical. Soft tissue techniques to the muscles and fascia of the limb, scapula and cervicothoracic region can be used while another practitioner extends and holds the forelimb to reduce excessive movement of the limb during the procedure (Figure 13.36).

In this position the mobility of the thoracic spine, particularly that of T6 to T14, can be improved. Putting both hands on the upward-facing lateral aspect of the spinous process, a downward pressure can be applied to encourage movement in these joints. This can be continued from the withers down into the mid- to lower thoracic spine and is a manoeuvre that is particularly useful when treating elephants! The technique can be refined when another practitioner exerts a degree of traction through the forelimb. By changing the angle of this traction, the paravertebral tissue can be tensed and the vertebrae stabilised at particular levels. The force then applied to the spinous process is concentrated at a specific intervertebral joint complex rather than dissipated into the surrounding tissue (Figure 13.37). Care should be taken with the amount of force used on the spinous processes at the withers as they are long, slender structures.

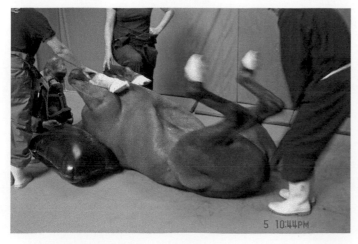

Figure 13.35 Spinal traction: with one practitioner holding back on the head, traction can be exerted from below by rhythmic pulling through the tail. The body may begin to roll to one side or the other.

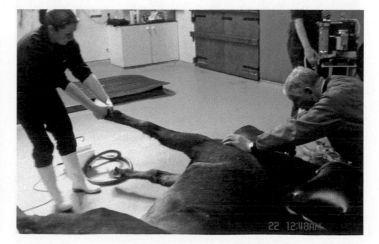

Figure 13.36 Thoracic girdle: in a partly sidelying position, soft tissue to this area can be applied while another practitioner steadies the forelimb.

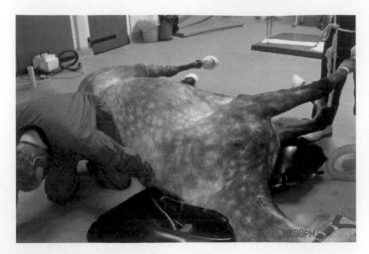

Figure 13.37 Thoracic spine: articulation is possible using the spinous processes. Traction on the forelimb focuses forces at a specific level.

The horse is then rolled on to the opposite side, and the process is repeated.

Sacrum, pelvis and hip

With the horse lying on its side, it is also possible to affect the hip and pelvis. Taking the foot lying uppermost, the hindlimb is articulated slowly in an oscillating movement to release any tension in the soft tissue of the hip, pelvis, sacrum and even the lumbar spine (Figure 13.38).

Tail traction can also be performed in this position and has the added advantage that a second practitioner can palpate the lumbar spine to identify levels of poor function and to assess any changes that are made in this region in response to treatment (Figure 13.39).

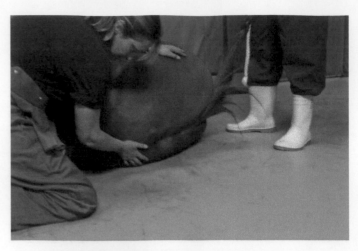

Figure 13.39 Lumbar spine: tail traction performed in the side-lying position allows a second practitioner to monitor changes in the lumbar spine.

Cervical spine

The horse is returned to the supine position. Rhythmic traction through the tail is used while a second practitioner monitors the cervical spine, rechecking the stretch through the whole spine. Again, there may be a tendency for the horse to roll to one side. The person stabilising the thoracic girdle in the supine position should allow, rather than push, the thorax to rotate in the appropriate direction as soon as this tendency becomes apparent (Figure 13.40).

Ensuring that the occipito-atlanto-axial region functions normally is vital. This area can be reassessed by lifting the horse's head on to the hand and palpating the response of the soft tissues and joints to passive articulation in flexion, extension and rotation. If the region is not moving freely,

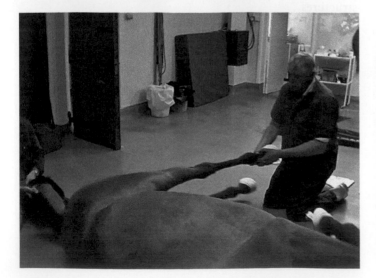

Figure 13.38 Pelvis: the hindlimb is articulated slowly in an oscillating movement to release any tension in the soft tissue of the hip, pelvis, sacrum and even the lumbar spine.

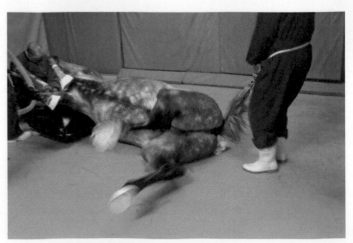

Figure 13.40 Spine: the stretch generated by rhythmic traction through the tail is monitored at the cervical spine. If the thorax tends to roll to one side, it should be allowed to do so.

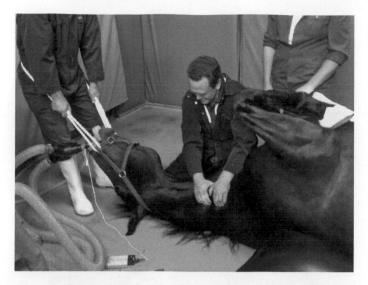

Figure 13.41 Cervical spine: rhythmic cervical traction may be augmented by local sideshift of vertebral joints to ensure full neck mobility.

the temporomandibular joint should be rechecked, and, if mobility is still reduced, traction and articulation should be applied again.

Rhythmic cervical traction is repeated by means of the rope, and if any blocks to movement are identified a tug release can be used. In order to ensure full mobility of the neck, a second practitioner can sideshift the joints of the cervical spine while the head of the horse is held above the floor and traction is applied (Figure 13.41).

Cervicothoracic spine

It is at this point that residual stiffness in the lower cervical and upper to mid-thoracic spine needs to be addressed. The cervicothoracic junction is not easily accessible by techniques other than those performed under anaesthetic. It is therefore important to make sure that this region is functioning normally at the end of the treatment, as there is less chance of influencing mobility in the standing horse.

Two practitioners squat either side of the horse's head and hold the headcollar at the cheek and under the jaw. The anaesthetic tube is disconnected and an assistant should steady the thorax to keep the front legs pointing upwards (Figure 13.42). On the count of three, both practitioners lift the head and neck straight upwards to produce a vertical traction through the lower cervical and upper thoracic spine (Figure 13.43). The thorax may rotate one way or the other.

If this is ineffective in releasing restriction in that the traction is not transmitted through the spine, this technique will need to be extended to incorporate other ranges of movement. Initially, however, the head is lowered, the tube reconnected and a few minutes taken to re-establish the anaesthetic at the appropriate level.

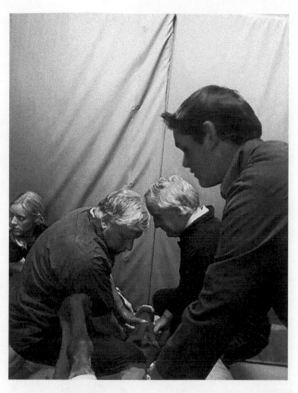

Figure 13.42 Cervicothoracic spine: two practitioners squat either side of the head, holding the headcollar at the cheek and under the jaw. An assistant supports the thorax to keep the front legs pointing upwards.

The practitioners again lift the head and neck vertically, but this time introducing an element of sidebending. As this occurs, the body will gradually rotate to the side opposite that of the sidebending, and the head and neck are taken alongside the body (Figure 13.44). The movement can be reinforced by pulling the head gently along the side of the horse (Figure 13.45). While in this position a very focused intervention can be made at the lower cervical level by pushing at the level of the transverse processes in the direction of the pull at the head (Figure 13.46).

The horse is brought back to the supine position and the level of anaesthetic checked. The process is repeated with sidebending to the other side.

Traction via the headcollar and the tail are then used to establish whether there is freedom of movement through the long axis of the spine. Any restrictions remaining at this stage are usually at the occipito-atlantal and atlanto-axial levels, with or without temporomandibular dysfunction. The tongue is used to recheck for hyoid involvement, and the temporomandibular function is reassessed and, if necessary, treated as described previously.

If the occipito-atlantal joint is still restricted, the head is lifted on to the practitioner's hand to assess the soft tissue state. Articulation may be used to improve mobility

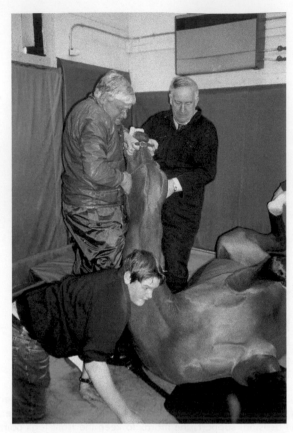

Figure 13.43 Cervicothoracic spine: the head and neck are lifted straight upwards to produce a vertical traction through the lower cervical and upper thoracic spine.

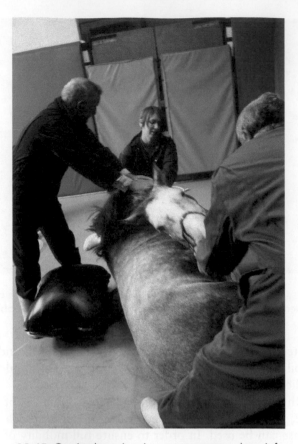

Figure 13.45 Cervicothoracic spine: movement can be reinforced by pulling the head gently along the side of the horse. Photo courtesy of Jonathan Cohen MSc (Ost).

(Figure 13.47). Where necessary, a tug release technique can be applied.

Articulation of the atlanto-axial joint may be performed, which can be extended into a thrust technique. With the horse's head in the midline and positioned on the neck midway between flexion and extension, the ears are held in each

hand. Pulling up rapidly on one side will take the head in a rotational movement in the opposite direction to mobilise the atlanto-axial joint and reverse some of the changes that often occur in a fall or pull-back on a halter (Figure 13.48). Alternatively, the head can be rotated to one side with a

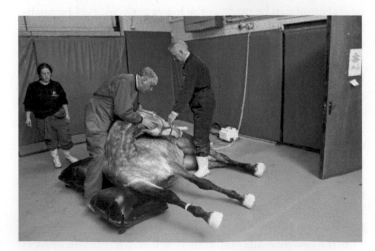

Figure 13.44 Cervicothoracic spine: on lifting, an element of sidebend is introduced. Photo courtesy of Jonathan Cohen MSc (Ost).

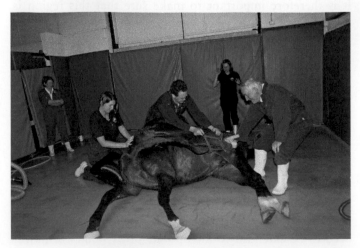

Figure 13.46 Cervicothoracic spine: localised movement can be produced in the lower cervical region by pushing at the level of the transverse processes in the direction of the pull at the head.

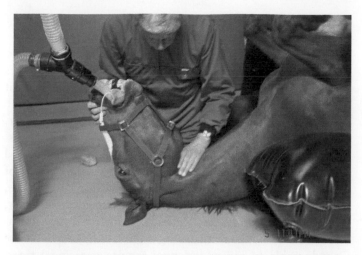

Figure 13.47 Occipito-atlantal joint: articulation may be used to improve mobility.

degree of flexion or extension, depending on which gives a sense of greatest tissue relaxation, and the thenar eminence used to deliver a short thrust against the wing of the atlas to encourage rotation (Figure 13.49).

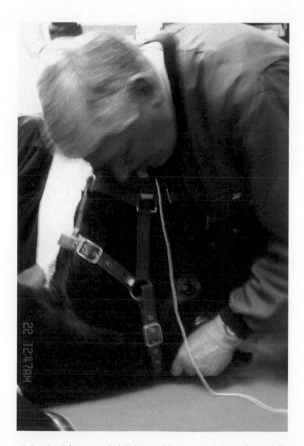

Figure 13.48 Atlanto-axial joint: with the head in the midline, the ears are held in each hand. Pulling up rapidly on one side will take the head in a rotational movement in the opposite direction to mobilise the atlanto-axial joint.

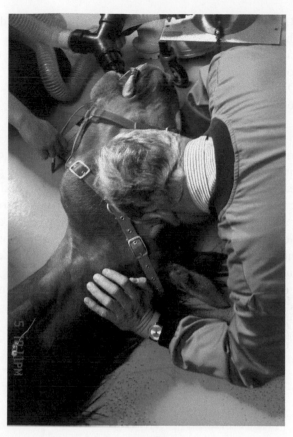

Figure 13.49 Atlanto-axial joint: the head is rotated to one side with a degree of flexion or extension. The thenar eminence is used to deliver a short thrust against the wing of the atlas to encourage rotation.

Final Check

Once treatment has been given along these lines, a reassessment of the function of the whole spine should be undertaken and further treatment given if necessary. Particular attention should be paid to the occipito-atlantal joint complex, especially if any compression still remains, and also to the cervicothoracic region. These are difficult areas to treat in the standing horse but are vital for efficient biomechanical function during locomotion. A second chance to access these areas may not present itself.

The final assessment should consider the following:

1. Cervical traction, which should be easy and sequential.
2. Tail traction with the second practitioner palpating at the subocciput to ensure full mobility through the long axis of the spine.
3. Soft tissue of the cervical paravertebral tissue should be relaxed.
4. Range and ease of motion of forelimb peripheral joints and soft tissue tested.
5. Range and ease of motion of cervicothoracic and scapulothoracic movement tested.

6. Range of movement of peripheral joints of the hindlimbs should be full.
7. Lumbar spine, sacrum, pelvis and hips should be tested for ease and symmetry of movement.
8. Occipito-atlanto-axial and temporomandibular joint movement should be tested.

Post-general anaesthetic

Comprehensive osteopathic notes should be made of the findings made and treatment performed during the procedure. In some cases the problem is so widespread and complex that it may appear that there has not been a full resolution at the end of the final check while under general anaesthetic. This should be noted on the case sheet and should be borne in mind on subsequent consultations. Clinical examination and diagnostic tests such as infra-red thermography will establish whether these slight reservations on outcome translate into physical dysfunction. A second treatment under general anaesthetic is occasionally necessary.

Following general anaesthesia the horse is transferred to a recovery box and is generally on its feet around 20 minutes later. As a precaution, the horse is generally kept overnight at the veterinary practice.

Post-treatment care should be discussed with the owner. The changes made during treatment under general anaesthetic are significant and far reaching, and the owner should be aware that time is needed to adapt to a different way of moving. Ideally, the horse will be turned out for 4 weeks, followed by reassessment. If this assessment is satisfactory, then the horse can be brought back into work slowly. Owners should be warned that during the first 6 months the horse is vulnerable to injury and may require occasional treatment for acute dysfunction, which is usually short-lived and responds well to osteopathic intervention.

14

Post-treatment Care and Management

Annabel Jenks

The osteopathic approach to treatments is always a holistic one. It is very important to ensure that the horse receives the most appropriate treatment and management to achieve optimum performance and lifestyle.

The unsedated osteopathic treatment on a sound athletic horse can be performed at competitions with successful results. If the presenting restrictions are minor musculoskeletal dysfunctions, response can be immediately very positive and the horse can be ridden and competed on that day, even winning the Hickstead Derby! These horses are regularly examined so the practitioner is familiar with their conformation and muscular structure. If a horse is performing well, it is very important that compensations are not disturbed as this will change proprioception and affect performance. Golden rule: if it is not broken, don't 'fix' it!

Ideally, consultations and treatments are applied in advance of any competitions and early in the horse's career to prevent biomechanical changes that may result in musculoskeletal problems leading to unsoundness.

The well being of the horse requires a team of experts who are knowledgeable in their individual field. As osteopathic practitioners it is important to build a team of professionals around the practice, approved by the veterinary surgeons one is working with.

The subjects covered in this chapter will require further study in depth using the relevant literature available. The British Horse Society bookshop has an excellent catalogue. Go to www.britishhorse.com to order on line. At the end of each of the following sections, websites have been listed for further information and references.

EXPECTATIONS OF THE OWNER/RIDER

Throughout the consultation, examination and treatment, the breed, age, temperament, and physiological and psychological suitability must be considered for the equestrian discipline the horse is being asked to participate in.

It is important to establish the ambitions of the owner/rider as this may surpass the horse's capabilities at that specific moment in time. Younger and older horses will need different considerations from those that apply to the athletic competition horse. Certain breeds and conformations are more suitable than others for a chosen equestrian discipline such as show jumping or dressage, although there are always those that surprise us all with their unexpected talent. The riding school horses and ponies will obviously have more difficulty attaining their optimum equilibrium and balance than the horse with one rider, simply because they have to adapt to different levels of riding. These are all aspects that the osteopath must consider when giving post-treatment advice.

It is very common for a horse's temperament to improve after treatment as pain is relieved. Owners will often comment on how much happier their horse is post-treatment and this is very rewarding for the practitioner and a good guide to treatment progress and success.

SHOEING

This is a huge subject, and the old saying, 'No foot, no horse', is as true today as it has ever been. Foot balance and correct shoeing are paramount if biomechanical problems are to be prevented. Good farriers are essential; they often recognise signs of locomotion and postural changes that will lead to lameness before the rider feels any limitation of movement.

The osteopath should familiarise themselves with the function of the foot and foot balance. Conformation of the limbs will greatly affect the placement of the foot and co-ordination of the stride. The wearing of a shoe must be noted during examination. During active observation the practitioner should always listen to the footfall as well as observing the horse's gait.

A basic knowledge of the practice of shoeing, foot care and the different types of shoes used for corrective shoeing is essential. Horses that are unfit, young or tired may have abnormalities within their gait that improve with fitness and corrective shoeing. After osteopathic treatment, the farrier will often notice an improvement in footfall. They may comment that the difficulties the horse had when being shod, such as stretching and holding a limb as the shoe is fitted, or standing with the weight on a dysfunctional limb and balancing correctly, have improved post-treatment.

The teamwork of the vet, farrier and osteopath is ex-tremely important to the horse's welfare.

For further information consult the Farriers Registration Council, www.farrier-reg.gov.uk, and the Worshipful Company of Farriers, www.wcf.org.uk.

RECOMMENDED READING

Brega J (1995) *The Horse – The Foot, Shoeing and Lameness*. JA Allen, London.

Curtis S (1999) *Farriery – Foal to Racehorse*. Hoofcare and Lameness, Gloucester, MA.

Hickman J, Humphrey M (1999) *Hickman's Farriery*. JA Allen, London.

Williams G, Deacon M (2006) *No Foot, No Horse*: Foot Balance – The Key to Soundness and Performance. BHS Bookshop, Kenilworth.

TACK

Always, on the initial treatment, assess the balance and fit-ting of the saddle, bridle and bit. The fitting and balancing of saddles is an enormous subject. Osteopaths should famil-iarise themselves with the basic rules, and be able to assess the abnormalities in the tissues and recognise behavioural problems associated with incorrectly fitted saddles. Knowledge of different types of saddles and their particular uses and balance on the horse is important (see Figure 14.1). Certain trees and fittings have advantages and disadvan-tages. To name just a few, there are dressage, jumping, general-purpose, sidesaddle, showing, close contact, western and racing saddles. They can be leather, synthetic, treeless, panelled, wool flocked or air filled. The most important

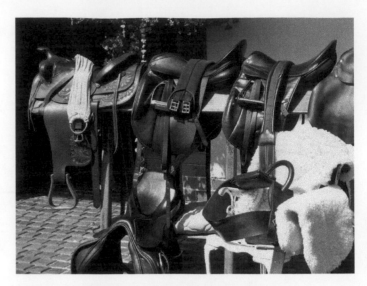

Figure 14.1 Examples of different types of saddle.

factor is that the saddle must fit both the horse *and* the rider.

Horses are constantly changing their muscular shape and structure as they mature and develop and become fitter. Like-wise, as they become older, the muscular tone changes and the back can become swayed. A qualified master saddler who is trained to fit and rebalance saddles must continu-ously assess the width and shape of the saddle. Ideally, the saddle should be assessed every 6 months, at the beginning and end of the competition season or in the autumn and spring.

A new saddle should be reassessed within 2 months of the initial fitting. It may need rebalancing and flocking (see Figure 14.2) as it moulds and shapes to the horse's back. Riders often forget how long they have had a saddle, and when asked think it is new but find that they have actually owned it for a couple of years and have never had it checked.

It is important to ask the owner/rider to place the sad-dle on the horse's back. Often a well fitted saddle is placed too far forwards on to the withers and shoulder or too far back on to the thoracolumbar spine. This may occur be-cause one's eye is drawn to the front of the numnah or pad instead of concentrating on the placement of the saddle and points of the tree. Incorrect positioning of the saddle will cause pressure, pinching and friction to the soft tissue and underlying structures.

The saddle should be assessed initially on its own. Then position the numnah and pad to reassess the balance. Quite often a well fitted saddle is unbalanced by the numnah or pad placed underneath! However, with a younger or older horse, an appropriate pad will allow the development of the correct musculature and reduce the concussive forces when ridden. This allows it to work up through the dorsal topline and lift the abdominal ventral line.

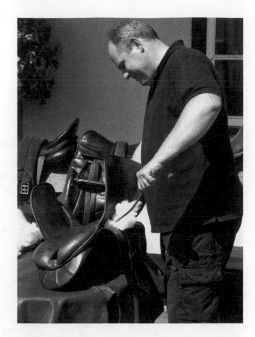

Figure 14.2 Reflocking of a saddle by a master saddler.

RECOMMENDED READING

Harman J (2006) *Horse's Pain-Free Back and Saddle-Fit Book*. Kenilworth Press, Kenilworth.

Lyndon-Dykes K (2005) *Practical Saddle-Fitting*. JA Allen, London.

BRIDLES AND BITS

The fitting of a bridle and bit is very important. Badly fitted bridles and misuse of bits can greatly influence the positioning of the head, the acceptance of the rider's hands and relaxation through the jaw. Any discomfort around the head and mouth will cause the horse to toss and head shake, have a high head carriage, and tilt the head, which may result in biomechanical dysfunction throughout.

It is important to check that the bit is not too high, causing pinching and even cutting the sensitive lips, or too low so that it bounces off the teeth. If the bit is too big, it will be pulled out to the side causing discomfort, and the rider will have difficulty influencing the direction they wish to go in.

In a recent radiographic study of bit position within the horse's mouth by Manfredi et al. (2005) some interesting observations were made. Areas where the bit crossed a bony surface, such as the hard palate or the interdental space (bars) of the mandible, were found to be particularly vulnerable to injury due to pressure from the bit.

Differences between bits in shape and orientation of the mouthpiece affect the proximity of the bit to the palate and cheek teeth. Bit movements in response to the application of a standard amount of bilateral rein tension support the suggestion that bit type affects pressure distribution on the different oral structures. These differences may explain the apparent preferences of individual horses for certain types of bit, and may affect the likelihood of injury to specific oral tissues (Manfredi et al. 2005).

Oral anatomy, including the position of the commissure of the lips relative to the interdental space, the width of the mandible, the shape of the palate, and the size of the tongue, may affect the size and shape of the mouthpiece that can be accommodated comfortably (Engelke and Gasse 2003).

When using a double bridle the positioning of the curb chain must be correct within the chin groove. The mandibular nerve extends down the underpart of the jaw and enters the bone just above the horse's chin. A badly fitted curb chain, or one that does not suit the particular animal's jaw conformation, can exert pressure close to the mandibular nerve (Crawford undated).

To help prevent soreness at the corners of the mouth, Vaseline can be applied to the lips as this will lubricate and ease the movement of the bit.

The headpiece and browband must allow room for the ears, and some headpieces are now padded to take

The numnah or pad must be correctly positioned so that it does not put pressure on the withers. It should not be too small or it may rub the supraspinous ligament, causing inflammation and acute discomfort. This can also occur if the pad or numnah's edges or stitches are worn and threadbare, or if it is washed irregularly.

A badly fitting saddle can cause circulatory changes and tissue damage that result in areas of white hair at the point of pressure. There may be palpable nodules in the connective tissue, which are caused by any number of factors such as unwashed sweaty patches, fly bites or pressure from the saddle. If the nodules are not tender, it is always advisable to ignore them, as treating the region with creams or ointments can cause adverse reactions and soreness. However, when fitting the saddle, these damaged areas must be taken into consideration in respect of concussion from the saddle and rider.

The girth must be of a correct length and suitable for the type of saddle. If the girth is too long, the saddle tends to slip from side to side. By examining the hair either side of the spine it is often possible to see by the positioning of worn patches how the saddle is positioned on the back and if it is slipping to one side. Girths with elastic must never be overtightened.

Racehorses can benefit from being exercised in light general-purpose saddles instead of being ridden continuously in the racing saddle.

For further information consult the Society of Master Saddlers, www.mastersaddlers.co.uk, and the Worshipful Company of Saddlers, www.saddlersco.co.uk.

pressure off the poll. The noseband can be too low, restricting breathing, and there may be a tendency to overtighten it in an attempt to control the horse and influence the head carriage. There is no substitute for correct schooling, and overtightening the noseband may just result in tension in the jaw and the horse resenting the restriction.

RECOMMENDED READING

Hartley-Edwards E (2004) *Complete Book of Bits and Bitting*. David & Charles, Newton Abbot.
Vernon H (1999) *The Allen Illustrated Guide to Bits & Bitting*. JA Allen, London.

DENTISTRY

It is obviously difficult to resolve musculoskeletal dysfunctions if there are presenting dental problems. Uneven, sharp, jagged molars lacerate the mucous membrane of the mouth, often resulting in ulceration. A wolf tooth may cause discomfort when a bit is in place and, in order to prevent problems occurring, will often be extracted as it appears. The inability to optimise chewing and cropping of food will also affect condition and muscular development. The following words were written at the beginning of the last century, and yet, still, many riders and owners fail to recognise the signs:

'Amongst the many dangerous and disagreeable vices contracted by horses, owing to defective teeth, may be mentioned, holding the bit, carrying the head on one side, rearing, plunging, bolting, incessantly tossing the head (especially when bridled), profuse foaming at the mouth, star gazing, irritability and bad temper generally' (Vahey 1928).

The troublesome period of tooth eruption occurs between 2 and 4 years of age. During this period it is a good idea to have the horse's mouth examined two or three times a year. If necessary, the premolar caps and wolf teeth should be removed and any sharp edges rasped (Hayes 1988). From then on a yearly examination and rasping by a vet (see Figure 14.3) or equine dentist should be adequate, unless there are complicating factors that need to be addressed more regularly. Ten years ago most owners couldn't tell you when their horse's teeth were last examined. Now they can tell you to the day! This has been a huge improvement in the welfare and management of horses.

For further information go to the British Association of Equine Dental Technicians site, www.equinedentistry.org.uk.

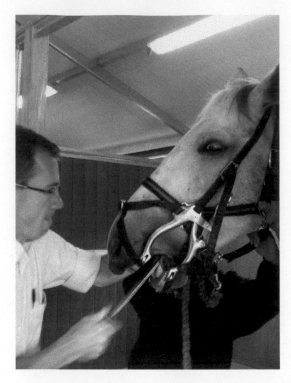

Figure 14.3 Dental examination and rasping of the teeth by a veterinary surgeon.

RECOMMENDED READING

Kreling K (2005) *Horse's Teeth and Their Problems*. The Lyons Press, Guilford, CT.

FEEDING AND STABLE MANAGEMENT

Always discuss with the owner their feeding regime and what supplements they give to their horse. There is a tendency to overfeed with high-energy mixes, resulting in avoidable behavioural problems.

Hay should be available ad lib as horses are natural grazers and therefore need to keep their digestive system quietly digesting food instead of sporadically receiving large feeds.

Some horses are dehydrated and may have an electrolyte imbalance. A simple indication is to take a pinch of skin in the cervical region: it should release easily. If it remains tight and wrinkled on release, the horse may be dehydrated. Veterinary advice is then required. Electrolytes are as important in the winter as in the summer. Most owners do not realise this and only give them when temperatures are high. Travelling can also greatly affect hydration. Ponies are often forgotten where supplements are concerned. Pony club rallies and camp easily exhaust ponies that probably at other times are only ridden two or three times a week during the school term.

The positioning of hay nets or racks, if too high, can cause cervical restrictions and hollowing through the spine as the horse reaches up. However, if the net is too low, a foot could become caught up in the hay net as the horse rolls. Feeding hay on the floor is preferable and much safer. Hay buckets can be fixed into the corner of the stable to prevent the hay being dragged and wasted through the bed.

An anti-cast roller is often used if the horse is prone to becoming cast. The problem with an anti-cast roller is that it applies a lot of pressure on the withers which may cause discomfort and tissue damage. It may also reposition resulting in pressure on the ribs and even on the abdomen if it slips completely round the rib cage.

RECOMMENDED READING

Frape DL (2004) *Equine Nutrition and Feeding*. Wiley-Blackwell, Oxford.

Vogel C (2003) *Complete Horse Care Management*. Dorling Kindersley, London.

TURNOUT

Horses are naturally herd animals and grazers. If it is safe to turn out in company, there is no better environment for the horse to mentally relax and this should be encouraged. On the same theme, they also need to have free time and a kick and a buck, so loose schooling can also provide this outlet of energy! None of us can be disciplined all the time, and horses must be allowed to develop their character and have the freedom to express themselves. The act of grazing allows stretching of the topline and movement of the limbs without the pressure of a training routine (see Figure 14.4).

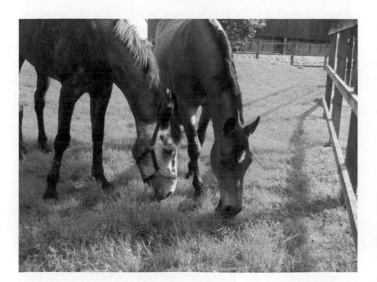

Figure 14.4 Horses are naturally herd animals and grazers.

THE SCALES OF TRAINING

It would be advisable for the osteopath to familiarise themselves with the way a horse should be ridden, known as the 'correct way of going'. A day or two spent with a local trainer or riding instructor watching them teach their pupils would be very beneficial and certainly time well spent. It is also a good networking exercise!

Before discussing horses being worked on the lunge or ridden, it is important to remember the Scales of Training as advised by British Dressage and the Fédération Équestre Internationale (FEI). These are the foundations for training of the horse and are accepted by both national disciplines and the FEI.

- Rhythm
- Suppleness
- Contact
- Impulsion
- Straightness
- Collection

The common denominator throughout these six stages is balance, which must be achieved at each and every phase.

The topline needs to stretch and lengthen while the abdominal musculature must be strengthened to give lumbar stability and support the rider. First, horses must stretch over the topline and acquire balance and rhythm. As they mature and develop the abdominal musculature, they can begin to engage the quarters and become lighter in their cadence and off the forehand. This applies to every discipline within the equestrian field and not just to dressage training!

It is the practitioner's role to ensure that, biomechanically, the horse can develop to optimise achievement within the limitations of its conformation, talent and mental ability. It is the aim of the rider to form a relationship and build up a harmonic partnership with the horse, who will then be willing and obedient and happy to work. These are the principles of good horsemanship.

Further information can be obtained from www.britishdressage.co.uk, www.horsesport.org, and www.bhs.org.uk.

LUNGEING AND LONG-REINING

Working horses from the ground is an excellent opportunity to observe how they are moving and developing. A good rapport and trust can be achieved by the use of the voice. However, there is an art to lungeing and long reining, and they will be beneficial and effective only if the trainer is experienced and competent.

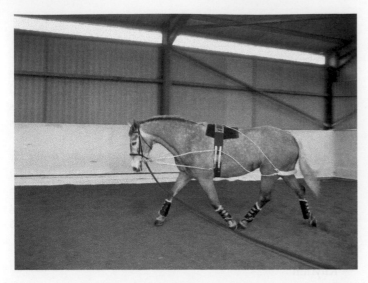

Figure 14.5 Encouraging the horse to both stretch and work from behind – lungeing using the Pessoa training system.

The horse must never be forced into an outline or pressured into working in a posture they are unable to maintain dynamically. Care must be taken when using lungeing equipment. Incorrect use may result in uncoordinated work, which leads to anatomical strains and stresses. The horse must work harmoniously to develop correctly.

Initially the horse should be lunged free of any restraints so that it can loosen and warm up the muscles, finding its own rhythm and balance, stretching over the topline and lowering the neck. Side reins or the Pessoa (see Figure 14.5) or Chambon can then be used to encourage development towards a correct outline into the bridle. These should only be used for a very short period on each rein until the horse is muscularly mature enough to work for longer periods. Continuous work on a circle can be detrimental, causing musculoskeletal strains, so the horse should be lunged up and down the arena utilising the long sides as well as the corners. Lungeing should ideally never be more than 10 minutes on either rein, and at the end of a session time should be allowed for the horse to stretch and relax. Cooling down after exercise is often ignored. Riders are often seen dismounting immediately after a dressage test or showjumping round, instead of walking the horse around for some time to allow relaxation and to encourage the elimination of lactic acid.

Pole work on the lunge is beneficial to sharpen proprioception and coordination, and free jumping down a jumping grid allows the horse to bascule without the restriction of a rider.

There are many books on lungeing and schooling, and osteopaths must familiarise themselves with the different methods that trainers use so that they can advise on any specific regime they feel may be beneficial to the horse.

RECOMMENDED READING

Bayley L (2004) *Ground Work Training for Your Horse*. David & Charles, Newton Abbot.
Loriston-Clarke J (2006) *Lungeing and Long Reining*. Kenilworth Press, Kenilworth.

RIDDEN WORK

Harmony between horse and rider is the key to success. Post-treatment advice and regimes given for individual horses depend entirely on the presenting biomechanical and orthopaedic problems and the response to osteopathic treatment.

Ideally, with the sound athletic horse, exercise and schooling can continue immediately if there are no issues to be addressed such as a badly fitting saddle. The horse should be ridden in a soft outline to encourage it to stretch over the topline. The rider should rise in the trot and keep the seat light in the canter so that they do not restrict the movement in the thoracolumbar region. Large circles and serpentines with transitions and simple lateral movements will engage the hindquarters. Once the horse is supple and loose through its back, more advanced exercises can be introduced depending on the level of training.

The aim of the rider is to educate the horse, encouraging correct biomechanical development and maintaining soundness of the limbs. This avoids unnecessary concussive forces, which require compensation and cause uneven gait and eventual lameness.

Horses should be exercised on different terrains to aid proprioception and coordination. Hacking and hill work are ideal for developing muscular tone and balance. In all disciplines, they must be encouraged to work freely and forward and so the work must be varied and interesting, not continually working in arenas and on surfaces!

A recent study by Rachel Murray (2006–2007) from the Animal Health Trust looked at factors that affect the risk of injury to horses. The results suggested that lungeing, hacking, jumping and turnout were protective against lameness. It is likely that this protective effect is related to adaptation of the musculoskeletal system to different types of exercise and proprioceptive conditioning using a variety of surfaces and movements (Murray 2006–2007).

At this point it is helpful to remember the herd instinct and how it can be very beneficial to ride with others, especially when riding young horses, to encourage them to be forward throughout their work and gain confidence.

Poles and jumping grids (see Figure 14.6) are used to provide gymnastic work for establishing balance and elevation. The rhythm of the paces can be established and the entire limb joints encouraged to flex and extend, depending on the

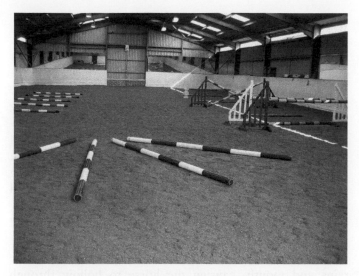

Figure 14.6 Poles and jumping grids are used to provide gymnastic work for establishing balance and elevation.

distances at which the poles are set. This gymnastic work is especially beneficial in opening up the shoulders as well as mobilising the cervicothoracic and lumbosacral junctions.

Poles can be raised alternately to facilitate elevation and raise the forehand. Canter poles to grids will assist the rider to establish the correct stride. Grid work also focuses the rider's mind and promotes balance and rhythm. If the rider does not enjoy jumping, they can still be encouraged to use trotting and canter poles to help the horse optimise performance using these exercises.

It is very important to reward the horse when it works correctly and to ride positively. For example, when the horse has been cantering disunited due to musculo-skeletal problems that are then addressed, it may still canter incorrectly through habit and compensation. The rider must remain very balanced and as soon as the horse strikes off into canter correctly, give lots of praise so that the horse understands this was the correct response to the aids.

When mistakes are made in any schooling, the horse should never be punished. The rider must first consider whether they are balanced and coordinated and whether the correct aids have been applied. A moment of contemplation can prevent tension and stress within the partnership. The movement can then be repeated quietly without pressurising or disturbing the harmony required for successful performances. A pat or stroke on the neck is far more effective than a sharp aid that can easily be misinterpreted.

The muscular structure must never be fatigued as this leads to uncoordinated and unbalanced movement, eventually resulting in changed biomechanics and possibly even lameness. Warming up the horse correctly is essential and should begin with walking followed by trotting and cantering with a light contact before progressing on to more intricate movements.

It is a mistake to perform suppling exercises at the start of the warm up while the tissues are cold, because the fibres in the muscles, tendons and ligaments are more susceptible to overstretching injuries (Clayton 1991, p. 137).

Every training and exercise session must finish by warming down the horse before returning it to the stable or into a horsebox if at a show. The maintenance of low intensity exercise (trot or canter) for 5–10 minutes allows a gradual redistribution of the blood flow and enhances lactate removal from the muscles by using it as an energy substrate for the continuing aerobic activity (Clayton 1991, p. 137).

Some invaluable advice given to me by a great friend and mentor, Yens Mumme, was to look at my watch and always begin the warm up and end the warm down with a 10-minute walk. It is amazing how long 10 minutes can feel!

In some cases, it may be advisable to have an experienced rider to ride the horse for the initial post-treatment training sessions. This enables the horse to respond and develop its potential, unhindered by the lack of experience and balance of the novice rider. In other situations, a good trainer on the ground can guide and give confidence to the rider and horse.

Horses must understand what they are being asked to do, especially as we are constantly increasing the demands in training throughout their careers. They must never be over-faced or forced to perform beyond their ability and talent.

RECOMMENDED READING

Bartle C (2009) *Training the Sport Horse*. JA Allen, London.

Diggle M, Raynor M (2002) *Basic Schooling Made Simple*. JA Allen, London.

McBane S (2007) *From Warming Up to Cooling Down*. JA Allen, London.

GROOMING, MASSAGE, STRAPPING AND STRETCHING

The practitioner can demonstrate to the owner how to massage the horse using a suitable grooming tool such as a long-toothed rubber brush and generally remind them of the importance and benefits of grooming, a forgotten art!

Beginning at the top of the neck, use circular movements with the groomer and then descend down the cervical spine to the pectorals and chest. Horses respond by scratching against the brush and lifting up through the withers. Proceed with gentle stroking movements under the sternum to encourage the horse to flex the thoracic spine. Owners must be cautioned that some horses resent their abdomens being groomed and may bite and kick. However, if they start very gently, most horses will respond positively. To

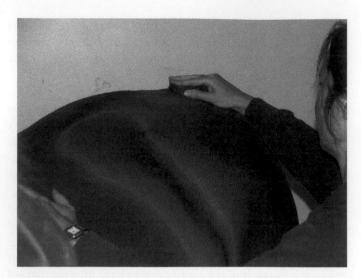

Figure 14.7 Massaging the gluteal musculature using a rubber grooming brush.

finish, the gluteals are massaged with the grooming brush (see Figure 14.7), which also encourages the horse to flex the lumbosacral junction. This is such a beneficial grooming and massage routine, and the horse really enjoys and responds to it; it also results in a positive bonding between groomer and animal.

The medial gluteals are often weak, and strapping this area can be very effective. Strapping is an old-fashioned term describing the use of a wisp or pad, which one bangs and slides on the selected region in the direction of the lay of the hair. This promotes better circulation and neurological stimulation. The horse flexes and contracts its muscles in anticipation of the contact of the wisp or pad, thereby toning the muscle fibres.

Stretching can be prescribed as required, although it must be stressed to the owner that this can only be applied when the muscles are warmed up after exercise or grooming and massaging. Some examples of passive and active stretches for the limbs and neck are described in Chapter 12.

RECOMMENDED READING

Blignault K (2003) *Stretch Exercises for Your Horse*. JA Allen, London.

Bromiley MW (2010) *Massage Techniques for Horse and Rider*. Crowood Press, Marlborough.

Hourdebaigt J-P (2007) *Equine Massage – A Practical Guide*. Wiley, Hoboken, NJ.

Meagher J (1985) *Beating Muscle Injuries for Horses*. Hamilton Horse Associates, Hamilton, MA.

Stubbs NC, Clayton HM (2008) *Activate Your Horse's Core*. Sport Horse Publications, Mason, MI.

Sutton A (2001) *The Injury-Free Horse*. Trafalgar Square Publishing, London.

RIDER'S FITNESS AND ABILITY

The rider's position, their suppleness in the saddle and their ability to execute the aids and ride the horse into a soft contact is paramount to the development of posture and balance throughout training. Postural stretching and strengthening exercises will improve the rider's seat and balance. The abdominal muscle tone is as essential to us as it is to the horse!

The rider must sit in the centre of the saddle and not hinder the horse's movement by sitting heavily or collapsing to one side. It is especially difficult when riding the lateral movements such as half-pass to keep the balance central. There is a tendency for the rider to collapse the hip and body weight to the outside as if to push the horse over.

Some riders balance themselves by hanging on to the reins and mouth, causing the horse to hollow through the cervicothoracic junction and poll. The horse's spine becomes extended, and thoracolumbar restrictions prevent the pelvis from flexing correctly, resulting in uncoordinated movement.

When the horse comes up off the forehand and carries the rider, it should be easier to sit and absorb the movement. However, some riders may find that the elevation and cadence may push them up off the saddle and unbalance their position.

Lungeing the horse with the rider will enhance and improve the position in the saddle and the 'feel' for the correct movement and balance required. The rider is able to concentrate on his or her own posture and stretch and exercise accordingly while trusting the trainer to work the horse through different paces.

Apart from going to the gym and seeing an osteopath, a useful innovation, which also improves a rider's posture and balance, is training on a mechanical horse (see Figure 14.8). Obviously there is no substitute for the living beastie, but the muscle memory and coordination learnt from the mechanical horse can then be applied when riding to great effect.

RECOMMENDED READING

Bromiley MW (1999) *Fit To Ride? Train Your Horse – Train Yourself*. Blackwell Science, Oxford.

Inderwick S (2003) *Lungeing the Horse and Rider*. David & Charles, Newton Abbot.

Swift S (2006) *Centred Riding*. JA Allen, London.

Wanless M (1999) *For the Good of the Rider*. Trafalgar Square Publishing, London.

ALLIED PROFESSIONS

The osteopath should build up a rapport with allied professionals in their area as the different approaches to restoring

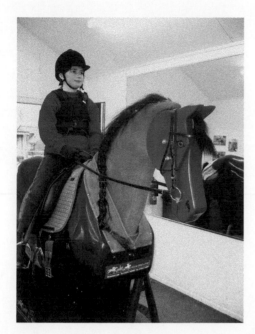

Figure 14.8 Improving the rider's posture and balance on a mechanical horse.

the horse's well being all complement each other and can be combined in the treatment programme (see Figure 14.9). It is essential that the practitioners all work as a team so that the horse receives the optimum treatment at the correct time.

With veterinary guidance the osteopath, chiropractor and physiotherapist can have a working regime that can greatly enhance the progress of the horse's rehabilitation.

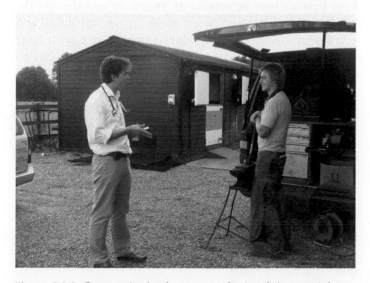

Figure 14.9 Communication between professionals is essential.

Acupuncture has always complemented physical treatments but this can only be applied by a veterinary surgeon.

Other complementary practitioners and therapies include healers, behavioural trainers, sports massage and hydrotherapy such as swimming or treadmills.

Networking and attending seminars and lectures on all relevant subjects is as important when treating horses as it is with our human patients.

Further information is available from the British Equine Veterinary Association, www.beva.org.uk; the British Association of Homeopathic Veterinary Surgeons, www.bahvs. com; the Association of Chartered Physiotherapists in Animal Practice, www.acpat.org; McTimoney College of Chiropractic, www.mctimoney-college.ac.uk; the Equine Behaviour Forum, www.gla.ac.uk/External/EBF; and the Equine Sports Massage Association, www.equinemassage association.co.uk.

RECOMMENDED READING

Bromiley MW (1991) *Physiotherapy in Veterinary Practice*. Blackwell Publishing, Oxford.

Bromiley MW (2007) *Equine Injury and Therapy*. Wiley-Blackwell, Oxford.

Sutton A (2003) *The Injured Horse*. David & Charles, Newton Abbot.

REFERENCES

Clayton H (1991) *Conditioning Sport Horses*. Sport Horse Publications, Mason, MI, p. 137.

Crawford P (undated) *The Society of Master Saddlers Essential Guide to Selecting and Fitting Bridles*, 5. www.mastersaddlerss. co.uk.

Engelke E, Gasse H (2003) An anatomical study of the rostral part of the equine oral cavity with respect to position and size of a snaffle bit. *Equine Veterinary Education* 15, 200–205.

Hayes MH (1988) *Veterinary Notes for Horse Owners*, 17th edn, revised by Peter D Rossdale. Stanley Paul, London, p. 697.

Manfredi J, Clayton HM, Rosenstein D (2005) Radiographic study of bit position within the horse's oral cavity. *Equine and Comparative Exercise Physiology* 2, 195–201.

Murray R (2006–2007) Identifying horse and rider, management, training and surface factors that affect the risk of injury in our horses. The Animal Health Trust/British Dressage/British Equestrian Federation Dressage Questionnaire.

Vahey W (1928) Horse dentistry. In: Lyon WE (ed.) *In My Opinion – Being a Book of Dissertations on Horses and Horsemanship*. Constable, London, p. 298.

Differential Diagnosis

Christopher Colles

Diagnosis of musculoskeletal problems in the horse is restricted by law to veterinary surgeons, and so the differential diagnosis should have been resolved prior to the horse being referred for osteopathic treatment. None the less mistakes can occur, more than one condition may be present, or conditions may develop during the course of treatment. For this reason it is important that osteopaths undertaking treatment of horses should have a good working knowledge of conditions that may be encountered that are unresponsive to physical treatment, that have signs similar to conditions that will respond to physical treatment, or where physical treatment is contraindicated.

MECHANICAL PROBLEMS

Teeth

As a grazing animal, the horse's teeth are subject to considerable wear. They are gradually 'extruded' from the upper and lower jaws throughout life, to compensate for wear, finally being lost at about 30 to 35 years of age. The lower jaw is slightly narrower than the upper, and so as the teeth wear there is a tendency for sharp edges to form on the outer edges of the upper teeth, and on the inner edges of the lower teeth. In addition, the surfaces of the teeth (the tables) may become irregular and form sharp points, especially at the back of the molars and the front of the premolars. These sharp edges and points can cause discomfort, and the horse may resent the presence of the bit or bridle when ridden. Tossing the head about or throwing it up or down is often a sign of discomfort, and soreness in the mouth should not be overlooked. These signs can be confused with pain in the upper cervical area. As with humans, abnormal tension in the upper neck can lead to uneven or restricted movement in the temporomandibular joints, which may also lead to uneven tooth wear.

The first premolar in the horse is often absent, or only present in the upper jaw. When present it is vestigial (termed a wolf tooth). It may lie under the gum, and frequently is thought to cause soreness. Associated traditionally with many equine ailments, it is usually removed when the horse first starts coming in to ridden work.

Foot Balance

Foot balance may be defined as 'trimming and shoeing the foot in such a manner as to result in normal stride and movement'. Assessment of balance and shoeing are a huge subject, and although the reader would be well advised to obtain a basic understanding of these topics, developing a working relationship with a knowledgeable, competent farrier will prove invaluable. Trimming the foot and shoeing have a major influence on limb flight and placement. As a result, poor balance may predispose to pathological changes in the limbs, and may lead to mechanical dysfunction over time. It may also make treatment of mechanical dysfunction much more difficult if foot balance is not corrected simultaneously. It must also be borne in mind, when assessing movement, that abduction, adduction, changes in stride length, and foot and limb placement may relate to problems with shoeing/foot balance as well as to mechanical dysfunction higher in the limb.

Saddle Fitting

As with farriery, this is a specialised area in its own right, and a lifetime's knowledge is really required to advise riders satisfactorily in this area. The saddle is the interface between rider and horse, and can play a major part in affecting movement and function. It can cause changes in stride length if badly fitting, and can lead to change in mechanical function by placing pressure incorrectly or unevenly on the back musculature. Saddles may be twisted, asymmetrical, and unevenly padded, faults that are reasonably easy to detect. Width of fitting, depth of the channel, and poor construction are more difficult to determine, and once again a good working relationship with a saddle fitter will prove invaluable. Owners frequently assume that back pain is the result of a poor saddle, and may change saddles two or three times before getting the back properly investigated. In fact, poorly fitting saddles are seldom a primary cause of back pain, but they may add to other problems and, as with shoeing, a poorly fitting saddle may contribute to the development of mechanical dysfunction and may well compromise attempts at treatment. It is important to realise that, as backs are treated, the musculature alters, and will often continue to change for up to two years after a back is treated. For this reason it is important that saddles should be checked, and adjusted or 're-stuffed' regularly after treatment.

NEUROLOGICAL CONDITIONS

Incoordination

A number of horses with muscular pain, or with bruising to the spinal cord as a result of trauma, may appear incoordinate. Before considering manipulation of such cases, however, it is important to differentiate them from other known causes of incoordination in the horse. Differentiation is not always easy, or even possible, but the necessary veterinary examinations should be completed before beginning manipulation of horses that might be mildly ataxic or incoordinate.

Cervical Stenosis (Wobbler Disease)

Incidence

Cervical stenosis is more common in colts than fillies, and in the UK is usually seen in thoroughbreds although it is becoming more common in other breeds. The onset is usually sudden, occurring in young horses and often associated with increased activity or possibly trauma, e.g. when broken in. Clinical signs may progress as work continues but often, if work ceases, signs stabilise or regress.

Pathology

There is narrowing of the cervical spinal canal, which causes compression of the spinal nerves. This interferes with motor and sensory nerves to all four limbs, and results in permanent damage by the time clinical signs are evident.

Clinical signs

Normally there is no pain associated with this condition, and horses seem unconcerned about it even if, in severe cases, they fall over. The horse moves with a rather straight-legged hindlimb gait. The hind end may drift to either side when trotting or, if trotted and stopped suddenly, the hindquarters may sway or the horse may even fall over. In severe cases there may be a hypermetric forelimb gait. If the tail is pulled to either side when standing or walking, the hindquarters will sway to the side and the horse does not resist the movement. When moved back, the horse will sink back on the hind legs before stepping backward. If cantered (usually on a lunge), both hindlimbs tend to be used together (bunny hops).

If the horse is turned short, it pivots on the inner hindleg and usually throws the outer hindleg wide. Frequently it will fail to cross the hindlegs correctly, or this is inconsistent.

Confirmation of diagnosis

X-ray and measurement of the sagittal section of the spinal canal may help in the diagnosis of this condition. Occasionally myelograms are made, but the technique is usually carried out under general anaesthesia and this, as well as reactions to the contrast agent required, may well make the condition considerably worse.

Endoscopic examination of the larynx can be helpful, making use of the 'slap test'. This makes use of a reflex that exists in the normal horse. When the horse is patted on the saddle area, the arytenoid cartilage on the contralateral side is momentarily adducted. This can be viewed through the endoscope, and the reflex is absent in cases of cervical stenosis.

Treatment

Steroids and NSAIDs have little or no effect.

Surgery to stabilise affected joints by fusion of the joint improves the condition by one or two grades. Although well established, the surgery remains controversial and many cases are destroyed on humane grounds.

Manipulation is contraindicated as movement of the cervical joints will increase pressure on the spinal cord.

Cauda Equina (polyneuritis equi)

Incidence

This is a relatively uncommon condition, occurring equally frequently in both sexes. It is normally seen in mature or teenage horses.

Pathology

The aetiology and pathology are still uncertain, but generally there is chronic inflammation of the nerve roots of the cauda equina (the last part of the spinal cord). Other nerves may also be affected, principally the cranial nerves. The cause is unknown, but it has been suggested that cauda equina may be associated with trauma. The prognosis is poor, but occasional cases do recover.

Clinical signs

Clinical signs are slowly progressive over several weeks, although cases are often presented as being of sudden onset. (This may be true, or probably the early signs are not detected.)

The condition is basically one of slowly ascending paralysis, so there is loss of sensation and motor tone initially causing a flaccid tail, but gradually creeping forwards. The next symptoms may be of bizarre lameness, or retention of faeces, or dribbling of urine. Frequently, affected animals will rub the base of the tail, and may be hypersensitive over the gluteal muscles.

Confirmation of diagnosis is generally made on clinical grounds. Serum samples can be checked for myelin degradation products, but a fairly high percentage of false negative and positive results makes this test relatively unreliable.

Treatment

High doses of steroids may be associated with resolution of symptoms. If this occurs, the dose is then gradually reduced. Unfortunately a large number of cases will then relapse, but treatment may well be worth considering.

DMSO (dimethylsulphoxide) has also been used. The numbers of cases treated by either means are too small to allow results to be seriously assessed.

Physical treatment is not beneficial.

Equine Protozoal Myelitis

Incidence

Equine protozoal myelitis does not naturally occur in the UK, but it is seen occasionally in imports from USA and Canada, where it is becoming much more common. It is most frequent in 1- to 4-year-olds, but can occur at any age from 2 months to 14 years. It may not give clinical signs until several years after importation.

Pathology

This is a protozoal infection of the CNS (the organism is probably a type of *Sarcocystis*, but is still not definitively identified). It may affect any part of the nervous system, and may spread with time. It is probably not infectious between horses, and requires an intermediate host – almost certainly the opossum.

Clinical signs

Clinical signs can be very variable, and may mimic almost any CNS problems. Generally signs begin as an obscure lameness, progressing to ataxia. There may be slight muscle wastage, and this, together with other neurological signs, is generally not bilaterally symmetrical.

Progression may be slow or rapid, often leading to recumbency in days or months.

Ante-mortem diagnostic tests are available in the USA, but there is a very high percentage of false positive and negative results making tests relatively useless.

Treatment

Treatment is with sulphonamides, NSAIDs and sometimes DMSO. The response to treatment is very variable. Occasional cases do recover. Others show no change, progress, or respond and relapse.

Fractured Vertebrae

Incidence

May occur in any age, sex or type of horse.

Pathology

Fracture of a vertebra or dislocation of an intervertebral joint usually results in paralysis or death. Hairline fractures without displacement or partial fractures may be compatible with life, but usually cause severe ataxia or recumbency depending on the severity and position of the lesion.

Clinical signs

Fractures are usually associated with a fall or other trauma. They occur most commonly in the neck. They are associated with acute pain, muscle spasm and stiffness in the affected area. There may be associated ataxia, which may be progressive to recumbency. The exact clinical signs depend on the site and severity of the fracture. Confirmation may be possible by X-ray. Fractures of the thoracic and lumbar spine are very difficult to identify, however, even with powerful X-ray machines, and may only be diagnosed by scintigraphy.

Treatment

Fractures of the spine seldom lend themselves to surgical fixation, but may heal in some instances if given time, usually with the use of painkillers and anti-inflammatory drugs to reduce oedema and swelling within the spinal canal.

Movement and exercise will need to be restricted, and food and water may need to be available above floor level.

DO NOT MANIPULATE, at least until the fracture is stable and healing, when cranial work to relieve associated muscle spasm might be considered.

Equine Herpes Virus Type 1

Incidence

EHV1 can occur in any age, sex and type of horse.

Pathology

EHV1 is a viral infection.

Clinical signs

This is an infectious viral disease with an incubation period of about 7 days. The principal clinical signs are of respiratory infection, although 2–3 days prior to onset of signs there may be a temperature of 39–40°C.

Although this is primarily a respiratory virus, there are sporadic outbreaks of neurological signs, and it may also be associated with abortion in late gestation. Neurological signs generally occur 2–3 weeks after respiratory signs have been seen in the affected animal or other associated horses. They generally have a sudden onset, which may be associated with apparent stress or trauma.

Ataxia may be mild, or severe enough to cause recumbency. There is sometimes associated urine retention and incontinence, and there may be loss of perineal sensation.

Confirmatory laboratory tests

- There are changes in the white cell count, but this may takes several days to occur, and they are not specific.
- A complement fixation test for rising antibody titre can be carried out, and will confirm the infection with good reliability. It requires two samples taken 14 days apart.

Treatment

Treatment is only by supportive therapy. There is no specific treatment.

Very mild cases may recover in 2–3 weeks but more severe cases may take up to a year, whilst recumbent cases frequently do not survive.

Current vaccines for EHV1 and EHV4 do not claim to prevent paralytic signs. They do, however, diminish shedding of virus by infected horses and so might help to reduce the incidence of disease in this manner. *Vaccination should not be used on in-contact animals in the face of infection.*

Manipulation is ineffective, and probably contraindicated as stress exacerbates the condition.

Motor Neurone Disease

Incidence

Motor neurone disease has been reported in the horse but the condition is probably very rare and the incidence is currently unknown. It occurs at any age (2–20 years) and in any sex and type of horse. It is considered to be most common in older horses, with a peak incidence of about 16 years. Usually at onset the horses have no access to grass, or are on very poor grassing.

Pathology

Neurological degeneration with ceroid lipofuscin inclusions. The lesions are primarily in the ventral grey matter and brain stem nuclei. It may be associated with low levels of alpha-tocopherol.

Clinical signs

Neurological signs usually have a gradual onset, accompanied from early on by muscle tremors. There are often increased periods of recumbency, but these should not to be confused with colic. There is gradual weight loss. Signs consistently involve the forelimbs (medial head of triceps), hindlimbs (vastus medialis, lateralis and intermedius muscle) and the tail head. Ataxia may be mild but tends to be progressive, leading to recumbency. Pigmentation of the retina often occurs.

Confirmatory laboratory tests

- Muscle biopsy may show atrophy of type II muscle fibres.
- Vitamin E levels may be less than 1.0 μg/ml (normal 1.5–4.0 μg/ml).

Treatment

Treatment is only by supportive therapy. There is no specific treatment.

Motor neurone disease is a rare condition in horses that is difficult to diagnose specifically other than at post-mortem. Cases frequently do not survive, and if they do are unlikely to return to normal work, 30% or more of the grey matter neurones being absent. It is not infectious.

Manipulation is ineffective.

PHYSIOLOGICAL CONDITIONS

Ataxia should be relatively easy to diagnose, although its cause may be more obscure. The following conditions may mimic ataxia on preliminary examination:

- Bilateral hindlimb lameness, e.g. spavin, bone cysts, osteochondritis dissecans (OCD)
- Rhabdomyolysis
- Exhaustion
- Hypocalcaemia

Equine Rhabdomyolysis

Equine rhabdomyolysis is the term used to describe non-traumatic myopathies. It covers such terms as azoturia, paralytic myoglobinuria, exertional myopathy, exertional rhabdomyolysis, tying up, set-fast and Monday morning disease.

The pathophysiology is open to much discussion, and there are undoubtedly several different conditions involved.

This should therefore be referred to as a syndrome (a collection of conditions or diseases giving similar symptoms).

Clinical signs

The incidence of the condition is higher in young fillies than in older animals, colts and geldings, but it can occur at any age and in any breed or sex. It is more common in winter than in summer, but any stress can precipitate attacks in susceptible animals. Cold and wet conditions predispose to attacks.

Clinical signs most commonly start during work (65%). Fifteen per cent may occur before real work is commenced, and about 20% show signs when resting after exercise. The signs are principally stiffness, which may be so slight as to be hardly detectable, or may be so severe as to prevent walking completely. There is muscle spasm, usually of the back, loins and hindlimbs, but potentially of any muscle mass(es). Although usually bilaterally symmetrical, this need not be so. Muscle fasciculations are often present. There is considerable pain and sweating. In severe cases there may be temporary paralysis of gut muscle, and colic. In a few very severe cases, recumbency and death may occur.

Differential diagnosis is not usually too difficult, but the most commonly confused conditions are colic, iliac thrombosis, laminitis, acute back pain, and tetanus. Confirmation of the condition can be made by measuring muscle enzyme levels in the serum (aspartate transaminase (AST) and creatine phosphokinase (CPK)). These levels may be raised to more than 10 times their normal resting levels 24 hours after an attack. In animals suspected of being prone to the condition, measuring the enzyme levels before, immediately after and 24 hours after a known amount of exercise may be helpful in confirming the diagnosis and ensuring that management precautions are effective in preventing recurrence.

Management plays a large part in the occurrence of the disease, and 90% of cases have been subjected to overfeeding and irregular work. There are a small number of cases, however, which show recurrent attacks despite carefully controlled nutrition and exercise, and these require more in-depth investigation.

Pathophysiology

The end point of rhabdomyolysis is that there is breakdown of the muscle cell integrity with resultant release of muscle enzymes into the blood stream. The pathophysiology is not understood. It has been shown that in many cases (especially those associated with poor management), there are excessive levels of glycogen stored in the muscle, and it has been suggested that this undergoes rapid anaerobic breakdown to release excessive amounts of lactic acid, which cause damage to the muscle cells. Whilst this is a nice theory, the levels of lactate measured in these cases have not been proven to be high enough to cause harm.

In 70% of cases (especially those with recurrent attacks but apparently good work regimens), fractional excretion measurements of electrolytes in the urine have shown electrolyte imbalances in susceptible animals. It has proved possible in most cases to prevent recurrence by adjusting the diet accordingly. It is currently suggested that changes in electrolyte concentrations lead to failure in the cell ATP pumping mechanism to maintain the normal high intracellular levels of potassium and phosphate. This may allow an increase in intracellular calcium with a resultant increase in activity of neutral protease and resultant cellular damage.

There is subjective evidence that horses may be predisposed to rhabdomyolysis after viral infections, which possibly leave muscle cells in a damaged state. There are also indications that mild hypothyroidism may be involved in some cases. Muscular ischaemia may also be a contributory factor, and in some instances cold wet conditions may stimulate vascular spasm, leading on to secondary muscle damage.

Treatment

Treatment will depend on the severity of the attack. Management initially entails not moving the horse, and keeping it warm and dry. Once an attack has begun, any exercise may result in exacerbation of the condition. If an attack occurs away from stables, it is advisable to transport the horse back to shelter rather than walking it. Feed should be reduced to good hay and little or no concentrates for the initial period. Blood samples are usually checked for muscle enzyme levels to confirm the diagnosis and also as an aid to determining how soon a horse can recommence work. Whilst enzymes are raised, no work should be attempted or a relapse is likely to occur. Some trainers insist on walking horses to try to maintain a level of fitness. This delays recovery, and is usually self-defeating. Blood and urine samples may be taken about 14 days after the attack to assess the electrolyte status of the horse, and the diet can then be adjusted accordingly.

Depending on the severity of the initial attack, the horse will require treatment with NSAIDs (and possibly steroids in severe cases). Very severe cases may need intravenous supplementation of electrolytes, fluids, and possibly vasodilators or sedatives. Some horses are very shocked, and the condition can result in recumbency and even death in rare cases.

Prevention of recurrence is essential. This will rely primarily on regular feeding and exercise. It will probably also require investigation and probably supplementation of the rations. In very persistent recurrent cases, medication with drugs such as dantrolene may be required. In a small percentage of cases, it is not possible to prevent recurrence, and such horses may have to be retired to a less athletic activity.

Idiopathic Rhabdomyolysis

Acute rhabdomyolysis has been seen in horses (or more commonly ponies) at grass with no history of work and often no supplementary feeding. A large percentage of these cases become recumbent, and subsequently prove fatal despite very extensive support and treatment. At the present time, the cause of this condition is unknown.

Malignant Hyperthermia

The pathophysiology of this condition is still not understood. It appears to be a hereditary condition, giving behavioural problems as well as chronically raised muscle enzymes and exercise intolerance. Work to date has shown no cure although it may be possible to help control symptoms in some cases by reducing the carbohydrate in the feed and compensating with an increase in oil. The condition is rare and poorly understood.

Iliac Thrombosis

Thrombosis of the iliac arteries gives signs of pain and muscle spasm in the hindlimbs when a horse is working. It is associated with high worm burdens, with resultant larval migration causing damage to the arteries. It used to be a relatively common condition in young horses but with better parasite management its incidence is now quite rare. Diagnosis can be confirmed using ultrasonographic examination of the distal end of the dorsal aorta and iliac arteries.

BACK PAIN/DYSFUNCTION

Back pain in the horse is a problem frequently diagnosed by riders but often doubted by vets. This is because of the difficulty of assessing backs in an objective manner. Many cases are chronic and show signs of change in function or gait quality rather than frank pain. Clinical signs are largely the same whatever the cause of the problem, and have been discussed in previous chapters. Bone and joint problems can be seen on x-ray or scintigraphy and so lend themselves to a positive diagnosis although they may well be the cause of less than 10% of cases. As in humans, relating radiographic changes directly to back pain is very difficult, and interpretation of the significance of radiographic changes should be tempered with a greater than normal degree of caution.

BONE AND JOINT CONDITIONS

Over-riding Dorsal Spinous Processes (Kissing Spines)

Arguably this condition is most commonly a symptom of another problem and not usually a primary disease entity although currently a very popular diagnosis. It normally occurs under the saddle region, although it may sometimes be seen in the lower thoracic or very rarely lumbar areas.

Diagnosis

As with most causes of back pain, diagnosis on purely clinical signs is not possible. The area will be painful on palpation, but this is not limited to the spinal processes themselves as adjacent soft tissues are also involved. Radiographically, significant cases show a number of adjacent dorsal spinous processes that are either touching or even overlapping. When this is clinically significant, there is evidence of porosis and sclerosis (remodelling) of the adjacent edges of the spinal processes. This should not be confused with cases where the spines are closely packed but no bone remodelling has taken place as these are seldom painful (this situation is very common in thoroughbred and thoroughbred cross horses).

Pathophysiology

There is no information on the cause of this problem. Certain breeds such as thoroughbred and thoroughbred cross horses normally have limited space between the dorsal spinous processes, but it is unlikely that this would be painful in normal circumstances. It has been suggested that some other cause of back dysfunction causes the horse to hollow the back when working, thus bringing the dorsal spinous processes into closer and more direct contact. This may then result in pain as a result of the change in positioning of the back, and increased trauma to the processes.

Treatment

In many cases no treatment is needed if the primary problem is addressed and the horse lifts the back and moves more correctly. In some cases, however, the bone reaction set up, and creation of new bone around the dorsal spinous processes may be so severe that it becomes a self-perpetuating problem. In these cases it is common practice to infuse the area with corticosteroids, or to resect surgically the summits of alternate processes in the area of overriding. Once a relatively common surgical operation, it is becoming less frequently practised as other treatments are introduced.

Arthritis of the Facet Joints

Arthritis of the facet joints usually affects the vertebrae in the lumbar region first, with the joints under the saddle region also being affected in some cases.

Diagnosis

There are no clinical signs specifically pointing to this diagnosis. As with arthritic changes in other joints it tends to occur in older horses. Diagnosis relies on good quality radiographs, or scintigraphy.

Pathophysiology

As with arthritis elsewhere, this is assumed to be a degenerative disease of the joints and as such to be slowly progressive. As mentioned above, relating pain directly to radiographic changes is very difficult, but radiographic changes accompanying back pain must give rise to a more guarded prognosis.

Treatment

Palliatives such as NSAIDs or joint injections may be used. Whether these are as effective as cranial osteopathy is uncertain. When manipulating these cases, care should, however, be taken not to exacerbate the underlying arthritic problems. The long-term prognosis must, of course, be guarded

Ossifying Spondylitis

Ossifying spondylitis is normally seen in the thoracic region, once again under the saddle region.

Diagnosis

Diagnosis can only be made radiographically, although it may be seen on scintigraphy when actively forming. The condition may be present without obvious clinical signs, making its significance difficult to determine. It seems likely, however, that it does cause reduced flexibility of the spine and so must adversely affect the prognosis when treating cases with spinal dysfunction.

Pathophysiology

Very little is known about the pathophysiology of this condition in the horse.

Treatment

Palliative treatments are used in this condition, but their benefit is hard to assess. Cases are generally retired to less demanding activities.

Fractures

Fractures of the vertebrae are not uncommon, generally as the result of severe trauma. Clinical signs range from death, through incoordination, to pain, depending on the area involved and the severity of the fracture. Complete fractures through the body of a cervical or thoracic vertebra generally lead to death or paralysis, whereas fractures through lower thoracic and lumbar vertebrae may only result in incoordination, or in rare cases partial fracture may only cause severe pain. Fractures of the spine are generally accompanied by acute muscle spasm in the affected area. See previous section for treatment.

Fracture of pelvis

Pelvic fracture is relatively common. In the adult it is usually caused by severe trauma such as a fall. In 2- to 3-year-olds it may occur as a 'spontaneous fracture' when the horse jumps off at the start of a race or training gallop.

Pelvic fracture results in severe, non-weight-bearing lameness, with rapid and marked muscle wastage of the gluteal muscles. The exact symptoms and prognosis depend on the site of the fracture. There is often a reasonable prognosis other than for dressage, provided the fracture does not involve the acetabulum. Box rest is essential, and exercise will severely affect the prognosis.

Confirmation is by x-ray, ultrasound, or scintigraphy.

Hip dislocation

Hip dislocation is very rare in the horse. In a small pony, immediate reduction may be possible, but it requires general anaesthesia within 2 or 3 hours. In larger ponies and horses the prognosis is very bad. Luxation generally results in rupture of the straight ligament, and also severe damage to the head of the femur. If reduction of the dislocation is possible, it is likely to be unstable, and damage to the head of the femur generally results in rapidly progressive arthritis.

Other Causes

Other causes of bone pathology underlying back pain are rare and include tumours, tuberculosis, and infectious osteomyelitis. These are too rare to give any guide to diagnosis on clinical grounds, and diagnosis is initially on radiographic evidence.

SOFT TISSUE CONDITIONS

It is likely that at least 90% of back pain cases in horses have a soft tissue origin. Although there are no published figures relating to the differential diagnosis, it is important in acute cases to eliminate muscle strain and ligament strain.

Muscle Strain

Strain of the back muscles can occur, usually with an acute onset. Palpation of the affected area reveals hot, swollen and painful muscle. Pressure applied to the area will result in a strong response from the horse. Cases are usually easily diagnosed on clinical examination, but might be confirmed using diagnostic ultrasound. These cases usually resolve satisfactorily with rest, possibly aided by physiotherapy.

Ligament Strain

Strain of the supraspinous ligament has been described, giving signs of heat, pain and swelling of the involved area of the ligament. This can be confirmed using diagnostic ultrasound. There may also be separation of the ligament from the summits of the dorsal spinous processes, usually over the withers or lumbar region, which can be seen on x-ray as small 'flakes' of bone separated from the summits of the processes. Ligament strain will normally settle down over a period of several weeks.

Sacroiliac Strain

Acute strain

This is a strain of the collateral ligaments of the sacroiliac joint, effectively a ligament holding the pelvis to the sacrum. It occurs after severe trauma, such as a fall. It usually presents with severe pain and with tilting of the pelvis, which can be assessed by looking at the tubera coxae from behind. The pain is exacerbated by pressure applied to the tuber coxa (especially in a dorsal direction) of the affected side. There is usually rapid gluteal muscle loss, especially on the affected side. The condition is best confirmed by scintigraphy, which often shows that it is accompanied by a hairline fracture of the wing of the ilium.

Treatment of acute sacroiliac strain requires box rest for at least 3 months, and possibly up to 6 months. Sensible animals may be able to receive some hand walking, or to be turned out after 3 months. The condition is usually accompanied by other marked soft tissue injuries, which may require rehabilitation once the sacroiliac joint is stable. If kept in work, or given inadequate rest, these cases become unstable and chronically lame.

Chronic strain

'Chronic sacroiliac strain' has a history of gradual onset, probably with no obvious trauma. There is a tilt of the tubera coxae when viewed from behind, which is the basis of the diagnosis. Frequently one tuber coxa will feel pulled forwards relative to the other. Generally pressure on the tubera coxae is not severely resented, but may show some soreness and may trigger muscle spasm in the longissimus dorsi muscles. There is progressive loss of muscle in the gluteal region, which may be unilateral or bilateral to a greater or lesser degree. The horse starts to develop a weak hindlimb action, fails to work from behind, and may 'bunny hop' when cantered.

It seems likely that this is a rotation of the lumbar spine rather than a strain of the sacroiliac joint itself.

These 'chronic strains' may respond to osteopathy. It is important to be sure of the differential diagnosis, and not to risk manipulating an acute strain.

Glossary

Abduction Movement of a body part away from the mid-sagittal plane.

Acute Term applied to a disease in which the attack is sudden, severe and of short duration.

Adduction Movement of a body part towards the midsagittal plane.

Bascule Shape or line a horse takes when jumping.

Break Also known as breaking-in. Train a young horse to obey commands and accept direction and control.

Breastplate A wide leather strap that encircles the horse's chest and attaches on both sides of the saddle and on to the girth between the forelegs.

Browband Part of the bridle that lies flat across the forehead below the ears and above the eyes of the horse.

Cadence Shown in trot and is the result of the proper harmony that a horse displays when it moves with well marked regularity, impulsion and balance.Cadence must be maintained in all different trot exercises and in all the variations of trot. The rhythm that a horse maintains in all the paces is fundamental to dressage.

Cast Describes a horse that has become lodged on the ground between a vertical surface and the withers. It occurs when a horse falls, rolls, or lies down in too small a space or too close to a fence, wall or manger and is unable to get up without assistance. The more strenuously it struggles to right itself, the more prone it is to injury.

Caudal Towards the tail end.

Chambon An advanced piece of schooling/training equipment designed to lower the head and upper neck while simultaneously raising the base of the neck to obtain a rounded topline and improved engagement of the hocks under the body.

Chestnut Horny growths or calluses located on the inside of the horse's leg, above the knees on the forelegs and below the hocks on the hindlegs.

Chifney bit A circular bit developed in the late 1700s by Samuel Chifney after whom it is named. May have a reversed half-circle mouth in which case it is used to prevent rearing.

Chronic Of long duration; the opposite of acute.

Collect To shorten the pace of the horse using light hand contact on the reins and steady pressure from the rider's legs to make the horse flex its neck, relax its jaw, elevate the back and bring its hocks well under its body. The impulsion created by the hindlegs is contained by the rider's hands.

Collected canter A pace in which the horse is ridden at the canter into the bit with the neck flexed and arched, jaw relaxed, hindquarters engaged and active, forehand light and shoulders supple and free. The stride is shorter than at other canters but lighter and more mobile.

Collected trot A pace in which the horse is ridden at the trot into the bit with the neck flexed and arched, jaw relaxed, hocks well under the body with energetic impulsion and the weight over the haunches. The horse is moved forwards from behind; the steps are shorter, but lighter and more mobile than at other trots.

Collected walk A pace in which the horse is ridden at the walk into the bit with the neck flexed, jaw relaxed, hocks well under the body with good action and the weight over the haunches. The horse is moved forwards from behind, and the pace is vigorous with each step placed in regular sequence. The stride is shortened and shows greater activity than at the medium walk.

Collection Also known as self-carriage and engaging the hindquarters: a learned weight-bearing posture of the horse. The increased and energetic engagement of the hindlegs, elevation of the back and lightening the fore-hand result in improved balance. The degree of desired collection varies greatly from sport to sport.

Combinations A term used in jumping competitions. The distances between two elements of a combination of jumps, whether it is a double, treble or multiple com-bination, may be of any length between a minimum of 7 metres to a maximum of 12 metres. The distance is at the course builder's discretion and the decision will be in-fluenced by factors such as the standard of competition, height, spread and nature of the fences and the surface conditions.

Contralateral Occurring on the opposite side.

Correct canter lead Also known as true canter: said of a cantering horse that leads with his foreleg on the side to which he is turning.

Cow kick A type of kick in which the horse strikes forward and to the outside with one of his hindlegs, enabling a horse to strike a rider or handler standing beside him.

Cranial Towards the head end of the body.

Cribbing (also known as wind sucking) This is a vice: the aspiration and swallowing of air by the horse through the mouth. The horse arches his neck and inhales air. May be facilitated by the horse biting or setting his teeth against a firm object. It is an acquired habit that may be controlled by the use of a cribbing collar.

Curb chain A small metal, metal and elastic, leather, plastic or nylon chain attached by hooks to the cheeks of a curb or Pelham bit; passed under the lower jaw and twisted clockwise until it lies flat in the chin groove.

Daisy-cutter Said of a horse who, when moving at the trot, appears to skirt the surface of the ground, predisposed to stumbling.

Dehydration Reduction in body fluids that occurs when fluid losses exceed fluid intake. The reduction in circu-lating blood volume lowers the horse's aerobic capacity due to poor muscular perfusion and hinders heat dissipa-tion through reducing the cutaneous circulation.

Dishing Also known as winging or paddling. Out-ward/lateral deviation of the foot during flight in which the foot breaks over the outside toe and lands on the outside wall.

Distal Away from centre of the body, the opposite of prox-imal.

Disunited canter Said of a cantering horse who changes leg sequence taking one lead with the front legs and the op-posite lead with the hind. This may be due to a lack of balance and/or back stiffness.

Draw reins Two leather or synthetic straps or ropes at-tached to the girth, saddle or harness which run through the bit rings to the hands of the rider. Used as a training aid to encourage the horse to lower the head.

Electrolyte Substance that dissociates in solution into elec-trically charged particles called ions. Electrolytes are lost in sweat and must be replaced in appropriate quantities to maintain the body's fluid and electrolyte balance.

Ewe neck Said of a horse's neck when the topline is concave and the lower line is more heavily muscled and outwardly bulging.

Extension The lengthening of the stride at the walk, trot or canter whereby the movement of the front legs is more forwards than upwards; the horse should demonstrate equal extension in both the fore- and hindlegs.

Flexion Bending or moving a joint so that the two or more bones forming it draw towards each other.

Flying change An advanced movement in which the horse changes leading legs simultaneously during the moment of suspension following the third beat of the canter. The horse springs from one pair of leading legs to the other in one fluent movement with the fore- and hind-legs chang-ing concurrently. This may be executed in a series such as at every fourth, third, second or first stride. The horse should remain calm and straight with lively impulsion and a consistent rhythm and balance.

Forge Known as click, clicking or forging. Limb contact in which the hind foot hits the sole of the forefoot on the same side. Recognized by the clicking noise that occurs when one shoe strikes the other. Indicates the horse is moving too much on the forehand, which delays the fore-leg break-over. This occurs in tired, green or immature horses, those with a short back and long legs or when shod incorrectly.

Gait Characteristic limb coordination pattern recognized by the sequence and timing of the footfalls and other kine-matic characteristics.

Galvayne's groove Also known as Galvayne's mark. A lon-gitudinal, dark-coloured groove in the upper third in-cisors. Appearswhen the horse is about 10 years of age. Begins at the gum line of the upper corner incisor at about 10 years, moving halfway down the tooth by 15 years, covering the entire length of the tooth by 20 years, seen in the bottom half of the tooth at 25 years and disappearing at about 30 years. It is less reliable than other indicators for estimating age in the young horse but is quite valuable in placing the age of the older horse.

Girth gall A gall that develops in the belly area behind the el-bow of the horse where the girth generally passes. Caused by dirty, stiff or badly fitting girths, and those that are too tight or too loose. Similar to a blister. Horses with thin, sensitive skin are most prone.

Grid An excellent means of schooling horse and rider. This can consist of a row of fences, possibly the first few as bounces or poles on the ground, then one, two or three strides between the following fences. At the beginning of the lane the fences should be small, progressively increasing towards the end of the row.

Half-pass A lateral dressage movement performed free of the track, in which the horse bends uniformly on two tracks throughout his body in the direction in which he is moving; the horse's shoulders move slightly in advance of the hindquarters, the outside legs pass and cross in front of the inside legs; the horse is looking in the direction he is moving. He should maintain the same cadence and balance throughout the whole movement.

Hollow back A dressage term: a fault in which the horse drops his back resulting in a concave topline as opposed to a convex one. May result when the horse fails to move from behind and/or evades the action of the bit by raising his head above the vertical.

Ipsilateral Occurring on the same side.

Lactic acid Acid produced as a toxic by-product of anaerobic lactic metabolism. Lactate accumulation in the muscles leads to fatigue.

Lateral work Also known as lateral movements, work on two tracks, or side steps. Any movement in which the sequence of steps in the walk, trot or canter remains unchanged, the hindfeet do not follow in the path of the forefeet and the horse moves forwards and sideways. The legs involved in the movement cross over in front of those that are on the ground.

Leg-yielding A lateral movement performed on two tracks, forwards and sideways, in which the horse moves away from the rider's leg applying pressure, i.e. if the rider applies pressure with his off-side (right) leg just behind the girth, the horse will move in the direction of the near side (left). Together with shoulder-in it is invaluable in making the horse supple, loose and unconstrained for elasticity and regularity of the paces and the harmony, lightness and ease of movements.

Lungeing To exercise or train the horse on a single long line attached to the bridle, lungeing cavesson or halter in a circle around the trainer on the flat or over jumps.

Martingale Any auxiliary rein or strap used to assist the action of the bit by restricting the position of the horse's head and neck. It consists of a strap, or arrangement of straps, fastened to the girth at one end, passed through the forelegs and, depending on the type, attached on the other end to the reins, noseband, or directly to the bit.

Napping Describes a horse demonstrating any form of resistance. This may include rearing, bucking, running away, failure to obey the aids, e.g. failing to move forward off the leg.

Near side The left side of the horse when viewed from the rear of the horse and the right side when facing it from a standing position on the ground.

Noseband A part of the bridle that consists of a slip head to which is attached a round nosepiece that lies across the bridge of the nose and buckles under the jaw, approximately 5 cm below the cheekbones yet above the bit.

Numnah A saddle-shaped pad cut slightly larger than the saddle, placed between the saddle and the back of the horse to absorb sweat and provide protection. May be made from felt, sheepskin or cloth-covered foam or rubber.

Off side The right side of the horse when viewed from the rear and the left side when viewed from the front.

Over-reach boots A bell-shaped protective covering for the hoof and coronary band made of leather, rubber and/or synthetic material used to protect the heels of the forelegs from injury by the toe of the hind shoe or hoof.

Oxer A parallel fence utilising two sets of standards and any combination of poles, angles, or spreads which is jumped as a single unit.

Parrot mouth A congenital malformation of the mouth in which the upper jaw is longer than the bottom jaw and the teeth in the top jaw overshoot or protrude beyond the teeth of the lower jaw, thought to be inherited. It may cause the horse to have difficulty eating.

Passage A shortened, very elevated, cadenced and collected trot with accentuated flexion of the knees and hocks and an extended movement of suspension as each pair of diagonal legs is raised. The hindquarters are more engaged than at other trots.

Pessoa The Pessoa training system encourages muscle development from the lumbar region to the top of neck. The system should be introduced gradually so as to avoid muscle stiffness.

Piaffe A ground movement in which the horse performs a cadenced trot in place. The trot has no forward movement and has moments of suspension between each diagonal step. The forelegs are light and elevated higher than the hind feet. This is the most collected of all dressage movements.

Piebald Refers to coat colour: a horse that has splashed asymmetric patterns of black and white. The lines of separation between the colours are well defined.

Pirouette A high school dressage movement similar to the volte performed in a circle in one place. The horse's forehand and outside hindleg make a 360° turn around the inside hindleg, the radius of the circle equalling the length of the horse. Ridden in collected walk, collected canter or piaffe. Lightness of the forehand is essential.

Plaiting A gait defect in which the horse moves in such a manner that the hooves are placed in front of each other through a twisting of the striding leg around the supporting leg in a manner similar to a person climbing a rope or plaiting two pieces of rope together. Common to horses wide at the base or having broad chests, or in the hindlegs of pacers; may be corrected with shoeing.

Poll The occipital crest – the highest point of the horse's head, just between the ears.

Poor doer A horse having a picky appetite who goes off his feed easily. May be undernourished; generally influenced by psychological causes.

Prophet's thumb Also known as thumbprint of the prophet. A pronounced dimple or indentation in the shoulder muscles.

Proprioception The reception of stimuli produced within the organism enabling the horse, especially when moving over obstacles, to know the position of his legs in relation to his body and the object jumped.

Proprioceptor One of the sensory end-organs that provide information about movements and positioning of the body. They occur chiefly in the muscles, tendons, joint capsules and labyrinth.

Protraction Pertaining to moving a body part forwards.

Proximal Towards the centre of the body, the opposite of distal.

Quarter horse An American-bred horse breed with massively muscled, large, rounded hindquarters. It is compact, agile, fast, and well balanced, with quick reflexes.

Quidding In this condition, the food is rolled and shifted about in the mouth and then finally ejected into the manger. In most cases the cause is due to dental irregularities which produce pain when attempts are made to masticate.

Related distances This term applies to jumping a course where, to test the horse's abilities and the horsemanship of the rider, the course builder may deliberately cause difficulties, without being unfair to the horse, by means of slightly widening or shortening the distances between some of the fences. In such a case it is up to the rider to decide how to deal with the problem set, in order to jump it clear. Depending on whether the horse has a long or short stride, it will either try to lengthen or shorten the stride between the fences accordingly.

Retraction Pertaining to moving a body part backwards (caudally).

Roach back A conformation defect. The spine of the horse is convexly curved on the dorsal aspect, between the withers and loins.

Roarer A horse with paralysis to one or both sides of the larynx due to the obstruction of the larynx by the arytenoid cartilage and vocal folds, resulting in a characteristic roaring noise during inhalation.

Rowelling To insert a piece of leather or other material under the skin of a horse to cause a discharge.

School To train or educate a horse, with or without a rider. It involves teaching the horse movements and gaits required for future use or refining those movements and gaits previously taught through specific exercises. Schooling techniques differ for each riding style.

Scoliosis Lateral curvature of the spine.

Shiverer Generally regarded as a nervous disease. Symptoms are that on lifting a hind leg, or on backing, the limb is suddenly raised, semi-flexed and abducted, shaking or shivering in suspension. The superficial muscles of the thigh and quarters quiver and the tail is raised and tremulous. Symptoms may be shown whilst the animal is being shod, or if made to move over smartly in the stall or box.

Shoulder-in A lateral movement performed on two tracks in which the horse travels forwards while bent uniformly from head to tail away from the direction in which he is travelling. Correctly executed, the angle should not exceed 30°.

Side reins Two rigid or elasticated and/or adjustable auxiliary reins attached on one end to the roller or girth and to the bit rings on the other end. Used to teach the horse head carriage. May be attached as high as the withers or low, as behind the shoulder.

Skewbald Refers to coat colour: a horse that has splashed asymmetric patterns of brown and white. The lines of separation between the colours are well defined.

Splint Enlargement of the splint bones. Usually occurs in the forelegs of young horses in the early months or years of training, on the medial aspect of the forelimbs between the second and third metacarpal bones. Associated with hard training, poor conformation, improper hoof care, or malnutrition. Characterised by swelling, heat and lameness that are only observed during splint formation.

Star gazer A horse that holds his head too high.

Stringhalt The sole symptom of stringhalt is an involuntary and exaggerated hock action, which is jerked upwards during the act of progression. This may not be presented at every step, and when slight may only be noticed when the animal is turned around suddenly.

Stud guard Leather pad or flap on the ventral aspect of the girth, which protects the sternum from possible injury by the studs placed in the shoes as the forelimbs are tucked up when jumping a fence.

Studs Metal heads screwed into the bottom of a conventional horseshoe to increase traction on slippery or deep surfaces such as grass, snow or asphalt.

Sway back Said of the horse's back when concave along the dorsal aspect between the withers and loin as caused by old age, faulty conformation, mineral imbalance, or in brood mares, by the weight of foals.

Sweeney Atrophy of the muscles of the shoulder resulting from disuse following lesion of the leg or foot that leads to prolonged diminished use of the limb or damage to the suprascapular nerve.

Travers A dressage movement performed on two tracks. The horse's head, neck and shoulders follow a straight track along the wall, while the loins and quarters are bent around the rider's inside leg and follow a track approximately 1 yard (91 cm) off the wall at an angle of around 30°. The horse's head is flexed in the direction of the movement.

Tucked up Said of a horse whose loins are drawn up tightly behind the ribs due to illness, overwork, lack of water or bulk in the diet and/or underfeeding rather than conformation.

Twitch A device used to distract the attention of a horse, or to restrain it for a specific purpose such as clipping, covering, shoeing, performing minor operations or administering medication.

Vertical An upright or vertical jump. Any show-jump or cross-country fence built vertical to the ground.

Warble fly Lays its eggs on the lower extremities of the horse. When hatched, the larvae migrate beneath the skin towards the subdermal tissue of the back where they secrete an enzyme to make a breathing hole through the skin. Within 4–6 weeks the larvae emerge through the holes and drop to the ground.

Weaving A vice: the rhythmic swaying of the horse from side to side in which the horse shifts his weight from one foot to the other while nodding or swinging his head and neck back and forth. This usually results from boredom, is most common in stabled horses and is generally corrected when the horse is turned out to pasture.

Wisp An egg-shaped grooming brush without a handle, made of horsehair, straw, rope or hay coiled in the form of a figure eight to make a tight pad. Used to massage the horse to stimulate circulation and tone the muscles.

Wobbler A group of diseases of the spinal column and spinal cord characterized by various defects of coordination and movement. May be caused by pressure on the spinal cord exerted by a malformed or injured spine.

PHRASES

Accepts the bit Said of a horse that holds the bit confidently in the mouth and responds to the contact and influence of the rider's hands on the reins without resistance or hesitation.

Aids, the Aids The rider influences his horse by giving aids with his weight, legs and hands. The co-ordination of the various aids controls the horse's posture, the quality of the paces and his overall obedience. The intensity of the aids is determined by the horse's sensitivity, his stage of training and the purpose for which the aids are given. The rider's feel and tact are shown by his ability to time and co-ordinate the various aids correctly and to apply them with the appropriate intensity.

Behind the bit Also known as behind the bridle, overbent or below the bit: an over-responsiveness to the bit in which the horse evades rein contact by refusing to take hold of the bit in the mouth and draws the chin in to the chest and also tries not to accept the bit by creeping behind it, escaping backwards.

Behind the leg Said of a horse that may respond to the rider's leg in the sense that he will increase the speed and pace but is not allowing the energy to come through from the hindleg to the bridle.

Between hand and leg Also known as 'on the aids': a horse framed between the rider's hands and legs and who is fully responsive to the actions of the rider including natural and artificial aids.

Change the rein To change direction of travel from left to right or vice versa when riding.

Not between hand and leg A dressage term: a horse that is not sufficiently under control of the leg and hand aids of the rider.

Not enough collection Said of a horse who does not demonstrate sufficient engagement of the hindquarters, resulting in steps that are too long and in movement on the forehand.

Not enough extension Said of a horse who does not show sufficient lengthening of stride.

Off the forehand Shifting slightly more weight on to the horse's quarters, the engagement of the hindlegs and the balance on the haunches are facilitated for the benefit of the lightness of the forehand and the horse's balance as a whole.

On the bit A horse is said to be 'on the bit' when the hocks are correctly placed and the neck is more or less raised and arched according to the stage of training and the extension or collection of the pace, and it accepts the bridle with a light and soft contact and submissiveness throughout. The head should remain in a steady position, as a rule slightly in front of the vertical, with a supple poll at the highest point of the neck, and no resistance should be offered to the rider.

Overface Also known as overfacing. To encourage a horse to jump a fence that is either too large or too difficult for it to jump, that is clearly beyond its capabilities.

Peck at a jump When a horse stumbles, before a jump or on landing.

Quarters not engaged Said of a horse whose hindlegs are not sufficiently brought under its body. The horse may be on the forehand and have a hollowed back.

Take off A jumping term: the moment at which a horse leaves the ground in preparation to clear a jump. It is preceded by the approach and followed by flight.

Take off too early A jumping term: when a horse begins his jump of an obstacle too far away from the take-off point appropriate for his stride. The horse will therefore descend from his jump before fully clearing the obstacle and thus may contact the jump with his body or hind legs.

Take off too late Also known as jumping too deep. When a horse begins to jump an obstacle too close to the jump to allow a full jumping stride. The horse will generally hit the jump with his forelegs.

Work on the long reins To train a horse from the ground using two long reins attached to the snaffle bit to influence the rhythm, activity and lateral bend of the horse in all lateral movements as well as in forward movements. The trainer holds one rein in each hand and a 4 ft 6 in (1.3 m) whip, pointing forwards, in the right. Whether the trainer stands behind or to the inside of the horse, the reins will run from the bit along the sides of the horse to the trainer's hands.

Working in the hand To train the horse from the ground. The trainer, standing at the horse's shoulder, controls the frame and movement of the horse using the reins held in one hand and a dressage whip held in the other. Care must be taken to produce even results on either rein, as unbalanced training may result in a lack of symmetry.

Wrong bend A dressage term: failure of the horse to achieve and maintain the correct degree of bend when executing corners, circles, etc. May result in a loss of balance and rhythm in the movements.

SOURCES

Most of these definitions are taken from the following 2 sources:

Belknap MA (2004) *The Allen Equine Dictionary*. JA Allen, London.
British Dressage Rule Book www.britishdressage.co.uk.

Appendix A
Safety Aspects for Treating Horses, Unsedated and Sedated

Annabel Jenks

- It is important that one's own health and fitness are sufficient to practise.
- A general knowledge and understanding of horses are essential.
- Clothing needs to be comfortable and suitable, allowing movement and freedom to work. It must not be tightly fitting, but nor should it be so loose that it flaps.
- No noisy material should be worn that may distract or frighten the horse. Waterproof clothing including hats are best removed before treatment commences.
- For warmth, light layers are best; thermal silk underwear is light and allows movement. Waistcoats are easier to work in than coats.
- Good footwear is essential such as jodhpur boots, sturdy walking shoes or similar attire.
- A hard hat and gloves can always be useful. When treating young stock or horses renowned to be difficult, it is wise to wear a hard hat.
- When treating stallions, do not use perfumes or aftershaves as stallions are extremely susceptible to pheromones and aromas.
- Watches and jewellery, earrings and piercings, necklaces and rings should be worn with extreme caution and are best removed.

ENVIRONMENT

- Ideally, it is best to work from stable yards or veterinary practices one knows but this is not always practical.

- Active examination needs to be on a flat safe surface, where the horse can be examined walking and trotting in straight lines and on circles, away from any obstacles such as cars, other horses, dogs, children, pushchairs, wheelbarrows, etc. Riding arenas make very good examination areas.
- If trotting a horse on tarmac or concrete, be very careful that the surface is not slippery and be aware of the positioning of drains and manhole covers. The advantage of trotting on hard surfaces is that one can 'hear' each footfall, which is a very useful aid in diagnosing gait abnormalities.
- The treatment area, usually a stable, needs to be at least 12 feet ×12 feet (3.6m×3.6m) and light and airy with good headroom. Avoid low beams, ceilings and hanging wires and electric light fittings. Toy balls, licks and other hazards that owners may place in the stable to keep their horse amused should be removed. A non-slip surface is required: ideally rubber matting, but a clean woodchip or straw bed will suffice.
- The stable must be empty of any utensils or objects that could injure the patient or practitioner. Forks, brooms, rugs, water buckets, grooming kits and feed bowls are some examples.
- Dogs and cats are a hazard in the stable when treating horses.
- Only the practitioner and owner/handler should be in the area with the horse and they must always on the same side as each other when treating. The owner must be instructed to change positions with you and hold the horse on both sides but you will find that they will often subconsciously keep returning to the near side (left) of the horse and have

to be reminded to stay your side if you are working on the right.

- The handler must stand to the side of the horse, not in front as they all wish to do!
- Always have the horse facing the exit and against the wall. Never be caught trapped between them and the exit or wall. If the horse swings round, go with the movement, ensuring both handler and practitioner are together at the horse's head to reorganise themselves before resuming treatment.
- Care must be taken with observers standing in the doorway in case the horse barges out. Children must never be allowed to be in a position of danger, and babies in pushchairs must be kept well clear of the vicinity.
- The door can be pulled to but never shut or bolted as there must be an easy escape route if needed.
- If a platform of some sort is needed to attain height, a crate, triangular feed bowl or sturdy water bucket with no handle may be used. Chairs, stepladders or any other implement which you or the horse could become caught on or in should never be used.
- If there are no stables or barns available, a quiet safe corner of the yard or field may be sufficient, with the practitioner and handler always at the 'open end'.
- *However, never compromise your own safety or that of those around you. There is always another place or day to treat safely.*

THE HANDLER

- It is the practitioner's responsibility to ensure the handler is safe and competent.
- The handler must be competent, with the knowledge and experience to anticipate the horse's reaction to treatment. They must be correctly dressed and if necessary wear a riding hat.
- The owner of the horse is not always the best person to hold the horse.
- The handler must always stand on the same side that the practitioner is working. It is up to the practitioner to monitor where the handler is positioned at all times. The handler should hold the horse by the headcollar rope in a secure manner, without restricting the horse, and should never stand directly in front of the horse.

Common Faults

- Kissing the horse's nose is very dangerous! The horse may throw their head up hitting the handler on the face. Some owners have to be constantly reminded.
- Giving titbits, unless instructed by the practitioner, can be distracting to the horse's concentration whilst it is being treated.
- The handler holds the horse too tightly.
- He or she fails to stay on the same side as the practitioner.
- The handler stands in front of the horse.
- Generally not concentrating on the treatment in progress is another common fault.

THE HORSE

- Horses can be very unpredictable and the practitioner must be constantly aware of the horse's reactions and of predicted reactions to the osteopathic techniques used.
- Observation and experience are the key.
- Allow the horse to 'settle' to you and the environment it finds itself in.
- If the horse is particularly nervous, allow them time to relax. Stand back yourself, quietly talking, before approaching gently and slowly towards the left (near) side, not making any sudden movements. Stroke the horse and familiarise yourself with them before even attempting an examination.
- Some horses are very suspicious of strangers because they think they are going to receive an injection of some sort. Many only ever see their vet for the annual flu and tetanus booster. As most injections are administered on the left (near) side these horses are best examined from the right (off) side first.
- Some horses just behave in a spoilt/bullish manner and barge about the stable, having no respect for the handler and practitioner. These are often homebred horses or particular breeds.
- Thoroughbreds cannot be 'bullied'; they have a quick, sharp temper and will even throw themselves on the floor! Take time to allow the horse to settle. You may even decide to leave them in the stable for a time and go and have a cup of coffee with the owner until the horse is more receptive to treatment.
- Warm bloods on the other hand generally need firm handling!
- Ponies and general riding horses must also never be underestimated. They can overreact to a treatment technique if very sore, and become frightened and kick out unintentionally.
- If the horse is particularly nervous and intolerant, there is no benefit in upsetting them further. Remember there is always another day for treatment.
- It is very important that the horse is 'concentrating' on the practitioner during treatment.
- The headcollar used must be secure, and make sure the headpiece tongue is slipped into the buckle and not flapping.
- For further restraint, a bridle, chifney bit or twitch may be required.

- Travelling boots, bandages (including tail bandages) and boots must be removed before examination.
- Ensure in cold weather that the horse does not become chilled during treatment by having suitable rugs available to place on the quarters if needed. In ideal situations, infrared lamps can be used.
- It is impossible to examine or treat a horse if they are wet and muddy. It is advisable to instruct the owners, when making the booking, to keep the horse in the stable on the day of the appointment. Some horses need to be turned out. If this is the case, ask the owner to turn them out early with a New Zealand rug and ensure that they are back in their stable and dry by the time you arrive!
- To test cervical spine mobility, use carrots to encourage the horse to bend left, right and forward to stretch the neck.
- When using the thrust–spring techniques (as described in Chapter 12) there must be woodchips, straw or rubber matting on the floor. The horse should always be bandaged or booted behind and even in front, to prevent injury of striking into itself as the technique is performed. Overreach boots can also be used as added protection.
- Some horses are intolerant or unfamiliar with boots and may kick out and become irritated when wearing them.

The practitioner must weigh the risks of injury to themselves and the horse; there are always alternative techniques that can be applied.

- Ask the owners to bring their saddle/s for inspection. Great care must be taken when placing the saddle on and tightening the girth as the horse may react by kicking, rearing or shooting forwards and backwards.
- Remove the numnah and any pads before asking the owner to place the saddle on the horse. It is important to assess the position on which *they* place the saddle as often this may be the key to any problems experienced when ridden. The numnah and pad may also radically change the balance of the saddle and should be fitted afterwards. Girths should also be looked at. The girth straps used can affect the balance of the saddle. Commonly there are three straps on the saddle and but only two are actually used, either the front two, or the first and third strap, depending on the individual's preference.
- It is always good to end a treatment with praise and a reward for the horse. A packet of mints goes a long way towards cementing good rapport between patient and practitioner!

THE GOLDEN RULE TO SAFE PRACTICE IS **NEVER COMPROMISE YOURSELF OR THOSE AROUND.**

Appendix B

Referral for Osteopathic Treatment

Julia Brooks

AG Pusey DO FE Cert   Haywards Heath Osteopathic Practice

Awbrook Lodge, Lewes Rd, Haywards Heath, West Sussex RH17 7TB
Tel: 01444 831576
Fax: 01444 831211

Referral for Osteopathic Treatment

To: *(Name of veterinary surgeon)* ....

At: *(Address of clinic)* ....

A client of yours *(Client's name)* ....

Address *(Client's address)* ....

With a horse *(Name of horse)* ....

Kept at ....

has contacted us requesting a consultation to assess and, if appropriate, give osteopathic treatment to this horse which presents with *(short description of problem)* ....

....

We would be grateful if you could confirm permission to assess and, if appropriate, to treat this horse by signing and returning this fax, or referring by letter. A report will be sent to you following the consultation.

If you would prefer to meet us with the client or to discuss the case, we would be delighted to do so.

If you are able to help by sending details of any previous history of problems and veterinary care received, we would be very grateful.

I give permission for the above-mentioned horse to be assessed and treated

Name of veterinary surgeon *(please print name)* ....

Signature of vet ....   Date ....

Appendix C

Owner Consent Form for Osteopathic and Sedation Procedures

Julia Brooks

AG Pusey DO FE Cert   Haywards Heath Osteopathic Practice
Awbrook Lodge Lewes Rd Haywards Heath West Sussex RH17 7TB *Tel: 01444 831576*

<u>Owner Consent Form</u>
<u>for Osteopathic and Sedation Procedures</u>

Name of horse/dog_____

    Breed _____ Colour _____ Age _____ Sex _____

Owner/agent name _____

    Address_____

          _____

          _____

    Tel. (Home)_____ (Work)_____

    Any relevant clinical history / special precautions _____

    _____

Insured horses/dogs

    Where treatment is covered by insurance, it is the responsibility of the owner to settle our account and reclaim the fees from the insurance company. It is the responsibility of the owner to ensure that the terms of their contract with the insurer are not infringed, and that they have suitable cover. While we are always prepared to discuss insurance matters, it is on the basis that we have no specialist expertise in this field, our knowledge being purely based on experience of previous claims.

I hereby give permission for the administration of sedation to the above animal and osteopathic assessment and treatment, together with any other procedures which may prove necessary. I understand that all sedation techniques and osteopathic procedures involve some risk to the animal. I have been informed of and agreed to pay the cost of assessment and/or treatment. I agree to pay on the day of treatment or within 7 days. I have notified the insurers concerning the procedures planned for this animal.

Signature _____ (Owner/agent)

Name (*Block capitals*) _____ Date _____

Appendix D

Information Sheet, Osteopathy

in Practice

Julia Brooks

Musculoskeletal problems are common in animals, and osteopathy has been shown to be of benefit in treating this type of problem.

The case history is the starting point of the consultation. This will give an idea of the type of work the horse is expected to do and the level it is expected to attain. It will also highlight any past injuries and illnesses that the animal may have suffered. Further questioning may reveal idiosyncrasies in behaviour or movement which, while noticed by the owner, had not interfered with performance sufficiently to be a cause for concern. When considering the history and the function of the horse as a whole, these subtle disturbances in motor function may, in fact, be early warning signals for more serious problems later.

and the level of discomfort by the way it holds itself and the way it interacts with the environment. Quantity and symmetry of muscle development and distribution of weight through the limbs can also be assessed.

In movement it is balance and the fluidity with which movement is transmitted from head to tail, alongside stride length and foot placement, which give further clues. How the animal copes with complex movements such as turning will help to identify problems with balance and lateral flexibility.

Observation will give an impression of how the animal moves as a whole, and indicate which areas are functioning poorly. Looking at individual joint movements is also useful. Running the hands down the paravertebral muscles from the

---

AG Pusey DO FE Cert   Haywards Heath
Osteopathic Practice
Awbrook Lodge Lewes Rd Haywards Heath West Sussex RH17 7TB *Tel: 01444 831576*

Equine Case Sheet

Name of Owner	Name of Horse	
Address	Stable Name	
	Age	Breed
	Sex	Colour
Address to which account should be sent	Present Use	
Tel: (daytime)		
Tel: (evening)	Intended Use	
Name of Vet:	Length of Ownership	

Details of Problem

When was the problem first noticed?

In what way did the problem first present?

The case sheet: an important starting point

Osteopathy in practice

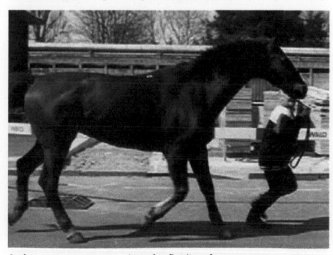

Active movements: Looking for fluidity of movement as it is transmitted from the head backwards along the spine.

Examination begins by looking at the static horse. Some impression can be gained of the temperament of the animal

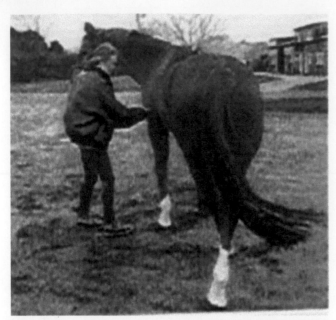

Observation of the short turn: Neck dysfunction will result in the early replacement of the foot or a rotation element to the sidebend as movement starts going through the region of discomfort.

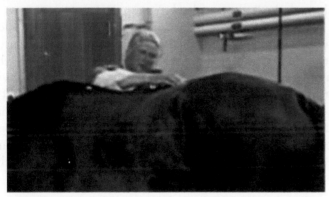

Palpation: Running the hands down the paravertebral muscles to locate areas of muscle spasm.

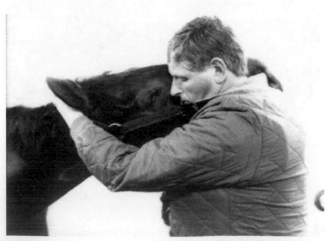

Treatment: Relaxing muscles and stretching joints at the top of the neck.

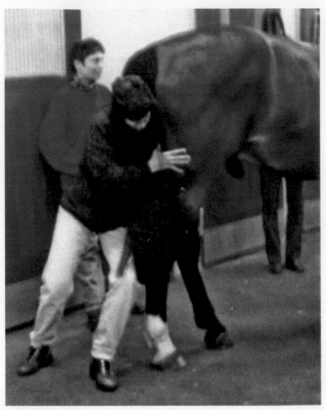

Treatment: Relaxing muscles of pelvic region.

occiput back to the tail, areas of muscle spasm and tissue texture changes can be felt. Moving the joints through the relevant ranges will identify those that are stiff.

Diagnosis requires consideration of past injuries, the way the animal moves overall and dysfunction in specific areas. Initially it will be a working hypothesis. Where problems have been present for some time, the horse will have had to develop patterns of posture and movement in order to work around poorly functioning areas, and there may be involvement at several levels. For this reason, clinical reasoning and application of the principles of biomechanics need to be developed to a high degree.

Once a diagnosis has been made, treatment involves using techniques adapted from human practice as well as those developed for the horse. During treatment and over the course of a number of treatments, response is carefully monitored. There may also be a need for contributions from allied professions such as farriers and physiotherapists. The owner is a vital part of this team approach as it is important to provide the appropriate care for the horse after treatment.

After treatment a small number of horses can resume normal work. The majority, however, require more care when reintroducing work, and, in particular, need to avoid jumping for as long as possible. Also worth noting is that some horses will, in the course of their recovery, suffer acute injuries while playing in the field, but these can be treated relatively easily. If there is any cause for concern, please contact us sooner rather than later.

Appendix E
Case Sheet

Julia Brooks

AG Pusey DO FE Cert   Haywards Heath Osteopathic Practice

Awbrook Lodge Lewes Rd Haywards Heath West Sussex RH17 7TB *Tel: 01444 831576*

Case Sheet

Name of Owner Address	Name of Horse Stable name
	Age Breed Sex Colour
Address to which account should be sent Tel: Name of vet:	Present use Intended use Length of ownership

Details of Problem

When was the problem first noticed?

In what way did the problem first present?

Please write in your own words how the problem started and how it has progressed.

Please try to answer the following questions.
Have there been any changes in temperament?
If yes, in what way?

Have you experienced any difficulties with shoeing your horse?
If yes, in what way?

Has there been any change in your horse's rolling behaviour?
If yes, in what way?

Has there been any change in your horse's urination pattern, including during riding?

Riding difficulties (*Please underline statements that apply*)
Difficulty with collection/Forming an outline/Reining back/Loss of propulsion/Lateral work/Leaning on one rein – left or right/Difficulty turning one way – left or right/Jumping to one side – left or right/Increasingly uncomfortable to ride.

Have you noticed any areas of stiffness? (*If yes, please underline area affected*)
Poll/Neck/Back/Pelvis/Throughout spine

Have you noticed any areas of sensitivity? (*If yes, please underline area affected*)
Poll/Neck/Back/Pelvis

Have you noticed any lameness?
If yes, which limb was affected?
Was a diagnosis made? If so, what was the diagnosis?
What treatment was given?

To your knowledge, has the horse suffered any accidents, falls, illnesses or traumatic incidents? If yes, please give details.

Current Problem

History

Examination

   Static

   Walk

   Trot

   Tight circle (left)

   Tight circle (right)

   Backing up

   Palpation

Diagnosis

Treatment

Advice

Vet contacted   *Letter*   *Telephone*

Appendix F

Case History Questions

Annabel Jenks

Address/phone numbers
Name of owner/rider
Veterinary practice details and referral
Name, age, sex of horse
Date teeth last rasped / examined

Period of ownership
Vetted or not at purchase
Brand marks and freeze marks
Colour and distinguishing markings
Breeding if known or type
Owner's ambitions for horse
Previous career history if known

Presenting symptoms
Stiffness/levelness of stride
Change in temperament
Bucking/rearing/napping
Difficulty in turning/circling
Difficulty going up or down hill
Lateral stiffness
Loss of extended work/collected work

Fussy in the mouth
Not accepting the bit
Head tilting
Hollow in work
Tucked in the neck so behind the bit

Any differences when other riders ride the horse?
Instructor's view of horse's way of going
Level of training and competition work
Any changes in tack when ridden or lunged

Does the horse go disunited in canter ridden and/or on the lunge?
Refusing to jump
Rushing fences
Unable to make the distance in combinations
Taking off too early or late
Hollowing over a fence
Unable to jump oxers or verticals

Resistance to being tacked up/rugged up/groomed
Acute resistance to the girth being tightened
Difficulty when mounting and/or dismounting
Last time saddle was re-flocked and balanced

Difficulty or resistance to being shod
Note any surgical shoes
Differences in foot size
Any known pathology in the feet

Previous history
Falls/accidents/illnesses/traumas/kicks
Muscular changes and atrophy

Previous veterinary clinical history
Lameness of any description
Any x-rays taken/lameness workup/scintigraphy/MRI scans
Operations
Joint injections
Blood test results
Any episodes of colic
Difficulty in passing urine or faeces
Episodes of azoturia
Viral infections, i.e. strangles/herpes/equine flu

Changes in feeding
Difficultly in lowering head to feed
Has the horse been cast in the stable?
Any entanglements with haynet or buckets
Pulling back when tied up
Difficulty or reluctance to roll
Does the horse go out in the field and/or loose-schooled?
Stable vices

Has the horse had osteopathic, physiotherapy or chiropractic treatment before?
If so, when and what was the outcome?

Keep on file a record of the owner's name, telephone numbers, addresses and directions to the stable yard, the veterinary practice they are associated with, and make sure these are easily accessible for quick reference.

Appendix G
Static and Active Examination

Annabel Jenks

Stand and just look.
What is the horse's general attitude to the handler and surroundings?
Alertness and temperament: are they relaxed or excited?

OBSERVATION FROM ALL ANGLES

- Observe unloading from lorry
- Observe in the stable
- Assess partnership between owner and their horse
- General health, coat sheen, weight
- Assess conformation/type/breed
- Suitability in type and shape for required work expected by owner
- General muscle tone
- Atrophy or lack of tone
- Position of head and neck relative to rest of body
- Height and shape of withers and quarters
- Abdominal tone
- Tail carriage

Observe straightness of limbs
Feet/shoes
Unshod or shod
Wear and type of shoes
Balance of feet and size of feet
Is the weight distributed through all four limbs evenly?
Obvious blemishes such as splints
Windgalls, thoroughpins and other signs of strain
Note any scars or signs of injury

Symmetry of sacro-iliac joints, hips, shoulders, eyes, nostrils
Length and shape of the back

White hairs in the saddle region denoting pressure points
Fullness or narrowness of chest
Is there the impression that there is 'a leg at each corner'?

These and much more are before the horse is even asked to move actively for examination! It is *very important*, as with all observations, to listen to your first thoughts and instincts and write them down, however trivial they first seem to be: they could be the key to the diagnosis.

GAIT AND POSTURE

- Request that the horse be walked away on level ground and back
- Observe from front/behind and side
- Repeat as many times as necessary

Then request that the horse is trotted away and back:

- *Listen* to the footfalls
- Watch the turns and transitions
- Levelness of gait
- Get the owner to turn the horse both ways if necessary
- Observe toe dragging, abduction, adduction or circumduction Protraction and retraction of each limb
- Limb swing and ease of movement in the shoulder and hip
- Positioning of head, neck and tail
- Fluidity of movement throughout the whole body

Turn the horse on a tight circle on both reins to assess limb placement and neck flexibility. The handler needs to stand on the inside of the circle and take care that they are not trodden on but push the horse over from the shoulder as it turns. There is more skill in asking the horse to circle than meets the eye!

In some cases, if weakness is suspected, the tail is pulled as the horse is circled.

Rein the horse back on flat ground.

- If you suspect sacroiliac joint problems, ask the horse to back up an incline.
- If neurological problems are suspected, ask the horse to step back and forwards, with the head positioned high and with the nose tucked into the chest (further tests should be under veterinary observation but these preliminary tests will indicate possible pathology).

Proprioception can be tested over poles and on different terrain.

Look for levelness of the stride, ataxia, weakness, toes dragging or scuffing, crossing over, and plaiting, dishing, and proprioceptive deficits. Which limbs are involved: front/hind, diagonal?

Look for evidence of pain:

- Abdominal muscles tucked up
- Reluctance to move or place weight on a limb
- Reluctance to turn the neck
- Position of head
- Signs of sweating

Observing the horse being lunged is very informative when assessing biomechanical dysfunction. The horse must be lunged on both reins in all paces.

In some instances it will be necessary to see the horse ridden to assimilate further the biomechanical function and assess the rider.

Repeat any active examination as often as you feel necessary, and take note of thoughts as they arise. Do not dismiss anything until an osteopathic working diagnosis is formed.

Appendix H

Drugs Used in Treatment with Sedation and Treatment under Anaethetic

Julia Brooks

Examination and treatment may be performed under a light sedation or general anaesthetic.

Sedation, where the horse is still standing but is more relaxed, may be helpful when dealing with an anxious horse or examining for deep-seated, long-standing dysfunction (Chapter 9).

General anaesthetic may be used in the treatment of cases with severe, long-standing problems (Chapter 13). Under these conditions, specifically directed forces can be applied in order to reverse effects of long-term injuries, without having to counter the muscular activity involved in keeping the horse upright. It also allows a slow, methodical examination of each joint complex to ensure that the articulation moves in the expected range rather than with a well established trick manoeuvre that involves accessory movements and participation of joints at other levels.

The following notes are guidelines only for administration of sedation and general anaesthetic for the osteopathic treatment of horses as anaesthetic practices evolve over time and new pharmaceutical agents are developed.

SEDATION

Ideally, this should be a combination of opioid to reduce sensitivity to pain and an α_2-adrenoceptor agonist to prevent sympathetic flight/fight behaviour. This does not abolish segmental responses to injury but it does make it easier and safer to identify local muscle spasm, joint asymmetry and tissue texture changes.

Butorphenol (Torbugesic)

- Butorphenol is an opioid analgesic.
- *Dosage*: 0.1 mg/kg body weight.
- *Action*: Modification of pain perception and behavioural reaction to pain. Induces drowsiness.
- *Receptor site*: It acts on opioid receptors which are distributed widely in the central nervous system (μ receptors in the periaqueductal grey, locus coeruleus and thalamus, and κ receptors in the thalamus and dorsal horn of the spinal cord).

Endogenous transmitter	Receptor site	Second messenger	Net channel effects	Action
Endogenous opiates*	Opiate receptor	Inhibit cyclic AMP	Increase K^+, Decrease Ca^{2+}	Inhibitory to pain transmission (analgesic)

*endorphins, enkepahalins and dyanorphins

Romifidine (Sedivet)

- Romifidine is an α_2-adrenoceptor stimulant.
- *Dosage*: 20 μg/kg.
- *Action*: Reduces alertness and arousal. Sedation, muscle relaxant and analgesic effects.
- *Receptor site*: α_2-adrenoceptors are presynaptic receptors or autoreceptors which act to inhibit further production of noradrenaline.

Endogenous transmitter	Receptor site	Second messenger	Net channel effects	Action
Noradrenaline	α_2-adrenoceptors	Inhibit cyclic AMP	Increase K^+, Decrease Ca^{2+}	Reduce arousal (sedation, muscle relaxant and analgesic)

GENERAL ANAESTHETIC

There are a number of ways to achieve general anaesthesia. This is largely determined by the environment, the availability of the equipment and the procedure to be carried out. The two principal forms of general anaesthesia are intravenous and inhalation.

Intravenous anaesthesia is not ideal for osteopathic treatment. It is shorter acting and limits the opportunity for methodical examination and more time-consuming techniques such as fascial unwinding

Inhalation anaesthesia is the preferred method as it can be maintained for longer to allow an unhurried, methodical examination and treatment.

Anaesthetics and their Effects on the Central Nervous System

- Neurotransmitters may be excitatory (ACh, 5-HT, NA), or inhibitory (GABA).
- General anaesthetics reduce sensation and response to stimuli such as touch and pressure.
- Not all are pain reducing so these may be combined with an analgesic.

Mechanisms

Inhalation

The mechanism is uncertain. There are two theories. In reality, the effect is probably a combination of the two:

1. Lipid theory, based on requirement for lipid solubility. Disruption of cell membrane resulting in loss of function of some or all membrane-bound voltage- and ligand-gated ion channels.
2. Protein theory: The anaesthetics interact directly with proteins within the cell membrane, notably ion channels and receptor proteins.

Intravenous

Here the mechanism is better understood. Benzodiazepines and the barbiturates midazolan and thiopentone enhance the effects of the inhibitory neurotransmitter, GABA. Some act as opioid receptor agonists, e.g. fentanyl.

Stages of anaesthesia

Stage I, analgesia: drowsy but still conscious

Stage II, excitement: inhibition is lost before consciousness (stage of potential risk of physical harm)

Stage III, surgical anaesthesia: loss of consciousness and reflexes

Agents

Intravenous: rapid onset but not prolonged in action.

Inhalation: maintain prolonged anaesthetic but slow in onset, prolonging the initial phases, notably the excitement phase.

Anaesthetic Practice for Osteopathic Treatment (Inhalation)

This form of anaesthesia is the method of choice for osteopathic treatment. It is administered in three stages, starting with premedication which is followed by induction and maintenance.

Premedication

This involves drugs administered before a general anaesthetic. An analgesic will reduce pain and a tranquilliser will reduce anxiety and facilitate handling.

Premedication is with 0.02 mg/kg intravenous acepromazine (ACP) followed 15–30 minutes later by 120 µg/kg romifidine.

Acepromazine

ACP is a phenothiazine-derived tranquilliser, which acts by blocking adrenoceptors. It has a marked potentiating effect of barbiturate anaesthesia.

Romifidine (Sedivet)

Analgesic and sedative effect by stimulating presynaptic α_2-receptors in the central nervous system. This reduces the synthesis and release of noradrenaline, so reducing alertness and arousal.

Induction

This is the stage occurring between the administration of the anaesthetic and loss of consciousness. The quickest way to produce loss of consciousness is by administration of intravenous agents, so reducing the amount of time in the excitement stage of anaesthesia.

Anaesthesia is induced 5 minutes after premedication by intravenous injection of ketamine (2.2 mg/kg) and diazepam (20 mg). The horse is intubated and anaesthesia maintained using a halothane or isofluorane and oxygen mixture. Where necessary, anaesthesia is maintained by ketamine and/or butorphenol.

Benzodiazepam (Diazepam)

Potentiates the effects of the inhibitory neurotransmitter, GABA, so reducing anxiety. It induces temporary amnesia, is a muscle relaxant and reduces alertness.

Ketamine (Narketan)

Dissociative anaesthetic agent inducing a state of cataplexy with amnesia and analgesia. Short acting. For induction prior to inhalation anaesthesia.

Maintenance

Prolonged anaesthesia is best achieved using a suitable inhalation anaesthetic agent such as halothane or isoflurane.

Halothane

This is administered with oxygen and provides deep anaesthesia but poor analgesia. Should the anaesthetic effect be reduced, it can rapidly be re-established by administering ketamine or butorphenol.

Isoflurane

Administered as for halothane.

Anaesthetic Risks

- Risk of physical damage during the excitable stage of anaesthetic.
- Risk of overdose, which may result in death.
- Risk to staff as the anaesthetic agents are excreted unchanged and the atmosphere may become contaminated with anaesthetic agent. This renders the staff susceptible to sedative effects and longer term consequences such as liver toxicity.

Index

Page numbers in *italics* represent figures, those in **bold** represent tables.